STRATEG

PUBLIC HE~~~~ ... ~~~~ ~~~~

SERIES

Advancing
Equity
and
Justice

For access to digital chapters,
visit the APHA Press bookstore (www.apha.org).

Strategic Skills for Public Health Practice Series
Series Editors: Michael Fraser, PhD, MS, and Brian C. Castrucci, DrPH

1. *Systems and Strategic Thinking*
2. *Policy Engagement*
3. *Resource Management and Finance*
4. *Community Engagement*
5. *Advancing Equity and Justice*
6. *Effective Communication*
7. *Change Management*
8. *Data-Informed Decision Making*
9. *Cross-Sectoral Partnerships*

STRATEGIC SKILLS FOR
PUBLIC HEALTH PRACTICE

SERIES

Advancing Equity and Justice

Jamila M. Porter, DrPH, MPH
Aysha Dominguez Pamukcu, JD

Illustrated by Jasmin Pamukcu

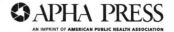
APHA PRESS
AN IMPRINT OF AMERICAN PUBLIC HEALTH ASSOCIATION

American Public Health Association
800 I Street, NW
Washington, DC 20001-3710
www.apha.org

© 2025 by the American Public Health Association

All rights reserved. No part of this publication may be reproduced, stored in a retrieval system, or transmitted in any form or by any means, electronic, mechanical, photocopying, recording, scanning, or otherwise, except as permitted under Sections 107 and 108 of the 1976 United States Copyright Act, without either the prior written permission of the Publisher or authorization through payment of the appropriate per-copy fee to the Copyright Clearance Center [222 Rosewood Drive, Danvers, MA 01923, (978) 750-8400, fax (978) 646-8600, www.copyright.com]. Requests to the Publisher for permission should be addressed to the Permissions Department, American Public Health Association, 800 I Street, NW, Washington, DC 20001-3710; fax (202) 777-2531.

DISCLAIMER: Any discussion of medical or legal issues in this publication is being provided for informational purposes only. Nothing in this publication is intended to constitute medical or legal advice, and it should not be construed as such. This book is not intended to be and should not be used as a substitute for specific medical or legal advice, since medical and legal opinions may only be given in response to inquiries regarding specific factual situations. If medical or legal advice is desired by the reader of this book, a medical doctor or attorney should be consulted. The use of trade names and commercial sources in this book does not imply endorsement by the American Public Health Association. The views expressed in the publications of the American Public Health Association are those of the contributors and do not necessarily reflect the views of the American Public Health Association, or its staff, advisory panels, officers, or members of the Association's Executive Board. While the publisher and contributors have used their best efforts in preparing this book, they make no representations with respect to the accuracy or completeness of the content. The findings and conclusions in this book are those of the contributors and do not necessarily represent the official positions of the institutions with which they are affiliated.

Georges C. Benjamin, MD, MACP, Executive Director

Printed and bound in the United States of America
Book Production Editors: Keira McCarthy
Typesetting: The Charlesworth Group
Cover Design: Alan Giarcanella
Cover Illustration: Jasmin Pamukcu
Printing and Binding: Sheridan Books

Library of Congress Cataloging-in-Publication Data

Names: Porter, Jamila M. author | Pamukcu, Aysha author
Title: Advancing equity and justice / Jamila M. Porter, DrPH, MPH, and
    Aysha Pamukcu, JD.
Description: Washington : American Public Health Association, [2025] |
    Includes bibliographical references and index. | Summary: "This book is
    a practical, values-driven guide for anyone working to improve community
    health. It's designed to inform, inspire, and equip readers with the
    knowledge, strategies, and tools needed to create meaningful, lasting
    change"-- Provided by publisher.
Identifiers: LCCN 2025024348 (print) | LCCN 2025024349 (ebook) | ISBN
    9780875533599 paperback | ISBN 9780875533605 adobe pdf
Subjects: LCSH: Public health | Health services accessibility
Classification: LCC RA425 .P67 2025 (print) | LCC RA425 (ebook) | DDC
    362.1--dc23/eng/20250811
LC record available at https://lccn.loc.gov/2025024348
LC ebook record available at https://lccn.loc.gov/2025024349

For everyone who envisions a more just world and dares to make it real: *Advancing Equity and Justice* is for you. May this book sharpen your thinking, deepen your work, and fuel your inner fire.

Contents

Strategic Skills for Public Health Practice Series Introduction

Over the last 15 years, governmental public health professionals and partners nation-wide have worked to define core competencies, essential services, and foundational capabilities of the public health.[1,2,3] Central to all these efforts is the public health workforce—the practitioners who work in local, state, territorial, tribal, and federal public health agencies to prevent disease and protect and promote the health of the public.

The governmental public health workforce is diverse and comprised of many technical specialties and professions. These professional identities have shaped public health practice and formed categories of work that comprise the organizational chart most governmental public health agencies utilize, such as maternal and child health, environmental health, epidemiology and surveillance, communicable disease control, administration and finance, school health, and several others.

These categories have served public health well by helping organize work and allowing for professionalization and leadership development within specific areas. Over 21 national professional associations represent categorical or function areas within state and territorial health departments alone, not to mention peer groups and affinity groups that are part of the Association of State and Territorial Health Officials and other allied organizations such as the National Association of County and City Health Officials, the Big Cities Health Coalition, CityMatCH (urban maternal and child health programs), the National Environmental Health Association, and others.

These specialty designations have also led to fragmentation within agencies at a time when government is attempting to align more nimbly to meet the needs of the jurisdictions they serve. Few public health professionals have formal training in the skills needed to successfully adapt their work to navigate these changes, especially the strategic skills needed to position their work to meet contemporary public health challenges that require inter- and intra-agency collaboration for success. For example, the pressures and challenges imposed on the public health ecosystem and its workers by the COVID-19 pandemic illustrate the urgency of preparing the public health workforce not just for technical challenges but also for strategic and adaptive challenges posed by novel health threats that require an "all of government" approach to resolve.

Several external forces in recent years, including the movement from Public Health 2.0 to Public Health 3.0 and the six-year-long, three-phased Public Health Workforce Interests and Needs Survey, have either advocated for or implied the need for complementing the workforce's existing discipline-specific expertise with developing a set of strategic skills.

In 2017, the de Beaumont Foundation spearheaded the development of the National Consortium for Public Health Workforce Development comprised of public health leaders from 34 national partner organizations representing a variety of disciplines and settings nationwide. The Consortium was established "to communicate the needs of the front-line public health worker to national partners and funders."[4]

By consensus, the Consortium identified the following nine "indispensable, high-performance skills applicable to the entire public health workforce regardless of specialty or discipline."[5]

- Systems and strategic thinking
- Change management
- Effective communication
- Data-informed decision making
- Community engagement
- Justice, equity, diversity, and inclusion
- Resource management and finance
- Policy engagement
- Cross-sectoral partnerships

These strategic skills are needed by specialty-specific, technical experts in order to realize the multisector, cross-cutting visionary leadership needed today. The Consortium's "call to action" paper asserted this challenge to public health educators: "While maintaining excellence in core scientific disciplines continues to be a priority, developers and deliverers of public health education and training need to act in new and different ways if the governmental public health workforce is to gain competency in the strategic skills needed throughout the entire public health workforce."[5]

Creating these "new and different ways" of building public health workforce competencies in the strategic skills should be a priority for academic programs, professional associations, and public health partners nationwide. This Strategic Skills Series presents a new way to expand the education and training of the public health workforce, equipping its members for multisector collaboration to create policies and programs intended to solve real problems.

To develop this series, we have recruited thought leaders and experts to serve as the authors of each volume. The consistent format applied to each book in the series is intended to facilitate the learner's absorption and retention of key concepts and applications. The practice-based objectives of each book in the series are described below:

- **Systems and strategic thinking:** Grasp patterns and relationships to understand systems contributing to public health problems and identify high-impact interventions.
- **Change management:** Scale programs in response to the changing environments and shape core elements that sustain programs in challenge and crisis.
- **Effective communication:** Convey resonant, compelling public health messages to broad audiences—the public, partners, and policymakers.
- **Data-informed decision making:** Leverage, synthesize, and analyze multiple sources of electronic data and use informatics to identify and act on health priorities, population impacts, evidence-based approaches, and health and cost-related outcomes.
- **Community engagement:** Describe the most effective methods of and the beneficial outcomes from engaging communities in promoting health and well-being. Promote the model of equitable distribution of decision-making power.
- **Justice, equity, diversity, and inclusion:** Understand and respond to the changing demographics of the US population and the public health workforce itself. Seek out, listen to, include, and promote underrepresented populations in reaching effective health solutions.
- **Resource management and finance:** Oversee recruitment, acquisition, and retention of the workforce and manage fiscal resources responsibly.
- **Policy engagement:** Address public health concerns and needs and engage effectively with local, state, and federal policymakers and partners.
- **Cross-sectoral partnerships:** Bring together two or more distinct fields (e.g., health care and transportation) for greater impact so that public health professionals can maintain long-term collaborations that combine a unique set of resources, experience, and knowledge to effectively address multifaceted issues (e.g., the social determinants of health).

As we aim to move public health forward to meet the challenges of contemporary practice, we are excited to edit each of these volumes. It is our fervent hope that each of the books in this series represents a significant brick in the foundation of developing your capacity to address today's urgencies as well as tomorrow's opportunities and challenges.

Michael Fraser, PhD, MS
Brian C. Castrucci, DrPH

REFERENCES

1. Public Health Foundation. Core competencies for public health professionals. 2014. Accessed January 22, 2021. http://www.phf.org/programs/corecompetencies/Pages/Core_Competencies_Domains.aspx
2. US Centers for Disease Control and Prevention. 10 essential public health services. 2020. Accessed August 30, 2024. https://www.cdc.gov/public-health-gateway/php/about/index.html

3. Public Health National Center for Innovation. Foundational public health services. 2018. Accessed August 30, 2024. https://phaboard.org/wp-content/uploads/FPHS-Factsheet-2022.pdf

4. de Beaumont Foundation. Building skills for a more strategic public health workforce: a call to action. 2019. Accessed September 26, 2022. https://debeaumont.org/wp-content/uploads/2019/04/Building- Skills-for-a-More-Strategic-Public-Health-Workforce.pdf

5. de Beaumont Foundation. Building skills for a more strategic public health workforce: a call to action. July 18, 2017. Accessed January 22, 2021. https://www.debeaumont.org/news/2017/building-skills-for-a-more-strategic-health-workforce-a-call-to-action

Foreword

As the extraordinary writer Audre Lorde taught us, "there is no such thing as a single-issue struggle because we do not live single-issue lives."[1(p138)] This book is a testament to that wisdom.

As a Palestinian American community organizer, this quote is the foundation of how I build power and solidarity to bring about transformative change on the issues most impacting the communities I love and am from. I see Audre Lorde's words in the essence of public health. For me, public health is more than just a field of study. It is a call to action. It is a declaration that every person is worthy of self-determination and care; that every community—regardless of who they are or where they live—deserves dignity; and that access to education, health care, and housing are not a privilege, but a human right.

For far too long, the systems that claim to serve us have failed us—especially those among us who are poor, working class, and people of color. We must all confront the reality that we continue to live with the consequences of structural racism, inadequate health care, and environmental injustice—often suffering in silence while our pain is normalized or neglected.

But the story doesn't and can't end there. We. Have. Power.

That's why this book speaks directly to our moment. In *Advancing Equity and Justice*, the ever-brilliant Jamila M. Porter and the exceptional Aysha Dominguez Pamukcu remind us that public health offers a powerful framework to not only name these injustices but also connect and dismantle them. I invite activists, organizers, teachers, and public health practitioners to remember that those closest to the problems are closest to the solutions. It is they who carry the keys to transforming their conditions, and yet they continue to be systemically blocked from resources and opportunity.

We can change that. Jamila and Aysha give us tools to trace the roots of inequity and chart paths toward repair together. Their words can help us move beyond reactive care and toward *proactive justice*—where safe neighborhoods, high quality public education, clean air, and accessible health care and services are seen as requisite to health and nonnegotiable.

This book is an unflinching reminder that racial justice and equity must live at the center of all public health endeavors. It invites us to think expansively and critically about what health actually means; it is not just the absence of disease or harm, but the overall well-being and the presence of opportunity, belonging, and liberation for our respective communities and our nation at large. It instructs us to listen to voices that have been sidelined and to design systems that serve everyone, not just the few.

In this generation, we are living in an unprecedented time of reckoning and reimagination. For decades, but especially since the COVID-19 pandemic, the cracks and limits of our public health infrastructure have been exposed, but so too has the power of solidarity, of organizing, of people who refuse to accept any of this as inevitable.

To everyone working at the intersections of health and justice: What you do matters. Your voice and work matters. And the future we are building together and that we all deserve is within reach. I believe in us.

Let this book be your motivation.

Linda Sarsour
National Racial Justice Activist and Organizer

REFERENCES

1. Lorde A. *Sister Outsider: Essays and Speeches.* Crossing Press; 2007.

Preface: A Time for Clarity and Courage

We are living in times that will demand courage. . . . I look back and I look at how my existence here today is owed entirely to the courage of people who came before me. And so, what do I owe myself . . . and to those who come after me? To exercise courage in this moment.

—Bree Newsome Bass, filmmaker and civil rights activist[1]

I have hope. I see the possibilities—how, despite the darkness, this is also a time when we can rebuild our societies, starting with what's right in front of us: our areas of influence.

—Maria Ressa, Nobel Peace Prize–winning journalist and democracy advocate[2]

We are publishing this book at a time when equity and justice are under coordinated, escalating attack. Across the country, campaigns are underway to bury our nation's long history of structural racism, strip civil rights protections, erase the achievements of marginalized communities, criminalize gender diversity, and silence advocates for equity and justice. Anti-immigrant policies and rhetoric seek to narrowly define who belongs and who doesn't. Attacks on civil society—including efforts to outlaw political dissent, weaponize the legal system, suppress voting, censor people and institutions, and deploy intimidation campaigns—threaten the very foundations of democracy.

This is part of a broader agenda to preserve existing hierarchies of power by redefining and narrowing who is allowed to participate, who is protected, and who deserves to thrive. Public health, by its very nature, is a threat to this agenda. When we take on the root causes of health inequities, hold governments accountable to communities, demand redress for harms past and present, and uplift health as a right and not a privilege, we challenge systems that profit from injustice and exclusion.

The backlash we are witnessing is not an isolated political event. It is part of a decades-long effort to permanently reorganize society to benefit those who already hold the most power—that is, those who are whiter and wealthier—while pushing everyone else further outside the boundaries of care, protection, and opportunity.

Just a few years ago, we were in a different moment. Amid the COVID-19 outbreak, protests against police violence, and the rising *Movement for Black Lives*, cities and institutions across the country took unprecedented action: They declared racism a public health crisis. Elected officials spoke out and introduced promising policy reforms. Corporations pledged support for racial justice initiatives. Donors and philanthropic institutions mobilized resources. For a brief time, structural racism and systemic inequities could no longer be ignored, and social changes that once seemed unthinkable felt within reach.

But now the pendulum has swung back. We see a wave of restrictions—bans on teaching history truthfully, dismantling of diversity and inclusion initiatives, attacks on reproductive rights and gender-affirming care, and attempts to punish those who speak truth to power. These are not simply policy fights—they are efforts to rewrite reality. History, facts, evidence, and even people's right to define their own identities are being invalidated and erased. Merely acknowledging that structural oppression exists is a political act that carries personal and professional risk.

But history teaches us that this backlash is not new. It's part of a recurring cycle in US history of progress and retrenchment, where advances in justice are met with fierce and even violent opposition.

While regressive forces have long been powerful, so too are movements that dare to push toward justice. We have always lived in a world where those who wield power over others seek to control narratives, hoard resources, and undermine change. What makes this moment different is the boldness, scale, and speed of these attacks—and the urgent need for clarity and courage in how we respond.

We are living through a defining moment in our nation's history—much like Jim Crow, the incarceration of Japanese Americans during World War II, and the government's deadly neglect during the height of the AIDS epidemic. Each chapter was marked by state-sanctioned cruelty—policies, inaction, and enforcement that targeted entire communities—as well as by the silence of people and institutions that could have made a difference. Lives were lost not just to injustice itself, but also because of the failure to name it, resist it, and act with courage.

Today, we face a different set of crises—some new, many enduring—and the stakes remain high. The backlash to equity and justice is growing, and neutrality is not an option. Equity and justice cannot wait for favorable political winds, positive public opinion polls, or permission from those in power. Those of us in public health have a choice: We can retreat behind the false objectivity of science and an exclusionary interpretation of health, or we can openly stand in solidarity with the communities we serve. This book is for those who choose the latter.

WHY WE WROTE THIS BOOK

Unfortunately, in public health, we have too often shied away from directly naming and addressing the root causes of poor health. Confronting racial injustice, economic exploitation, and structural discrimination has been routinely sidelined in favor of superficial interventions that appear "neutral" but fail to challenge systems that produce and maintain inequity.

These attempts at neutrality have kept us from fully grappling with public health's complicity in racism and oppression—from the 40-year Tuskegee Syphilis Study that deceived and irrevocably harmed Black men and their families; to the destruction of neighborhoods that people of color called home under the banner of "urban renewal"; to the forced sterilization of women, people of color, disabled individuals, and incarcerated people deemed "unfit" by eugenic ideology.

In moments of crisis, our field has not always risen to the occasion. At the turn of the 20th century, for example, San Francisco, California public health officials responded to a bubonic plague outbreak by scapegoating and quarantining Chinese residents based on racist fears, not evidence. Over a century later, during the COVID-19 pandemic, inconsistent data collection and government harm obscured the virus's deadly toll on communities of colour, particularly Indigenous and Black communities.

In public health, we cannot consider ourselves beyond politics or "above the fray." The fray is about us. Today, even the illusion of neutrality is no longer an option. Organized efforts to defund, discredit, and dismantle public health and social justice institutions make clear what's at stake. The very idea of equity is under attack—not because it has failed, but because it has made progress. And that progress has not gone unnoticed.

So the question becomes: *Will we meet this moment?*

Will we speak out as communities are stripped of their rights, denied health-affirming resources, and excluded from political discussions and policy decisions where their futures are decided? Will we reclaim the proud legacy of public health—a field forged by decades of bold, highly politicized fights for labor protections, environmental justice, reproductive freedom, and more? Or will we choose comfort over courage?

Yes, there are risks to standing for justice—to our employment, to our funding, even to our safety. *But what is the greater cost of staying silent?*

We are being targeted because our work matters. The backlash we're experiencing is not just repression—it's recognition. It's a sign that equity and justice efforts have been gaining ground, rewriting narratives, and challenging systems that depend on exclusion and oppression.

Public health is about improving health outcomes, and that means it's also about uncovering truth, protecting the public good, and ensuring that every person and community has an opportunity to thrive. This work is not easy, and it never has been. But history shows that collective action, grounded in courage and shared purpose, is where real change begins.

No one can do everything. But everyone can do something. We hope this book supports you in finding *your* something. We hope it offers clarity, resolve, and inspiration—to live your values, to advance equity and justice however you can, and to practice public health as a bold force for collective liberation.

OUR POSITIONALITY STATEMENTS

A *positionality statement* is a way of acknowledging that no one writes from a neutral perspective. Our insights and beliefs are informed by our backgrounds, professional experiences, and lived realities.[3] Every author brings their own lens, experiences, and worldview to their work, and this book is no exception.

Jamila's Positionality Statement

I always knew that I wanted to work in public health—even when I didn't know it by name. As a young girl growing up in the American South, I lost close family members and friends to chronic diseases and fatal injuries. These early life experiences nearly tempted me to become a physician. But I learned early that while medicine would teach me how to treat an individual, public health had the power to protect entire communities. That made public health more than an area of academic interest. For me, it became a personal passion.

I still remember the first day of class in my master of public health program. Our instructor said, both simply and factually, "Poverty is the greatest predictor of poor health." No one in our class questioned it, including me. And in those two years of graduate study, no one ever mentioned that structural racism and other systems of oppression were also major predictors of poor health. It still alarms me to realize that racism was never mentioned in any of my graduate public health courses at all.

Fast-forward a few years later, and I was conducting evaluation, programmatic, and advocacy work on behalf of state injury and violence prevention programs. Topically, much of my work involved pedestrian injury prevention, traffic safety, and road transportation policy, as well as community design. Practitioners in these spaces were proposing policies and initiatives to create safer streets for pedestrians and cyclists. Solutions focused on the "five Es"—education, enforcement, encouragement, evaluation, and engineering. But we failed to ask more fundamental questions: *Why were so many of our streets designed to be unsafe in the first place? And why did the most dangerous streets largely run through communities of color?* If we had asked these questions, perhaps we would have connected the dots sooner. Perhaps we would have realized—as many of my colleagues and I have since confirmed through our research—that policy decisions like Jim Crow, redlining, and neighborhood disinvestment had baked inequity into how communities were designed and built decades earlier, and these decisions continue to undermine our health to this day.

Having worked as a program director, evaluator, and researcher, this work is a personal passion—for me and for the many colleagues who I've had the honor to work with over the years. This book is a direct result of that passion: an opportunity for us to connect the dots between inequity, injustice, and the barriers that have kept us from realizing health for all. For I believe, in our efforts to make these connections, we will ultimately find the solutions we seek.

Aysha's Positionality Statement

I didn't find my way directly to public health. My career began in human rights and civil rights law, inspired by my upbringing in California's Bay Area as the child of immigrants from the Philippines and Türkiye. That experience taught me—long before I had the words for it—that our identities and circumstances unfairly shape our chances in life. We don't choose what "race," nationality, or class we're born into, yet those forces tip the scales for how long and how well we'll live. I became a lawyer to confront that injustice.

Early in my career, I worked for a war crimes tribunal and quickly learned the power and the limits of the law. We need legal advocacy to name harm and try to prevent it from happening again—but this can only go so far in the face of atrocity. That experience planted a central question for me: *What does true justice require?*

Later, while working on economic justice at a multidisciplinary civil rights organization, I found myself collaborating with colleagues in public health. I saw how we were struggling against the same systems but using different language. I talked about *disparate impact* and the *racial wealth gap*; they talked about *health disparities* and *social determinants*. That realization opened a new path for me—one focused on building connections across sectors and movements.

But when I entered the public health field, I was surprised by how rarely people were willing to name racism or speak openly about justice. Even the term *health equity* could spark discomfort. Years later, I coauthored a paper about the *civil rights of health* with critical race scholar Angela P. Harris that articulated what I had long sensed: that civil rights lawyers, public health practitioners, and movement leaders are natural allies, but have not yet come together in a truly transformative way. This book is the next step in that work: an invitation for public health to connect with other movements and disciplines and to make justice-driven practice more accessible, actionable, and aligned.

Across my career, I've had the privilege of working alongside brilliant leaders in climate justice, economic justice, civil rights, place-based organizing, and the fight for a multiracial democracy. These collaborations have made one thing clear: our struggles are linked, and our power is collective. If we want to build a healthy, abundant future, we need to move like a movement—one that draws strength from our differences and finds unity in shared purpose.

Jamila M. Porter, DrPH, MPH
Aysha Dominguez Pamukcu, JD

REFERENCES

1. Drake O. Bree Newsome leads Wesleyan's Martin Luther King celebration. *The Wesleyan Connection*. February 3, 2020. Accessed June 12, 2025. https://newsletter.blogs.wesleyan.edu/2020/02/03/bree-newsome-leads-wesleyans-martin-luther-king-celebration
2. Ressa M. *How to Stand Up to a Dictator: The Fight for Our Future.* HarperCollins; 2022.
3. Daly H, Martinchek K, Martinez R, Morgan J, Farrell L, Falkenburger E. Exploring individual and institutional positionality: A tool for equity in community engagement and collaboration. Urban Institute. December 2023. Updated March 2024. Accessed May 7, 2025. https://www.urban.org/research/publication/exploring-individual-and-institutional-positionality

Acknowledgments

We are grateful to the many people who helped bring this book to fruition.

We start by thanking our collaborator, illustrator, and cover artist—Jasmin Pamukcu of Cusp Consulting—whose phenomenal talent and vision infused these pages with life and meaning. You took on the daunting task of visualizing complex ideas—and did so with great creativity and patience. Your generous collaboration resulted in visual storytelling that engages both the heart and the mind. We are profoundly grateful to you.

To our trusted and brilliant reviewers who gave us feedback on early ideas and drafts: Thank you for challenging us to think more deeply, communicate more clearly, and ensure our words align with our values. Our reviewers are listed here in alphabetical order by first name, with titles and affiliations of their choosing:

- Ashley Chu, EdM, educator and curriculum writer
- Hannah Sheehy, MPH
- Ina I. Robinson, MPH, DrPH candidate, public health practitioner, health equity leader, and social justice advocate
- Jessica Hill, PhD, MPH, public health practitioner and artist
- Julian Drix, MPH, bridging community power-building and public health at Health in Partnership
- Motunrayo Tosin-Oni, PhD candidate, health policy scholar, and professional
- Phebe Gibson, MPH
- Sonja F. M. Diaz, JD, MPP
- Taren Evans, MURP, urban planning and environmental justice professional
- Zamir M. Bradford, MPH, FRSPH, Muslim, husband, son, brother, founder, and innovator

We are also grateful to Zamir for heroically providing formatting, glossary, and citations support. Additionally, we thank Dena Afrasiabi, whose keen editorial eye helped structure and sharpen this text through many revisions.

We thank the Strategic Skills Series editors, Brian C. Castrucci and Mike Fraser, as well as the teams at the de Beaumont Foundation and APHA Press for making this book possible and standing firm in a commitment to equity and justice.

We are grateful for the care and thoughtfulness each of our collaborators brought to this project. Any remaining errors or oversights are entirely our own.

To everyone who helped us refine, question, and create—thank you.

Finally, we have some personal appreciations.

Jamila: I am deeply grateful for many wonderful family members, friends, and colleagues—all of whom helped make this book possible. Their love, support, guidance, humor, and encouragement got me through seemingly countless nights and weekends that were consumed with writing, all while working full time. I could never have achieved this accomplishment without their love and support, and I am forever thankful.

I am honored to have two incredible people for parents—Shirley and Barry Sr.—who have loved and inspired me in more ways than I can count. Despite experiencing the trauma of Jim Crow, they survived and thrived. They went on to college and graduate school, and ultimately became accomplished professionals. My mother became an award-winning teacher with an illustrious 43-year career in education, and my father became a certified public accountant and successful business owner. They always told me I could accomplish anything I set my mind to achieve. This book is as much their accomplishment as it is mine, and I also share it with my grandparents—Earnestine, Woodrow Sr., Lula, and Carl Sr.—and all of our ancestors who came before us.

My siblings, Barry Jr. and Dara—an accomplished attorney and a user experience designer, respectively—have both made my life a wonderful adventure, as have my niece, Ariel, and my nephew, Aston. Their love and humor have been a constant, and I can't imagine my life without them. I'm also thankful for my best friend, Lauren, who has been a steadfast source of support, encouragement, and laughter since we were undergraduates at Wake Forest University.

I am thankful for my mentors, Joel Lee and Chris Kochtitzky, and my uncle, Earnest Curry—all of whom passed away far too prematurely. They encouraged, inspired, and uplifted me in so many ways. My Uncle Earnest once told me, "people don't do what you expect; they do what you inspect." His words have stayed with me and compel me to be worthy of others' high expectations. Although they didn't live to see this book published, their influence lies within its pages.

Finally, I want to thank all of my colleagues and collaborators, especially the people and communities that are part of the Modernized Anti-Racist Data Ecosystems (MADE) for Health Justice initiative. They are courageous trailblazers who are doing some of the most transformative work in the nation—perhaps the world—to advance health equity and data justice, and it is ever-inspiring.

I am immensely appreciative of so many others who I call friends, family, and colleagues. You have expanded my thinking and brought out the best in me. You continue to push me to see what's possible and to strive for even more.

Aysha: I must foremost thank my loving and fiercely feminist partner, Tom, who indulged my nerdy tangents and held it down through the evenings, weekends, and even across time zones and continents. Your unwavering support has been "the work that makes all other work possible"—this book exists because of you.

Love and gratitude to our children, Rio and Linden—three and five years old as of publication—who grew alongside this book and continue to teach me so much.

I also appreciate and honor my parents, who each took a leap of faith in coming to this country, and who see both its flaws and its promise with great clarity. And to my sister, Jasmin: Your brilliance of course shines through these illustrations—but my deepest gratitude is for traveling together through the many intersections we inhabit.

Special thanks to Angela P. Harris, whose partnership and mentorship helped shape my understanding of public health as a movement for justice. And thank you to my colleagues, past and present, at the San Francisco Foundation and the Partnership for the Bay's Future, who work shoulder to shoulder with me to change systems, build power, and support our government in fulfilling its aspiration of being truly by the people and for the people.

These acknowledgements are necessarily incomplete. So many others have inspired, educated, and supported me—if your name isn't here, know your influence is.

Introduction

This is precisely the time when [we] go to work. There is no time for despair, no place for self-pity, no need for silence, no room for fear.

-Toni Morrison, author and cultural critic[1]

Imagine a world where no neighborhood is considered the "good" side of town—where every community is vibrant, well-resourced, and full of opportunity. Where healthy food is abundant and culturally affirming. Where every school nurtures growth, confidence, and a love of learning in students. Where joy and connection are deliberately designed into the places where people live, work, and travel. Where health care is not just universal but also proactive, empathetic, and accountable. Where our lives, our livelihoods, and our health are understood as interdependent—with each other and with the planet.

And yet, despite all we know and the advances we've made, this vision feels far away.

Why? Why is the deck seemingly stacked in favor of injustice? Why do efforts to "move the needle" so often fall short—or, worse, perpetuate the very problems we've committed our careers to solving? Why, in spite of all our efforts, does it feel like we're always treading water and managing acute issues? Why are we unable to truly address the root causes of public health problems?

As we grappled with these questions—especially early in our careers—we longed for a resource that could help us name the forces continually undermining public health, explain why traditional public health approaches often miss the mark, and offer guidance for doing things differently.

So we wrote the book we wished we had.

In *Advancing Equity and Justice*, we make it clear that the challenges we're facing in public health aren't just problems related to implementation or underfunding. They're systemic and structural. Our field has been shaped by—and remains embedded in—systems that fundamentally, and often fatally, undermine community health. This has forced us to merely respond to the symptoms of injustice while leaving its root causes intact.

Public health interventions and funding models were never designed to address the root causes of unjust health disparities. They were created to manage risk, modify individual behaviors, and mitigate disease—not to prevent systemic inequities or rectify injustice.

This contributes to missteps in how we do the work. Even well-meaning public health efforts are designed and implemented in shortsighted, hierarchical ways that overlook the wisdom, power, and leadership of communities themselves. Health inequities persist not because individuals make "bad" choices but because community priorities and solutions are routinely ignored, unfunded, or overridden by systems that prioritize control over care.

Advancing Equity and Justice is a call for change—not just in achieving health outcomes, but in how we do the work to get there. It is an actionable, values-driven guide for anyone working to improve community health. It's designed to inspire and equip you with the knowledge, strategies, and tools you need to make a positive impact that is meaningful and lasting.

The book is structured in three parts:

- **Part I: Uncovering the Foundations of (In)Equity and (In)Justice** sets the stage by establishing core definitions and examining the historical and systemic roots of health inequities.
- **Part II: Seizing Opportunities for Change** explores how misleading mindsets and harmful narratives limit progress—and how our work to shift power and take an assurance-based approach to public health can create new possibilities.
- **Part III: Creating Flourishing Futures for All** offers bold visions and concrete steps to advance equity, justice, and community health in ways that are both aspirational and applicable.

Throughout the book, we invite you to engage both your heart and your mind. The ability to advance equity, justice, and community health is not just about learning and doing; it's also about feeling and being. That's why this book includes the following:

- Historical context and systems analysis that conveys why and how health inequities persist.
- Arguments and counterarguments to help navigate resistance and political pushback.
- Resources and research that provide reliable information, evidence, and entry points for further learning and exploration.
- Strategies and practical guidance to move from ideas to action.
- Insights from lived experience, including voices of community leaders, organizers, and scholars.
- Lessons from justice movements, visionary approaches to public health that unite and inspire, and enduring values to guide us toward a flourishing future.
- Graphics to bring complex topics to life and support different learning styles.

Quotes that appear at the beginning of sections are meant to set the tone and spark reflection. Illustrations throughout the book offer a way to engage with the material visually and creatively. We invite you to interact with them in any way you like—color them in, use them to center your thoughts, or simply take a moment to pause and breathe.

We also have made values-driven choices about how we refer to people's identities, including the following:

- We use *queer* to refer to people whose sexual orientation or gender identity is not exclusively heterosexual or cisgender. Though once used as a slur, it has been reclaimed by many as a proud and expansive identity. Today, *queer* is increasingly used in activist, academic, and cultural contexts to be inclusive of the many ways that people self-identify and actively resist rigid gender categories.[2] That said, the term is not embraced by everyone, and in some settings, terms like *LGBTQ+* may be more appropriate.

- We use *Latine* as a gender-neutral and non-Anglicized term to describe people with origins in Latin America. It is a newer identifier intended to affirm gender diversity while being culturally and linguistically respectful. We also recognize that no single descriptor is used by all members of this diverse community, existing alongside *Latino*, *Latina*, and *Latinx*—each reflecting different histories, preferences, and contexts.[3,4]

- We use *Indigenous people(s)*, *Native Nations*, *Tribal communities*, and *Tribal Nations* to refer to the diverse and sovereign peoples who have long inhabited lands now known as the United States and North America. These terms honor both cultural identity and the political status of Tribal Nations as distinct, self-governing entities with inherent rights to land, governance, and self-determination.

- We use *people of color* and *Black and brown people* to describe those who have been racialized—that is, people upon whom the construct of "race" has been imposed and who bear the burdens of racism. (Following the lead of many community leaders and scholars, we use a lowercased spelling of *people of color* and *brown* to reflect their use as broad political or social descriptors, not as specific ethnic or cultural identities.) This is not meant to oversimplify or flatten distinct identities, but to speak to shared experiences of racialization and systemic exclusion.

- We capitalize *Black* and lowercase *white* when we describe racial categories. The Associated Press explains, "people who are Black have strong historical and cultural commonalities, even if they are from different parts of the world and even if they now live in different parts of the world. That includes the shared experience of discrimination due solely to the color of one's skin." By contrast, "white people generally do not share the same history and culture, or the experience of being discriminated against because of skin color . . . [and] capitalizing the term *white*, as is done by white supremacists, risks subtly conveying legitimacy to such beliefs."[5]

We have also been intentional about how we name harm. Language shapes how people understand the origins of injustice, and throughout the book, we use words that highlight structural causes, rather than those that obscure:

- We place the word "race" in quotation marks to provide a visual reminder that "race" is an unscientific categorization with no biological basis—but one with profound life-and-death consequences caused by the system we call *racism*. This duality gives "race" its enduring and destructive power. The convention of and rationale for placing "race" in quotation marks is one that has been used by other scholars as well.[6,7]

- We say *climate disaster*, rather than "natural disaster," because the devastation that communities face is not natural. It has been created by human decisions—including those related to extraction, deregulation, and disinvestment—that have destabilized ecosystems and driven long-term, extreme changes we now experience as a climate crisis.

- We use terms like *cissexism* and *heterosexism* rather than "transphobia" or "homophobia" because the suffix "-phobia" inaccurately and inappropriately suggests fear and psychological conditions. In actuality, they are manifestations of deeply rooted systems of prejudice and discrimination that threaten the safety, dignity, and recognition of people's full humanity.

No terminology can fully capture the richness and diversity of people's lived experiences. Preferences and norms shift across time, place, community, and context. If we've used language that doesn't reflect your identity, we ask for your grace and forgiveness. This book is situated in a particular moment, and the language we have used will almost certainly evolve—a dynamic that we appreciate and welcome.

Finally, two notes on what this book is *not*.

First, this is not an exhaustive resource on equity and justice. These are vast and evolving fields with long histories, deep roots, and vibrant schools of thought. We acknowledge the value of related concepts like diversity, inclusion, and belonging, and note that this book is focused specifically on equity and justice within the context of US public health practice. While our focus is on the United States, we recognize that equity work and struggles for justice are global, and practitioners everywhere have much to learn from one another. To that end, we encourage you to look both within and beyond national borders for inspiration, strategy, and solidarity.

Second, this book is not a one-size-fits-all solution. Instead, it offers frameworks, guidance, and examples that can be adapted across roles and contexts—whether you work at the local, state, or national level; in government, nonprofit, philanthropic, or academic spaces; or outside of institutions as a grassroots advocate, social entrepreneur, or consultant.

This book is interdisciplinary and wide-ranging in its scope. But we also recognize that any resource about equity and justice is, in some sense, unfinished, because the struggle is ongoing. The work is collective and evolving—and this book is one of many contributions to a living, growing movement.

Advancing Equity and Justice brings together hard-won lessons we've learned through our training, on the job, in justice movements, and in community. It's shaped by questions we've asked ourselves, truths we wish we'd known, and tools we've discovered or created along the way. In that sense, this book is both a reflection of where we've been and a foundation for what comes next. We hope it not only informs and engages you but also sparks new ways of thinking. We hope it encourages you to do the work of public health in deeper alignment with social movements for justice. And, most importantly, we hope it inspires you to *act*. A more just, flourishing, and liberated world is possible—and your work can bring it to life.

Thank you for joining us on this journey.

REFERENCES

1. Morrison T. No place for self-pity, no room for fear. *The Nation*. March 23, 2015. Accessed May 7, 2025. https://www.thenation.com/article/archive/no-place-self-pity-no-room-fear

2. Collins C. Is "queer" OK to say? Here's why we use it. Learning for Justice. February 11, 2019. Accessed June 16, 2025. https://www.learningforjustice.org/magazine/is-queer-ok-to-say-heres -why-we-use-it

3. Gonzales E. Why we're saying "Latine." Chicago History Museum. October 24, 2023. Accessed June 26, 2025. https://www.chicagohistory.org/why-were-saying-latine

4. Baker C, Cabezas C, Lorenzino A. Hispanic, Latino/a, Latinx or Latine? Find out how to use the terms. *Temple Now*. Temple University. October 8, 2024. Accessed June 30, 2025. https://news. temple.edu/news/2024-10-08/hispanic-latinoa-latinx-or-latine-find-out-how-use-terms

5. Meir N. Announcements: Why we will lowercase white. The Associated Press. July 20, 2020. Accessed June 24, 2025. https://www.ap.org/the-definitive-source/announcements/why-we-will-lowercase-white

6. Jones CP. "Race," racism, and the practice of epidemiology. *Am J Epidemiol*. 2001;154(4):299–304. doi:10.1093/aje/154.4.299

7. Mukhopadhyay CC, Moses YT. Reestablishing "race" in anthropological discourse. *Am Anthropol*. 1997;99(3):517–533. doi:10.1525/aa.1997.99.3.517

I. UNCOVERING THE FOUNDATIONS OF (IN)EQUITY AND (IN)JUSTICE

We begin our journey by establishing a shared understanding of health, equity, and justice—and the interconnections between them. We explore foundational definitions, the root causes of health inequities, and how our nation's history shaped the unjust disparities we face today.

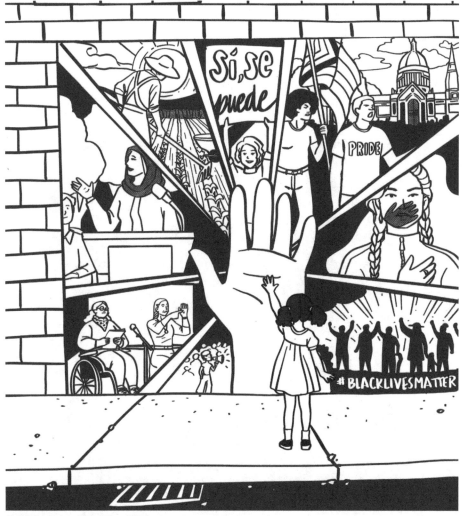

Artist Credit: Jasmin Pamukcu, 2025.
On Their Shoulders

Defining What's at Stake

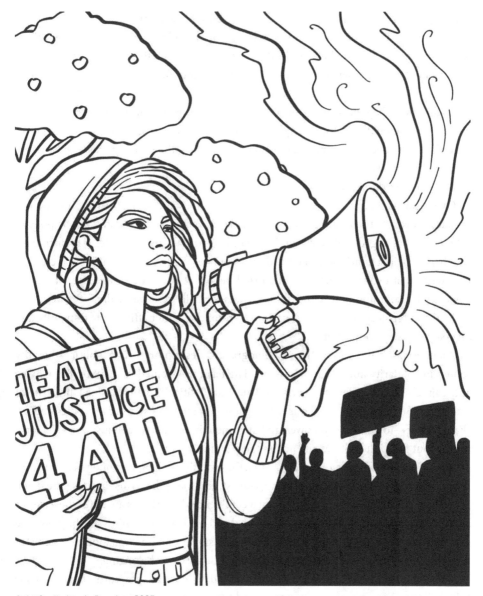

Artist Credit: Jasmin Pamukcu, 2025.
Our Health, Our Voice, Our Power

Your silence will not protect you. . . . What are the words you do not yet have? . . . What are the tyrannies you swallow day by day and attempt to make your own, until you will sicken and die of them, still in silence? . . . [W]e have been socialized to respect fear more than our own needs for language and definition . . . it is not difference which immobilizes us, but silence. And there are so many silences to be broken.

-Audre Lorde, poet and feminist scholar[1(p41,44)]

Language is one of the most powerful tools we have for making sense of the world and for shaping it. The words we choose express our thoughts and feelings. They reflect our values, convey our beliefs, and influence how we relate to one another. Language is never neutral. It carries the weight of our history and the spirit of the times in which we live.

In this first chapter, we present terms that are foundational for understanding the intersections of public health, equity, and justice. Some of these definitions may be familiar. Others have been reinterpreted or expanded to reflect the evolving nature of language and the shifting social contexts in which we use it.

But why does this matter?

Over time, language evolves to reflect shifting values and social norms. In just a few decades, words that once appeared in textbooks, government forms, and public policies have been challenged and replaced. The word "Oriental," for example, was once used widely in official records and in everyday discourse—despite being rooted in a colonial worldview that exoticized and dehumanized people of Asian descent.[2] After sustained advocacy by community leaders, the term was formally removed from US federal law in 2016 and replaced with *Asian American*,[3] a term that better affirms the humanity and diversity of Asian communities.

Asian American is more than a demographic descriptor; it is a political identity rooted in solidarity and collective action. The term was coined in 1968 by Emma Gee and Yuji Ichioka, founders of the Asian American Political Alliance at the University of California, Berkeley. Their goal was to bring together diverse Asian communities under a shared name—to build unity, power, and alignment in solidarity with justice movements throughout the United States and across the world.[4,5]

This example offers several insights: First, the evolution of language often begins within social movements, as communities claim, contest, and shape the terms that describe them. Second, language can reveal power. Language influences how stories are told, whose voices are centered, and whose experiences are valued and made visible. Third, shifting language can shift perspectives, moving people from exclusionary and assimilationist systems of thought toward those that are rooted in dignity, solidarity, and belonging.

This same evolution in language is evident in today's efforts to use words that reflect our values. Terms that were once commonly used have been and continue to be reevaluated, refined, and, in some cases, discarded. At the same time, new terms have emerged—or existing ones have been reclaimed—to more accurately capture people's lived experiences and to describe their identities and circumstances in ways that are authentic, inclusive, and respectful. Here are some examples:

- **Using the term *people of color* rather than "minorities":** The term "minorities" wrongly implies that people of color are numerically marginal or politically insignificant.[6] Today, *people of color* is more commonly used, recognizing both the shared experiences of structural racism and the demographic shifts reshaping the United States, where people of color will be the majority in coming decades.[7]

- **Describing forces that have oppressed communities over time:** Rather than blaming individuals for harms inflicted by systems and structures, terms like *disinvested*, *marginalized*, and *systematically excluded* draw attention to the policies, practices, and power structures that have oppressed entire communities over generations. This language appropriately places the focus and blame on the root causes of injustice.

- **Prioritizing person-centered language:** Person-first language puts humanity before conditions or circumstances. For example, instead of saying *homeless people*, a person-centered alternative could be *people experiencing homelessness*. This phrasing acknowledges that housing status is just one aspect of a person's experience, not their entire identity or a permanent characteristic. A person's housing status is something that can change over time and is shaped by broader systems and contexts.

- **Respecting people's pronouns and identities:** Asking for and using someone's correct pronouns is a basic practice of respect. It recognizes that gender cannot be assumed, and that *gender identity* (a person's internal sense of self), *gender expression* (how someone chooses to externally show their gender identity), and *sex assigned at birth* (a label given to infants when they are born) are distinct and may not align with the assumptions of the dominant culture. Rigid societal norms often erase the full spectrum of people's experiences. By inviting individuals to self-identify their pronouns and by using them, we help build a culture that affirms gender diversity and respects people on their own terms.

These changes to language reflect progress and are part of an ongoing effort to align our words with equity, justice, inclusion, and respect.

But not all language changes are made in good faith. Some terms have been deployed to insidiously divide us rather than nurture connection and empathy.

These terms are **coded language**: words that seem neutral on the surface but carry hidden meanings—often to invoke stereotypes, perpetuate prejudice, and reinforce power imbalances. Coded language operates under the guise of civility, professionalism, and common sense. It provides the speaker with plausible deniability while simultaneously allowing them to communicate ideas that would otherwise be called out as discriminatory, offensive, and socially unacceptable. As sociolinguist and language rights advocate Geneva Smitherman and others have shown, coded language allows people to speak about "race,"* class, and power in ways that maintain domi-nance because they avoid accountability.[10]

Coded language is often used to obscure the structural causes of harm and deflect responsibility for addressing them. Rather than explicitly using racist terms and stereo-types, coded language offers "race-neutral" or "colorblind"† explanations that shift blame to individuals or communities. Consider these examples:

- **Problematic geographic stand-ins for "race":** Terms like "urban" and "inner city" have been used as code for Black people, while the term "rural" has been used as code for white people.[12] These inaccurate generalizations mask both the racial diversity of all geographic regions[13] and the true drivers of inequity. For example, saying "inner-city schools underperform" blames the location—and its presumed residents—rather than the decades of underfunding, legalized racial segregation, discriminatory tax policies, and exclusionary school districting that have all perpetuated unjust differ-ences in "school performance."

- **Dehumanizing language for people with limited political and structural power:** Terms like "illegal immigrant" reduce people to a legal status and erase their humanity and personhood, making it easier to justify cruel policies that vilify them. This lan-guage simultaneously keeps us from recognizing our shared humanity while framing immigration as a criminal legal issue and a national security threat, rather than what it is: a matter of public health and human rights.[14]

- **Equating "bad" with Black and brown communities:** The term "bad"—in the con-text of phrases like "bad schools" and "bad neighborhoods"—carries a long history of being used to covertly and negatively describe Black people and other people of color.[15] "Bad" is used to implicitly blame people of color for adverse circumstances, ignoring the many policies that have ensured decades of segregation, disinvestment, and concentrated disadvantage.

- **Using "law and order" to justify subjugation:** Political calls for "law and order" have long been used to justify state-sanctioned violence against and mass incarceration of Black and brown people. Coined in the post-Civil Rights era to oppose movements

---

*Throughout this book, you will find the word "race" in quotation marks. This is a convention that has been used by other scholars as well (e.g., Jones,[8] Mukhopadhyay and Moses[9]) to provide a visual reminder that "race" and the categorization of people into "races" is an unscientific social construct with no biological basis. Never-theless, simultaneously, we must acknowledge that although "race" is false, it has a very real and damaging impact on our lives. It is a primary way by which people are categorized in the United States and across the globe. As you come across every reference to "race", we encourage you to keep these ideas in mind.

†**Colorblindness** is an ideology that downplays or denies the role of structural racism in shaping opportunities and outcomes for people of color. Colorblindness can manifest in ways that include (1) denying the concept of "race" altogether (e.g., "We are all the same"); (2) ignoring or dismissing blatant racial discrimination; (3) over-looking institutional racism, which includes the cumulative policies, practices, and norms that disadvantage people of color; and (4) disregarding the influence of *white privilege*: the unearned advantages and opportuni-ties that come with being classified as white.[11]

for racial justice, the phrase intentionally presents policing as neutral and necessary, while disguising state violence as protection for white communities. It also shifts attention away from actual structural drivers of violence—like poverty, disinvestment, and trauma—to focus on destructive forms of punishment and control.[16]

Our words shape how we perceive our reality, making language both descriptive and constructive. The words we use influence how we understand problems, assign responsibility, and imagine solutions.

Yet, language associated with equity and justice has become a political flashpoint. Terms like *woke*, *Critical Race Theory*, *DEI* (diversity, equity, and inclusion), and even people's pronouns have been distorted and weaponized—not because of what they actually mean but because of what they represent: efforts to name injustice and advocate for change. Vilifying these terms is part of a strategy to erase knowledge about racism and systemic oppression, demonize and silence people working to advance social justice, and fuel divisions to cement political power.

As community health advocate and scholar Tamarie A. Macon puts it, "Language matters because our words can reflect our heart and shape our mind."[17] Words convey histories, voices, and experiences. They shape our collective understanding of the world and influence what we believe is possible within it.

As public health practitioners, language is one of the most powerful tools we have, and we must speak with both precision and purpose. We don't always have to use the same words, but we do need to convey the same shared meaning.

EXPANDING OUR DEFINITIONS OF *HEALTH, PUBLIC HEALTH,* AND *COMMUNITY HEALTH*

What I care most about are definitions . . . as always, we need sharp words in order to articulate our ideas clearly . . . [I]t is impossible to find the right definitions by pure thought; one needs to detect the correct problems where progress will require the isolation of a new key concept.

–Peter Scholze, mathematician and author[18]

Let's start with the most fundamental concept of our work: **health**. As a field, we have long measured health by what threatens it: disease, injury, disability, and death. Although rooted in loss, these indicators have helped us identify inequities, inform policy, and save lives.

But when we define health only by what goes wrong, we risk telling an incomplete and inaccurate story. A deficit-based approach to health overlooks the importance of joy, connectedness, and belonging. It ignores the complexity of people's lives and reinforces a narrow, medicalized view of what it means to be healthy. Many people navigate physical and mental health conditions every day while leading fulfilling lives rooted in meaning, connection, and dignity. Yet our field's classic definition of health often fails to embody these vital and valuable lived experiences.

We see this limitation reflected in the World Health Organization's definition of health: "a state of complete physical, mental, and social well-being, and not merely the absence of disease or infirmity."[19] But the presence of illness or disability does not automatically negate health. What matters is that people have the ability to live fully, meaningfully, and on their own terms. As disability justice leaders remind us, health is not a binary state or a personal virtue. It is a dynamic, self-defined experience shaped by care, community, and having access to the resources we need to live well, both individually and in relationship with others.

To better reflect this broader vision of health, we use the term *flourishing*—having what we need, both individually and collectively, to lead lives of purpose, agency, connection, and possibility. **Flourishing** is about more than survival or longevity; it's about living a life that feels meaningful. The Health Equity and Policy Lab describes flourishing this way:

> [People who flourish are] living a good, fulfilling life, a life with a sense of purpose. They have the ability to do what they want to do and be who they want to be. . . . [They are] surrounded [by], supported by, and contribute collaboratively to strong support systems, institutions, resources, norms, and security.[20]

Flourishing invites us to move beyond deficit-based ideas about health and toward an expansive vision of thriving, connection, and self-determination.

We consider *health* and *flourishing* to be synonymous because health is ultimately about having the ability to lead a full and fulfilling life rooted in dignity and purpose—in other words, to flourish.

If *health* is *flourishing*, then what is *public health*?

In 1988, the Institute of Medicine defined public health as "what we, as a society, do collectively to assure the conditions for people to be healthy."[21(p19)] A widely used earlier definition comes from bacteriologist and public health scholar Charles-Edward Amory Winslow. First introduced in 1920 and refined by 1947, he described public health as

> the science and art of preventing disease, prolonging life, and promoting physical and mental health and efficiency through organized community efforts . . . and the development of the social machinery which will ensure to every individual in the community a standard of living adequate for the maintenance of health; organizing these benefits in such fashion as to enable every citizen to realize his birthright of health and longevity.[2(p396)]

We build on these earlier definitions to define **public health** as the science and art of ensuring that entire communities have what they need to flourish. As public health researcher and storytelling scholar David O. Fakunle puts it, public health is "anything

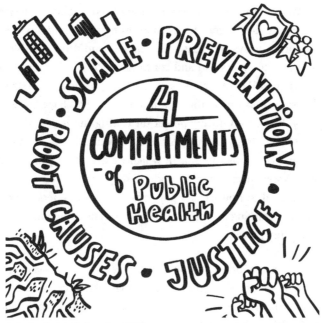

Artist Credit: Jasmin Pamukcu, 2025.

Figure 1-1. Four Commitments of Public Health

related to the acknowledgement, appreciation, understanding, and advancement of human health and well-being."[23] As a field, we fulfill this purpose through the *Four Commitments of Public Health* (Figure 1-1):

1. Scale—Promoting collective flourishing

Public health is fundamentally about people—not as isolated individuals but as interconnected communities. Whether we work across neighborhoods or nations, our goal is to promote health at the population level—to create conditions in which everyone can flourish. This charge includes the well-being of our families, coworkers, neighbors, and even future generations. It requires us to think beyond personal responsibility and focus on our collective capacity to thrive.

2. Prevention—Stopping problems before they start

Ultimately, public health is not about monitoring, describing, or treating illnesses and injuries—it is about preventing them in the first place. This involves addressing risk factors like housing instability or discrimination, while promoting protective factors such as dignified work and strong social support systems. Prevention spans policies, environments, and interventions that have the power to create healthier societies.

3. Root causes—Addressing the systems behind the symptoms
Public health goes far beyond promoting healthy behaviors to transform the systems that shape choices and drive health outcomes. As a field, we zoom out to understand and confront the forces that impact our lives and collective experiences. These include systems of oppression—like structural racism, sexism, and classism—as well as the laws and policies that shape our everyday lives.

 4. Justice—Building power for lasting change
Our health is and always has been political, subject to the social, legal, and economic systems in which we live. Who you are, what you look like, your family's wealth, and your zip code all shape your access to the resources and opportunities needed to flourish. As public health practitioners, we cannot achieve our goals without centering justice, and that requires us to help foster civic participation and community power.

Communities are more than just groups of people living in the same place. They are connected by shared experiences, identities, and geography. Because of its focus on entire communities, the term *public health* is synonymous with *community health*.

Community health emphasizes the well-being of communities overall, focusing on the interconnectedness of social, economic, and environmental factors and their influence on health and flourishing. *Community health* is a holistic, inclusive term that recognizes the complexity of our world and the interrelated systems we seek to transform. *Public health* and *community health* are synonymous and can be used interchangeably. That said, the term *community health* can be particularly useful when communicating with the public and with people working in other fields to emphasize the people-focused and community-centered nature of our work.

DEFINING *SOCIAL DETERMINANTS OF HEALTH* AND *SYSTEMS OF OPPRESSION*

Your health is as safe as that of the worst-insured, worst-cared-for person in your society. It will be decided by the height of the floor, not the ceiling.

-Anand Giridharadas, author and journalist[24]

To improve health for all—and to ensure that everyone can flourish—we must understand and address the underlying forces that shape health outcomes.

Health is often mischaracterized as the result of our genes or the choices we make as individuals. In reality, our health and well-being are shaped far more profoundly by the conditions in which we are born, grow, live, work, and age. These contexts and conditions—like access to affordable and desirable housing, clean air, safe and supportive

Box 1-1. Plain-Language Options to Describe the Social Determinants of Health

The social determinants of health are a cornerstone of public health. This book uses the term because it is widely recognized across various fields, including human rights, social work, health care, and policy. It also reflects the sociological nature of health, which encompasses multiple factors that influence health outcomes.

That said, the term *social determinants of health* doesn't always resonate with the general public. The FrameWorks Institute[28] and others have recommended several alternatives that can help convey this concept more effectively to a broader audience, such as these examples:

- The essential conditions for good health
- The foundations of community health
- What surrounds us shapes us
- The ways the world influences our lives and our health

It can also be helpful to share examples of what the social determinants of health are, like our ability to have healthy foods, safe and desirable housing, high-quality education, and dignified work.

More important than having the same words is having the same meaning. Use language that connects with your audience while staying grounded in this core idea: Health is far more than the effects of our individual choices or our genes. Our health—and the health of our communities—is shaped by the conditions in which we all live, work, grow, and age.

neighborhoods, quality education, and dignified work—are known as the **social determinants of health**.

These factors are referred to as *determinants* because they help determine how well and how long we live. For example, communities that lack access to fresh food and recreational spaces experience higher rates of chronic diseases like diabetes.[25,26] Families living in unsafe housing or in neighborhoods with polluted air experience elevated rates of asthma and other respiratory conditions.[27]

Although the term *social determinants of health* is widely used among those of us who are public health practitioners, allies, and partners, it may not always resonate with the general public. In Box 1-1, we offer alternative terms that can help make this concept more accessible while preserving its meaning.[28]

Still, no matter what language we use, one thing remains clear: Access to the social determinants of health is not distributed equally, and that inequality is not natural or fair. It reflects far more fundamental forces at work: interlocking **systems of oppression** that are the root causes of health inequities. These include *white supremacy, structural racism, racial capitalism, sexism, ableism,* and *classism.*

Together, these systems shape the conditions of our lives. They influence who has access to resources and opportunities in ways that unfairly advantage some and unfairly disadvantage others. These systems set the rules of the game, embedding inequity into our laws, policies, and institutions.[29] They give some a head start in obtaining health, wealth, and longevity, while leaving others to bear the burden of preventable illness and premature death. These systems of oppression will be discussed further throughout Chapters 2 and 3.

While the social determinants of health help explain how people's life conditions shape their health outcomes, systems of oppression explain why those differences are unfair and why they persist. To solve health inequities, we must confront the systems that create and sustain them.

THE APPLE TREE MODEL: A JOURNEY FROM INEQUITY TO LIBERATION

Our collective ability to improve community health and well-being comes down to how we understand and practice fairness. **Fairness** means ensuring that people are treated justly and have meaningful access to the resources and opportunities needed for health and flourishing.

The following sections explore the *Apple Tree Model*, a visual framework that helps us understand fairness in the context of public health by understanding *inequity*, *equality*, *equity*, *justice*, and *liberation*. These terms overlap and are not mutually exclusive. Each plays a critical role in shaping conditions for health and flourishing.

The first three concepts within the Apple Tree Model are *inequity*, *equality*, and *equity* (Figure 1-2).

An **inequity** is a difference that is avoidable, unfair, and indefensible.[30,31] These unfair differences are caused by long-standing and deeply entrenched forces, such as *structural racism* and *colonialism*. Inequities are not a natural result of differing needs or circumstances; they are produced by social, political, and economic systems that disadvantage specific groups of people.

Health inequities—like the disproportionate rate of pregnancy-related deaths among Black people—are preventable, unfair, and indefensible differences in health

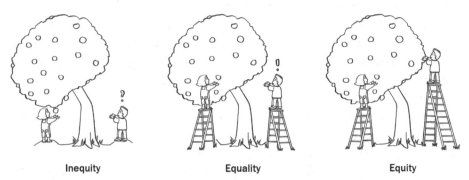

Inequity   Equality   Equity

Artist Credit: Jasmin Pamukcu, 2025.

Figure 1-2. Inequity, Equality, and Equity

outcomes between groups of people. They result from systemic barriers to respectful, high-quality care, as well as the broader conditions necessary to flourish.

It is important to distinguish *inequity* from *inequality*. **Inequality** simply describes a difference between individuals or groups. Not all inequalities are unjust. For instance, younger people typically have more years of life ahead of them than older adults, largely due to the natural aging process. **Disparity** is a similar term that also describes difference. A disparity or an inequality becomes an *inequity* when that difference is avoidable, unfair, and indefensible.

Inequities should provoke moral outrage because they result from unjust systems and structures. The racial wealth gap (discussed further in Chapter 2), for example, is not an innocuous or natural disparity—it is an inequity produced by the compounded legacies of slavery, Jim Crow laws,* redlining,† labor exploitation, white supremacy, and structural racism. This book uses the terms *inequity* or *unjust disparity* to underscore that these differences are neither accidental nor acceptable, and to highlight the role of systems in maintaining them.

From here, the Apple Tree Model moves to **equality**, which simply refers to the sameness of all people. As a value or principle, it means that people have the same inherent worth—for example, by asserting the right to equal protection under the law. In practice, equality means treating everyone the same—providing the same resources and opportunities regardless of people's starting points, needs, or circumstances. Equality, as an approach, assumes that everyone begins from a level playing field and requires the same support to succeed.

When applied in the context of addressing systemic oppression and structural inequity, this kind of uniform treatment can do the opposite of what we may expect: Treating

---

*Jim Crow laws** were state and local laws in the United States that legalized racial segregation and racial discrimination in all facets of daily life. Jim Crow laws restricted the movement of Black people in public spaces, including schools, public transit, parks, and hospitals, forbidding interaction between Black and white people and denying Black people access to community resources and services. Jim Crow laws were a form of racial terror used to deny Black people the right to vote, gain employment, obtain an education, purchase homes and land, and much more. If these laws were even perceived to be violated, Black people faced arrest, imprisonment, violence, and death. A discussion of Jim Crow laws can be found in Chapter 3.

†**Redlining** originated as a discriminatory federal policy that started in the 1930s, but the term has since come to describe the broader system of racialized disinvestment carried out across public and private sectors. Under the New Deal, the federal government—through agencies like the Federal Housing Administration and the Home Owners' Loan Corporation (HOLC)—designated neighborhoods as "hazardous" for investment if Black people, other people of color, and immigrants lived there. HOLC created color-coded maps to illustrate the perceived "desirability" of neighborhoods. These maps—informed and used by state and local government officials, bankers, realtors, appraisers, and others—determined where banks would issue loans, where businesses could invest, and where government resources would be allocated. The graded color codes were based on "race": White neighborhoods received the highest grades and were systematically approved for public and private loans and investments. However, neighborhoods where Black people and other marginalized people resided were color-coded red on maps and systematically denied public and private loans and investments. This came to be known as "redlining." A discussion of redlining can be found in Chapter 2.

everyone equally can actually reinforce injustice. Equal treatment within unequal systems cannot produce equal outcomes. In fact, offering the same supports to people—regardless of their specific circumstances and contexts—can perpetuate harm, widen unjust disparities, and exacerbate the root causes of inequity.

Equity, by contrast, recognizes that people face different barriers and circumstances and need different supports to achieve fair outcomes. Equity is the recognition that systemic injustices—such as discriminatory policies, unequal access to resources, and histories of exclusion—have created vastly different starting points for people and entire communities. Rather than treating everyone as if their needs are the same, equity is about meeting people where they are and making sure they have what they need to flourish.

As epidemiologist and antiracism scholar Camara Jones explains, equity has three requirements:

1. Valuing all people and populations equally;
2. Recognizing and rectifying historical and contemporary injustices; and
3. Providing resources according to need.[29]

In Figure 1-2, two children want to pick apples from a tree, with the apples symbolizing the resources and opportunities needed to flourish. The tree itself represents the systems and structures that shape people's lives. But the tree is bent and distorted: Its structure allows one child easy access to apples while preventing the other from reaching any apples at all. This situation reflects an inequity, so we are compelled to intervene.

An intervention based on equality would provide both children with the same ladder—failing to account for the distorted system that unfairly advantages one and unfairly disadvantages the other. Equity, on the other hand, is recognizing that the child farthest from the apples needs a taller ladder to reach them. By providing each child with a ladder that is specific to their needs, we can ensure that both children can access the apples. Whether the outcome is picking fruit or living a fulfilling life, equity means addressing the real barriers people face in their lives by providing the specific supports they need.

Health equity applies the principle of equity to health and flourishing. It means ensuring that everyone, no matter who they are or where they come from, has a fair opportunity to live a full, meaningful life. Achieving health equity requires us to confront historical and ongoing injustices, provide resources according to need, and actively dismantle social, economic, and systemic barriers to health.[32] In short, health equity is not about giving everyone the same thing; it is about ensuring everyone has what they need to flourish.

Despite equity's intrinsic connection to fairness, the concept is often misunderstood. This confusion has fueled backlash and even outright animosity toward advocates for equitable policies, processes, and systems. But that's all the more reason why we, as public health practitioners, must be courageous and unwavering in our commitment to equity.

Equity is not the endpoint; it is a necessary step on the path to justice and liberation. And because advancing equity lies within our collective power, we must deepen our understanding of what it requires and why it is essential for improving community health and well-being.

Taking a Deeper Dive on Equity

The Strategy and Practice of Equity

Equity starts with a **universal goal**—a fair and just outcome that we believe everyone deserves.

Because we equally value both of the children depicted in Figure 1-2, we want to make sure that both can achieve the universal goal: to pick the apples. The ladders represent a necessary intervention to meet the goal. In this case, the children must be given ladders of different heights—what we call a *targeted approach*—to account for their different needs and circumstances. This is an example of *targeted universalism*—a concept introduced by civil rights attorney and social policy scholar john a. powell.

Targeted universalism means setting universal goals that apply to everyone and using tailored strategies to help different groups achieve these goals based on their unique needs, circumstances, and contexts.[33] For example, a universal goal might be safe streets for all pedestrians, but achieving that goal requires targeted interventions like curb cuts, wider sidewalks, and audible traffic signals so that all pedestrians can experience that shared outcome.

Equity is not complex or overly idealistic. For some, it may sound counterintuitive to treat people differently to achieve fairness. But in reality, we practice equity in our lives every day. For instance, we're practicing equity when we take these actions:

- Retrieve a book that's just out of reach for a child. *(Universal goal: Everyone should have access to books.)*
- Graciously give up our seat for an older adult on the bus. *(Universal goal: Everyone should have a safe and comfortable ride while using public transit.)*
- Turn on closed captions during a TV show for a deaf or hard of hearing family member. *(Universal goal: Everyone should be able to enjoy the show.)*

Equity in the Law: Principle Versus Practice

Equity is already central to what we do routinely and instinctively to help people. But as public health practitioners and advocates, our challenge—and truly, our mission—is to translate this often instinctive and individualized understanding of equity to communities and groups who have different needs.

The idea of treating groups differently to advance fairness is not new or radical. In fact, US law and policy have long recognized that fairness often requires different approaches for different people—at least on paper. Civil rights protections in education, for example, acknowledge that students with different needs—such as English language learners or students with learning disabilities—are entitled to receive specific supports to achieve universal goals of learning and academic achievement. Other aspects of our daily lives, from workplace accommodations for pregnant workers to language interpretation in health care, also reflect a shared understanding: Fairness means acknowledging, valuing, and embracing our differences.

But even though equity in principle is commonplace in our laws and policies, it too often fails to translate into equity in practice. Consider the Servicemen's Readjustment Act of 1944, commonly known as the GI Bill: Adopted during World War II, the law aimed to assist returning veterans—many of whom it was anticipated would face unemployment, psychological trauma, and housing instability. To preemptively address this, the bill provided subsidized education, home loans, and other critical resources for veterans. The GI Bill was crafted around the principle of fairness: that those who served the country deserved structured help to reintegrate and thrive.

On its face, the GI Bill was "race-neutral"—but in practice, its implementation was deeply racist. Across the country, Black veterans were systematically excluded from receiving the full benefits of the bill—including educational opportunities and home loans—due to pervasive discrimination by banks, universities, and local officials.[34,35] The shut-out was virtually absolute. For example, in 1947, more than 3,200 home loans were issued to veterans across 13 cities in Mississippi—but only two loans went to Black veterans.[36] The intergenerational wealth-building effects of the GI Bill were reserved for white families, widening the racial wealth gap for decades to come.

Another example of equity in principle versus practice is the US tax code, which includes progressive features, such as marginal tax rates that increase with income. Yet the tax code also contains large loopholes and exemptions that disproportionately benefit the wealthy, reinforcing economic inequality across generations.[37,38]

These examples reflect a theoretical understanding in law that fairness requires acknowledging and addressing people's different needs and circumstances. But equity cannot be measured by intent alone; it must be assessed by impact.

Government plays a unique and essential role in acknowledging and redressing inequities—conditions that are preventable, unfair, and indefensible. Government is not only responsible for enacting laws and policies; it is also responsible for ensuring they are implemented with integrity and fidelity to core values. Because government is charged with safeguarding the well-being of the people it serves, it bears a heightened obligation to translate the principles of equity into tangible outcomes. The full promise of equity and justice can only be realized when government acts with transparency, empathy, and accountability—ensuring that fairness is not merely a legal ideal, but a lived reality.

Deliberate and Ongoing Action for Equity

Equity is a destination and a journey. This means it is both a process and an outcome. As an outcome, equity is about ensuring that everyone has a fair opportunity to achieve universal goals. As a process, equity requires these deliberate, ongoing actions:

- **Prioritizing marginalized communities:** Equity efforts must prioritize communities that have been systematically exploited and oppressed—particularly Indigenous and Black communities, given the enduring impacts of colonialism (see Chapter 2), chattel slavery,* Jim Crow (see Chapter 3), and redlining and disinvestment (see Chapter 2).
- **Shifting power to communities:** Those most affected by injustice must be decision-makers in shaping solutions and determining how shared resources are used. Government agencies—alongside other powerful institutions—must support community visions and remain accountable to community members.
- **Distributing benefits and burdens fairly:** Policies should direct the greatest benefits to communities harmed by disinvestment and discrimination. Conversely, the burdens of change should be carried by those with the resources and capacity to absorb them.
- **Rectifying past and present injustices:** Equity demands action to address and redress structural injustices—both historical and ongoing. This includes prioritizing protections and resources for communities long denied them, while also confronting systems that perpetuate harm.
- **Allocating resources according to need:** Equity is not about equal distribution but about ensuring communities receive the support necessary—based on their specific contexts and challenges—to reach universal goals.

Because equity requires treating people differently to achieve fairness, it is sometimes misunderstood as a form of discrimination—when, in fact, it is the opposite: Equity is a response to injustice that ensures those who have been marginalized have fair access to resources and opportunities. **Discrimination,** by contrast, involves treating people differently in ways that violate their dignity. Discrimination entrenches and exacerbates inequities—typically by benefiting already-privileged groups at the expense of those who have been historically excluded and oppressed. Equity seeks to rectify these imbalances by prioritizing those who have been left out or pushed aside, ensuring that everyone has the support they need to reach universal goals.

---

*Chattel slavery** was a colonial system of slavery, supported by the Transatlantic Slave Trade, that was practiced in all 13 British colonies in what would eventually become the United States. African people were purchased to become the personal property of their owners for all of their lives and for their descendants' lives. Through chattel slavery, enslavement was permanent and inheritable. Children of an enslaved mother automatically inherited her status and were also enslaved for life. Enslaved people were considered a commodity that could be bought, sold, bequeathed, and traded like livestock or furniture.[39,40]

Recognizing Fakequity: Equity in Name Only

Equity becomes real through acknowledgment, accountability, and—most importantly—action. We must *acknowledge* that historical and contemporary injustices have caused disproportionate harm, hold institutions and industries that have committed these harms *accountable*, and take *action* to repair damage and provide redress. Equity is not about checking a box or saying the right words; it is about honestly reckoning with the past and committing to meaningful change moving forward.

Too often, efforts labeled "equitable" are revealed to be superficial, performative, or even counterproductive. This false equity—also referred to as *fakequity*—can be deeply damaging, especially to the marginalized communities it claims to support. Rather than addressing systemic injustice, fakequity allows harmful structures to remain intact and unchallenged (Box 1-2).[41,42]

Consider terms like "equitable policing" or "equitable law enforcement." Modern policing in the United States is rooted in systems of racial control. Its origins trace back to slave patrols, which were created by white plantation owners and colonial legislatures to track, capture, and terrorize enslaved people who tried to escape or resist being enslaved. These patrols evolved into early urban police departments tasked with suppressing labor unrest, controlling Black and immigrant communities, protecting property owned by white people, and enforcing racial segregation through violence and intimidation. These systems were not built to protect everyone equally. They were built to enforce racial hierarchies through state-sanctioned violence,* intimidation, subjugation, and terror.[43-46]

While tools and techniques have evolved over time, policing's core functions remain racialized surveillance, violence, and punishment of marginalized communities. Today, policing continues to disproportionately harm Black and brown people, as well as people who are poor, disabled, immigrants, unhoused, or queer—often under the guise of maintaining public safety. In this context, applying the term *equity* to institutions like policing is not only misleading, it is inappropriate, irresponsible, and even dangerous.

Critiques of institutions like policing should not be conflated with critiques of individual police officers; it is about the system of policing itself. Our nation's most powerful institutions have evolved from deeply racialized and oppressive foundations, and these foundations still shape their structures, operations, and outcomes. Naming this history

---

*State-sanctioned violence—also referred to as *state violence* or *state-sponsored violence*—refers to violence that occurs when a government, through its authorities—such as police or the military—uses force, intimidation, and repressive actions against its citizens. The "necessity" of these actions is often purported to uphold law and order and to protect citizens' interests, even if such actions overtly violate human rights. State-sanctioned violence can also include the refusal of a government and its agents (including police, government attorneys, and judges) to uphold or enforce existing laws intended to protect marginalized groups from violence and intimidation, serving to further subjugate and oppress marginalized groups.

Box 1-2. Fakequity: The Harms of Performative and Inauthentic Equity

The adoption of the term *equity* across public health and other sectors marked a meaningful shift toward acknowledging that fairness requires more than simply treating everyone the same. But not every use of the word *equity* or every initiative labeled "equitable" truly reflects its meaning. Equity is not a feeling, a one-off pilot project, or a branding strategy. Any equitable effort must meet three requirements. It must (1) value all people and populations equally, (2) recognize and rectify historical and contemporary injustices, and (3) provide resources according to need.

Even when pursued in good faith, equity work can be constrained by **dominant institutions**—organizations and institutions in our society that concentrate power, resources, and authority, such as governments, philanthropic organizations, universities, and corporations.[41] If we aren't careful, approaches that were designed with even the best of intentions can be implemented in ways that are harmful and antithetical to the meaning of equity.

Coined by educators and systems change advocates Heidi (Schillinger) Sohn and Erin Okuno, **fakequity** refers to performative or inauthentic work that co-opts the language of equity without doing the work of shifting power, resources, or decision-making to those who have been marginalized.[42] These efforts protect the status quo while falsely giving the appearance of change. Ultimately, they deceive people, cause harm, and deepen distrust.

Fakequity is not just imperfect equity work; it is a wolf in sheep's clothing. It uses the language of change while upholding the same policies, processes, and systems that created the harms in the first place and continue to perpetuate them.

Here are some red flags that may indicate fakequity:

▶ **Lack of clarity:** There is no clear definition of what makes a process or policy "equitable," leaving the term vague and unaccountable.

▶ **Silence on systemic issues:** Systems of oppression, such as structural racism and colonialism, are never named or acknowledged.

▶ **Performative listening:** Marginalized communities are invited to participate in "listening sessions," but there is no commitment to implement any of their recommendations, or their feedback is ignored.

▶ **No real decision-making power:** Decision-making processes ask communities to "rubber stamp" pre-made plans and approaches already in progress, or they exclude communities from decision-making entirely.

▶ **Failure to value labor:** Community members and organizations are not compensated for their expertise and time.

▶ **Avoidance of difficult truths:** There is reluctance or refusal to have conversations about power, decision-making, and resource allocation.

▶ **Erasure of experience:** Historical and contemporary harms are glossed over or sanitized to make them palatable for more powerful groups.

▶ **Resource inequity:** Resources are not allocated based on community needs, perpetuating unjust disparities that already exist.

If you spot one or more of the above, what is being presented as equity may actually be superficial and detrimental. By contrast, real equity involves a long-term, intentional effort that must be grounded in acknowledgment, accountability, and action. Equity without these elements is not equity; it is simply maintaining the status quo.

and these harms does not automatically mean every police officer or institutional representative acts with bad intent. But equity requires us to focus on systems—not just intentions—because even well-meaning individuals who operate within harmful structures can and do perpetuate harm. This is why we must focus on understanding and transforming systems rather than applying personal blame.

Equity is foundational to our work as public health practitioners. But we can—and must—push ourselves further. To truly achieve flourishing for all, we must think beyond equity and reach for the final two concepts in the Apple Tree Model: **justice** and **liberation**.

Bridging Equity and Justice

Once implemented, equity-centered interventions can have an immediate, positive impact on people's daily lives. But even when equity efforts succeed, they typically operate within the constraints of existing systems. Rather than fundamentally transforming those systems, equity work often seeks to make them more inclusive, accessible, or responsive—improving conditions within established institutional boundaries.

This is not a flaw of equity; it is a reflection of the power dynamics that shape it. Public health initiatives are generally funded and guided by powerful institutions—namely, governments, philanthropic organizations, universities, and corporations. Because these institutions control resources and influence, their timelines, agendas, and strategic priorities shape what equity work is allowed to look like, how far it can go, and how long it can last.

What happens when these institutions shift priorities, face political opposition, or simply lose interest? Too often, the equity work that communities rely on is not just paused, it is defunded, dismantled, or erased entirely, making it virtually impossible to maintain or rebuild existing progress.

Unless systems and institutions are completely reimagined, they will continue to do what they were designed to do. While equity is necessary to create fairness within an existing system, transformational change—change that rewrites the rules of the system itself—requires justice.

Justice (Figure 1-3) embraces the three requirements of equity—valuing all people, addressing historical injustices, and redistributing resources based on need—while also transforming systems themselves.

If equity is about leveling the playing field, justice is about changing the game entirely. Justice is focused on making permanent changes to systems and structures, and is transformative in its scope and scale. Justice work creates policies and processes that cement shifts in power and generate conditions where opportunities to flourish are built into the very foundations of society.

In Figure 1-3, the children can more easily pick apples because of a structural intervention: The tree itself has been pulled upright. Once the tree is no longer bent away from one of the children, equality—providing the same-sized ladder to each child—becomes possible. But this shift did not happen on its own—it required intentional effort and significant intervention. The boards and wires propping up the tree represent

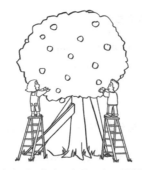

Artist Credit: Jasmin Pamukcu, 2025.

Figure 1-3. Justice

justice-centered tools for systems change, like policy and funding structures (explored further in Chapter 3), that hold the tree in place. These supports must be actively maintained. If they are weakened or removed, the system will become distorted again, returning to a state of inequity.

Equity and justice are not mutually exclusive—we need both, working together. Equity helps shift resources and support to those who need them now, while justice creates the structural change necessary for long-term transformation. Equity efforts are most effective when paired with bold justice strategies that dismantle and reimagine the systems that produce inequities in the first place. While equity can drive meaningful improvements within existing structures, it cannot, on its own, dismantle the deeper systems of oppression that shape our society. Justice is what enables us to fundamentally change those systems at their roots.

For example, equity-centered interventions that expand access to healthy foods or improve traffic safety are necessary, but they do not address the root causes of injustice in our food and transportation systems. These systems remain inequitable because of how they are designed, operated, and funded. Achieving lasting change requires more than working within existing structures—we must fundamentally transform them. When systems are so deeply rooted in injustice, they are beyond repair. In those instances, equity is not enough; we must reimagine and rebuild these systems entirely. While equity can support change within current systems, it cannot uproot or remake them. For that, we need justice.

And it matters who leads the work of equity and justice. Government agencies and other dominant institutions can lead equity efforts and make changes within existing systems, but they cannot lead justice work, which fundamentally transforms systems themselves. Justice is not a top-down initiative; it requires community leadership. The people most affected by inequities must be in charge of defining the problems and determining the solutions. Institutions can be valuable partners by offering resources, platforms, and expertise—but they cannot and should not control the agenda.

Health Justice and Liberation

To be truly visionary we have to root our imagination in our concrete reality while simultaneously imagining possibilities beyond that reality.

-bell hooks, feminist writer and activist[47(p110)]

The Cost of Abandoning Public Health's Social Justice Roots

In the 19th century, social justice movements—motivated by a desire to improve community health and well-being—demanded clean water, better working conditions, fair pay, and dignified housing. As public health scholars and advocates Nancy Krieger and Anne-Emanuelle Birn write, "Social justice is the foundation of public health."[48(p1603)] But in the 20th century, the field of public health distanced itself from the understanding that social reform is critical to preventing disease and death.[49] This shift proved costly. The field's voluntary transformation into an academic, clinical, and laboratory-based discipline[50] moved it far from its origins of championing social justice.

This decision, according to public health advocates and organizers Selma Aly, Asamia Diaby, and Julian Drix, "left public health without the political base and social justice movement ties that gave it power."[51(p9)] As a result, justice has largely been absent from mainstream public health discourse—rarely mentioned in public health academic programs, interventions, or practice settings.

This omission has led to a systemic shortsightedness, paternalism, and deep moral hesitancy within many public health organizations and academic institutions. By denying its strong, justice-focused foundations, the field of public health has struggled in at least three key ways to decisively—or even adequately—address the root causes of health inequity. Too often, public health (1) over-relies on behavioral interventions at the expense of addressing systems; (2) fails to hold powerful industries and institutions accountable; and (3) avoids evidence-based solutions because they are perceived as too politically risky.

1. **Over-reliance on behavioral interventions at the expense of addressing systems.** As a field, public health has overfocused on individual-level behaviors and interventions. Although behavioral interventions can be helpful in specific contexts, they are often insufficient on their own. Public health interventions that promote behaviors—like breastfeeding or eating healthier foods—can offer individuals useful guidance. However, when these strategies dominate public health approaches, they distract from the deeper, systemic forces that shape behavior, limit choice, and drive health outcomes.

   For instance, many neighborhoods lack access to affordable, nutritious food due to redlining, ongoing disinvestment, and businesses' refusal to serve areas they consider unprofitable—factors that suppress the development of essential community assets like grocery stores.[52] Similarly, many public health organizations promote breastfeeding without acknowledging that many working parents—especially those in low-wage jobs—lack access to paid parental leave and workplace accommodations like lactation rooms. In both examples, responsibility is unfairly shifted onto individuals, while systemic forces that make healthy choices difficult or impossible—like structural racism, labor exploitation, and systemic disinvestment—all go unaddressed.

2. **Failure to hold powerful industries and institutions accountable.** In the field of public health, our tendency to focus on changing individual behaviors—rather than systemic conditions—has contributed to a pattern of deflecting responsibility from powerful corporations and institutions. We have made meaningful progress in holding some industries accountable—such as the tobacco and motor vehicle industries— by using litigation, regulation, and public awareness campaigns to benefit community health.

But in other sectors, public health institutions have hesitated to challenge powerful systems head-on.

Take the criminal legal system and carceral system: Mass incarceration is widely recognized as a public health crisis[53,54]—with a 500% increase in the number of people who have been incarcerated over the last four decades.[55] Incarceration has well-documented links to illness, trauma, barriers to employment and housing, community disruption, and premature death, particularly among Black, low-income, and other marginalized communities.[56] Yet, public health practice has often stopped short of directly confronting this system or advocating for it to be dismantled. Enforcement-based approaches still shape public health interventions—from punitive responses for noncompliance (such as issuing fines or criminal penalties for violating public health orders[57,58]) to problematic surveillance-based interventions (such as GPS tracking of individuals during COVID-19[59] or requiring biometric data for access to services[60]). See Chapter 6 for more information on moving away from enforcement-oriented practices.

A similar pattern plays out in the realm of housing. Corporate landlords and private equity firms have become dominant forces in real estate, contributing to rising rents, mass evictions, and displacement—all of which directly jeopardize health.[61] Despite this, much of public health's engagement with housing remains focused on issues like mold or air quality. While important, this approach fails to confront larger systems that perpetuate unsafe housing conditions and profit from housing instability.[62]

When public health institutions do not direct attention and resources toward holding powerful industries and institutions accountable, they continue to operate unchecked and with impunity.

3. **Avoidance of evidence-based solutions because they are perceived as too politically risky.** Public health institutions have historically been slow to embrace interventions perceived as controversial, even when evidence strongly supports them.

Syringe services programs, for example, reduce the spread of infectious diseases from unsafe injection drug use,[63] yet they remain underused in many areas because of political and social stigma. Similar dynamics play out across many of today's most contested public health issues. Efforts to expand access to gender-affirming care, abortion services, comprehensive sex education, and housing-first approaches to homelessness are all backed by evidence and supported by many public health practitioners.

Yet because these issues remain politically charged, public health institutions have often sidestepped them to avoid controversy, backlash, and threats to funding. While bold leadership does exist in the field, a persistent tendency to retreat from politically uncomfortable terrain limits our collective ability to protect communities most impacted by systemic harm.

The Five Commitments of Health Justice

In public health, we have an opportunity and a responsibility to courageously pursue effective, long-term, and justice-focused solutions. This will require us to unite with other fields behind a shared banner of health justice.

Health justice is a community-driven movement to dismantle systemic barriers to well-being and ensure resources are distributed according to need, so that everyone has an equal chance to live a flourishing, fulfilling life. The health justice movement recognizes that health is shaped by social, economic, and political conditions and seeks to transform these conditions to eliminate unjust health disparities.

According to the San Francisco AIDS Foundation, health justice will exist "when all people have the power and resources to make decisions about their bodies and health—regardless of identities and experiences."[64] We build on this by outlining *Five Commitments of Health Justice* that should guide our practice:

1. Urgency

Health justice demands action—not someday, but now. Every delay in addressing inequities has a human cost: People are living shorter, sicker, less self-determined lives because of systems that can and must be changed. For communities that have been historically marginalized, the consequences stretch across generations. Urgency doesn't mean rushing or abandoning strategy; it means acknowledging that the status quo is unacceptable and responding to health inequity with the moral clarity and speed it demands.

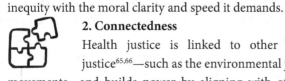

2. Connectedness

Health justice is linked to other interconnected struggles for justice[65,66]—such as the environmental justice and reproductive justice movements—and builds power by aligning with other movements and fields to address the full complexity of challenges that communities face. Health justice is also intersectional and acknowledges that people experience overlapping and compounding forms of oppression—like racism, sexism, ableism, and nativism—that interact to deepen harm.

3. Solidarity

Health justice is not only aligned with other justice movements; it is one. This builds on a long legacy of collective struggle—people organizing across "race," class, gender, disability, immigration status, and more to demand change. Health justice as a movement helps transform grief into action and isolation into solidarity. It expands what we believe is possible by challenging the status quo and activating our imagination about what flourishing can be. Health justice holds institutions accountable, demanding responsiveness, transparency, and alignment with community-defined priorities. When we organize and invite others to join the movement, we help translate community demands into durable shifts in policy, resources, and systems. As public health practitioners, we move in partnership, bringing institutional and technical expertise into alignment with the visions and demands of marginalized communities, to the benefit of all.

4. Law

Health justice draws from a long tradition of community organizing and advocacy to win major legal and legislative reforms—directly challenging the systems that produce health inequities. From the *Civil Rights Movement* to disability justice, communities have reclaimed the law as a tool to confront discrimination, redress harm, and expand protections. In practice, health justice builds bridges between spaces and sectors, combining the tools of advocacy with the power of community organizing. Health justice recognizes that legal systems can both uphold and dismantle oppression—and calls on us to pursue the full promise of justice through law and policy change that is grounded in community power.

5. Power

Health justice is grounded in the leadership, vision, and agenda-setting power of communities most harmed by inequities. Community power means ensuring that these communities are not only heard, but they hold the influence and authority to define problems, set priorities, and implement solutions. Communities should not be merely informed, consulted, or "engaged"; they are the decision-makers and agenda-drivers when it comes to governing. Health justice involves the alignment of public health's technical expertise, resources, and policy tools with community-defined visions and goals. When communities have the power to govern in partnership with responsive and accountable institutions, it creates the conditions for meaningful, positive, and sustained transformation.

Health justice is not only about fixing harmful and oppressive systems that drive health inequities but also about reimagining what is possible. It envisions a world where health is not a privilege but a fundamental right, where communities shape the policies and environments that affect their well-being, and where every person has the resources and opportunities they need to flourish.

The Endgame: Liberation

Health justice helps bring us closer to liberation (Figure 1-4). **Liberation** is the realization of self-determination, justice, and collective flourishing. A liberated future is one in which all people have the freedom, power, and resources to live with dignity, make informed choices about their own lives, and participate fully in shaping their communities and the systems that govern them.

In a public health context, liberation means people have open and abundant access to the resources, opportunities, and conditions necessary to lead a healthy and flourishing life on their own terms. It means making sure all communities can flourish in ways that embrace sustainability, empathy, connection, and mutuality. Liberation is about self-determination, dignity, and the ability to live well and in community with one another and the planet.

In Figure 1-4, liberation is depicted as not just one tree, but an entire orchard—a place of abundance where there is more than enough for everyone. Liberation still requires justice; the trees (symbolizing our systems) require active care and supports to keep them upright. But because empathy and care are central to how we live in a liberated future, there is also time to rest and appreciate the fruit of our labors.

Liberation is both a cherished ideal and a goal. In our current reality, we are surrounded by a great deal of injustice. We can face intense—and sometimes violent—resistance to small positive changes, let alone large transformative ones. Because of this, liberation may be difficult or even impossible for many of us to envision. And, like justice, liberation is not commonly taught or used in public health spaces.

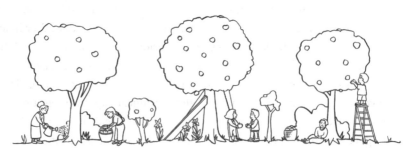

Artist Credit: Jasmin Pamukcu, 2025.

Figure 1-4. Liberation

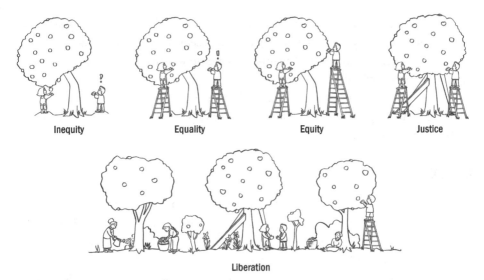

| Inequity | Equality | Equity | Justice |

Liberation

Artist Credit: Jasmin Pamukcu, 2025.

Figure 1-5. The Apple Tree Model: Inequity, Equality, Equity, Justice, and Liberation

But liberation is truly the endgame of our work in public health. It is the culmination of everything we do to make health and flourishing possible. Simply learning about the concept of liberation can help expand our imaginations. It can help us envision what liberation could be and how we can get there. And envisioning a liberated world is an important first step toward achieving it. With all of this in mind, the Apple Tree Model (Figure 1-5) is now complete and ready for us to apply.

APPLYING THE APPLE TREE MODEL: ACCESS TO HEALTH-PROMOTING FOODS

To convey how the ideas illustrated in the Apple Tree Model might function in the real world, let's explore an example related to a universal goal of providing everyone with access to healthy, fresh, and culturally relevant foods—and the actions a city might take to meet that goal.

Inequity

In this city, inequity is the status quo and is actively enforced. Wealthy, predominantly white neighborhoods have full-service grocery stores with fresh and affordable produce, while low-income areas—particularly those home to immigrants and communities of color—are left with limited options: fast food chains, liquor stores, and discount stores stocked mostly with processed goods. This contributes to higher rates of nutrition-related illnesses and chronic diseases like diabetes and hypertension. Families in the city struggle to access the ingredients central to their traditions, while culturally affirming food vendors are pushed out by restrictive zoning and enforcement practices. At the same time, the city invests in attracting high-end grocery stores to wealthy neighborhoods using tax breaks and public subsidies.

These are not neutral decisions. They reflect a pattern of valuing some communities while marginalizing others. In this scenario, the city perpetuates inequity through both neglect and active, unjust decision-making.

Equality

 City officials take action by changing zoning laws and offering incentives to build one new grocery store in every neighborhood, regardless of need. Each area—whether wealthy or low-income—receives the same level of funding and support.

While this approach treats all neighborhoods the same, it overlooks existing conditions and inequities. Some communities already have several full-service grocery stores within walking distance; others have none. Equal inputs do not guarantee equal outcomes—and neighborhoods that have long been excluded continue to face significant barriers to accessing healthy and culturally relevant foods.

Equity

 The city takes a more targeted approach. In partnership with local residents and community organizations, elected officials and city staff prioritize neighborhoods most affected by food insecurity. They invest in mobile food markets, subsidize culturally relevant produce, and support community-run farmers' markets. They also expand public transit to help people reach grocery stores and other destinations outside of their immediate neighborhoods. These actions are designed to meet communities where they are—addressing specific barriers and working toward fair access to nutritious, affordable, and culturally meaningful food.

These actions make important and significant improvements within the city and to residents' daily lives. But these approaches do not fundamentally change the underlying structures that created food access inequities in the first place.

Justice

 In addition to addressing issues of access, city residents and government agencies begin to address the root causes of the problem. Together, they pursue solutions that shift power.

In one historically disinvested neighborhood, residents reclaim vacant land and turn it into community gardens and urban farms. They form food cooperatives and develop models of collective ownership, reducing reliance on corporate grocery chains. City departments—like planning, zoning, and transportation—share power by deferring to community leadership and funding infrastructure and transportation options based on community members' preferences and aspirations.

Community members also organize to confront the industrial food system's influence in their neighborhoods. In response, elected officials begin to divest from large corporate food contracts and instead invest in local, regenerative food systems. Mutual aid networks grow, helping community members meet immediate food needs while building long-term alternatives rooted in community power and sustainability.

Liberation

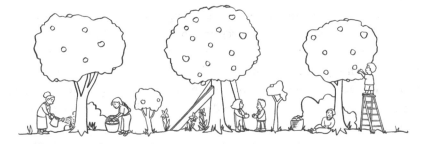

Over time, communities not only build food systems that meet their needs, they reclaim control over them. Residents govern shared land, shape local food policies, and ensure that culturally meaningful foods are grown, distributed fairly, and celebrated.

As cross-city coalitions grow, communities exchange knowledge and skills, creating networks of solidarity that transcend neighborhood boundaries. Urban farms, food cooperatives, direct-to-community models, and land trusts form the backbone of these systems, bypassing corporate control entirely. Inspired by Indigenous movements for food sovereignty, these efforts go beyond immediate food needs to holistic solutions that affirm identity, dignity, and collective self-determination.

The result is not just healthier meals but stronger, more connected communities where people have the power to shape systems to support culture and health.

Public Health as Liberatory Practice

This example shows how equity and justice are not only milestones on a path but also can exist side by side, reinforcing one another to address systemic barriers and open new possibilities. When practiced together, they expand our imaginations and strategies, pointing the way toward liberation.

Public health efforts can build on each other in powerful ways: from solving urgent problems, to shifting power, to repairing past harms and preventing future ones.

By responding to the specific needs and insights of communities, we can move closer to achieving universal goals like ensuring access to food that is nourishing, culturally meaningful, environmentally sustainable, and rooted in community.

YOU CAN STILL DO THE WORK WITHOUT SAYING THE WORDS

At this very moment, the word *equity* and related terms are being weaponized, vilified, and in many cases outlawed entirely.[67,68] In recent years, government agencies and businesses alike have rolled back policies to promote equity, defunded DEI programs,[69-71] prohibited the teaching of Critical Race Theory in schools,[72-74] refused to fulfill financial pledges to fund racial equity, and even scrubbed websites of photos and references to transgender people, women, and people of color.[75]

The backlash has been intense but unsurprising. It is part of the ongoing cycle of progress and retrenchment that has occurred throughout US history.[76,77] Momentum toward equity and justice often threatens those in power because it requires them to confront their unearned privilege, center those who have been marginalized, shift resources to others, and take responsibility for past and present harms. But this cycle of progress and retrenchment should not cause us to despair. As abolitionist and author Frederick Douglass said, "If there is no struggle, there is no progress."[78]

When it comes to discussing equity and justice, there are no magic semantic substitutes. But the work cannot disappear simply because the words we use to describe it are being targeted and legislated against. In fact, the work of equity and justice is even *more* important in such times. Whether or not we use the specific terms, we must ensure our work lives up to these principles. But doing this in the face of staunch opposition requires thoughtfulness, strategy, and adaptability.

It is possible to describe what equity and justice mean without using the exact words, but it does require having a solid understanding of their meaning. For instance, *equity* could be described using Camara Jones's three requirements that we discussed earlier in this chapter. Terms like *fairness* can be used as well, and we encourage you to use the Apple Tree Model to inspire additional ways to describe your work.

Determining the words you need to use, why, with whom, and to what end will require intentionality. Start by considering your audience's receptiveness to terms like *equity* and *justice*. Some people may fundamentally disagree with these principles, no matter what phrasing you use. Knowing this in advance can allow you to conserve time and energy.

That said, there are others who may misunderstand or feel discomfort with these specific words, but may still be open to their underlying values. In these cases, it may be helpful to describe your work by discussing intended outcomes, without directly using the words *equity* or *justice*.

This approach is not an abandonment of our values. It can be a useful and strategic choice—especially in challenging and hostile environments. Flexibility in our language also serves as a valuable exercise. All too often, we find ourselves using the term *equity* as a convenient shortcut for describing a more complex initiative. But by changing up the words we use to describe our work, we can sharpen our communication skills and find new ways to connect with different audiences.

If you are wondering whether to use or avoid specific terms like *equity* or *justice* at all, consider these five strategies:

1. **Know your audience.** Your language should resonate with the people you are engaging with, whether you are sharing information or seeking to persuade. For some audiences, explicitly using terms like *equity* and *justice* will build trust and solidarity—particularly among organizers and community members who may appreciate directness and clarity about your commitment. In other contexts, different phrasing may be necessary to secure support. When crafting a message or communication, ask yourself these questions:

   • Who is my audience? Are they advocates, policymakers, community members, business owners, or funders?
   • What values do they hold? What motivates them? What are they invested in protecting?
   • Who holds them accountable? To whom must they justify their actions?
   • What causes and initiatives have they supported or opposed in the past? Do equity and justice align with their track record?
   • What words already resonate with them? Can I make connections between my work and language they use?
   • What's in it for them? What do they stand to gain—or lose—by providing me with support?

2. **Clarify your communication goals.** This is the first step to prepare for a conversation or craft a message. Focus on conveying the *why*: the values, meaning, and significance behind your work. This can allow you to stay committed to deeper principles while adjusting language as needed. To identify your communication objectives, ask yourself these questions:

   • What universal goals am I working toward? How can I describe these goals clearly and simply?
   • Can the audience I'm addressing help me to advance these goals?
   • Will using the words *equity* or *justice* potentially persuade or alienate them?
   • How can I remain true to the principles of the words behind *equity* and *justice*?

3. **Put the focus on people.** Equity is about recognizing people's humanity and providing support according to their specific needs and contexts. For example, in road safety,

putting the focus on people may mean centering residents of Tribal communities that lack sidewalks or children in neighborhoods who must walk to school without safe crossings. We can't achieve our goals—such as stopping preventable traffic deaths and creating safer roads for everyone—without paying special attention to the people who most need support. As you consider how to center people in your messaging, ask yourself these questions:

- Who are the people most directly affected by the issue I'm addressing? What are their needs and wishes?
- How can we use data and evidence—not only numbers but also stories and lived experiences—to support the need for targeted interventions?
- What connections can I make between my audience and the people most affected by this issue? How can I generate empathy (rather than pity or sympathy) from my audience?

4. **Describe a universal goal you're working toward and the process for getting there.** Set a clear, universal goal that you want everyone to achieve and explain how the work you are doing can help accomplish it. Then get your audience on board with the process: Describe what the work entails, who needs to be involved, and how it will be thoughtful and fair. For instance, if you are addressing asthma prevention, the universal goal is clean air for all, which will benefit the whole community. The process for this work could involve creating an advisory group to act as decision-makers, with members recruited from the neighborhoods that suffer from the highest asthma rates. Ask yourself these questions:

- How can I describe the value and benefit of the universal goal in ways that are clear and compelling?
- What connections can I make between the universal goal and the values and interests of my audience? How can I describe the goal in a way that resonates with what I know about my audience?
- What steps will help us get closer to achieving the universal goal, and what can my audience do to help us get there?

5. **Emphasize the benefits to all.** It can be helpful to explain that our efforts to improve the lives of marginalized communities will ultimately help everyone. The *Curb-Cut Effect*, coined by equity advocate and public interest attorney Angela Glover Blackwell, is a helpful example. It describes disability rights advocates' successful efforts to get cities to build curb cuts—sloped areas on sidewalks originally meant to help people in wheelchairs. This innovation ended up benefiting entire communities, including caregivers pushing strollers, workers moving carts, travelers wheeling luggage, and pedestrians

seeking a smoother walking path.[79] Similarly, improving the air quality in communities that are most adversely affected by smog and industrial air pollution will improve the quality of the air breathed by everyone in the surrounding area.

By improving the conditions for health and flourishing for excluded and disinvested communities, we improve conditions in ways that are beneficial to everyone. Ask yourself these questions:

- Why does centering specific marginalized groups achieve broader benefits for my community and society as a whole?
- What other groups can I highlight that will benefit from this work?
- How can I describe the broader benefits of this work in ways that will resonate?

As discussed earlier in this chapter, we don't all have to say the same words, but we must have the same shared meaning. If we are working to ensure that all people— particularly those who have been historically marginalized and excluded—have the resources, opportunities, and environments they need to flourish, then we are advancing equity and justice, no matter what words we use to get there.

CONCLUSION

The words we use are powerful because they shape not only what we know and say but also what we are willing to name and change. One of the first steps on the path toward equity and justice is our language: understanding the full meaning of the terms we use and recognizing how our words can either reinforce harm or open the door to health, flourishing, and liberation.

Expanding our vocabulary is how we stay in conversation with the world and in relationship with the communities around us. Words give shape to our ideas, make space for new ways of thinking, and connect us to one another. They also allow us to articulate injustice more clearly and name the futures we are striving to create.

The world we want will require new systems, but first we must create and use language that makes these possibilities real—language that helps us name the harms we see and experience, honor our shared humanity, and envision a better world together. Banning words like *racism* and *inequity*—and punishing those who use them—does not make injustice disappear. Instead, it deepens and exacerbates the very harms these words describe.

Translating what we experience and observe into language will always be necessary. Terms and definitions that feel right today may shift tomorrow. These changes in our language are part of the natural course of evolution and growth.

We must be clear and intentional in our language. And because language is always evolving, our willingness to learn, adapt, and speak with intention must evolve alongside it. We will not always get our words exactly right. But we can stay open, continue to listen, and choose words that convey care, clarity, and respect. When our language reflects our values, it becomes a tool for solidarity, truth-telling, and transformation.

KEY TAKEAWAYS

The language we use matters. The words we choose shape how we perceive the world, how we define its problems, and how we envision potential solutions. The language of equity and justice evolves to ensure that we use words that reflect our values. Our ability to use language that respects people's identities, acknowledges their inherent dignity, and avoids harmful coded meanings allows us to engage more effectively and authentically with communities and with one another.

Health is about flourishing. Health is not solely the absence of disease—it is the presence of well-being. Flourishing captures this broader vision of health: a life of dignity, agency, and connection. It emphasizes quality of life, adaptability, and an ability to thrive both individually and as part of a community. As public health practitioners, we are working to advance community health and create a world where everyone can flourish.

The *Apple Tree Model* helps us journey from inequity to liberation. This illustrated metaphor shows two children attempting to pick apples from a tree that symbolizes our systems. We can use this imagery to better understand and describe the connections among *inequity, equality, equity, justice*, and *liberation*. It conveys how these ideas exist in relationship to each other, advancing from inequity (a difference that is avoidable, unfair, and indefensible) toward liberation (the profound, sustained presence of self-determination, justice, and collective flourishing).

Equity's focus on those who are systemically marginalized benefits us all. Equity is a necessary step toward justice and liberation that begins with a universal goal—a fair outcome that everyone deserves. Equity has three requirements: valuing all people equally, recognizing and rectifying historical and contemporary injustices, and providing resources according to need. Equity-centered work must be authentic and intentional in shifting power, resources, and decision-making to marginalized communities. Equity work means acknowledging harm from historical and contemporary injustices, holding institutions and industries that have committed harm accountable, and taking action to repair damage and provide redress.

We must still do the work, regardless of the words. Social justice is foundational to public health. Even when the language of equity and justice is vilified and suppressed, the work must go on. We may adapt our words for different audiences or settings, but the substance and purpose must remain. As we continue to uphold the meanings of equity and justice, we can find new and compelling ways to describe the purpose and value of public health and collective flourishing.

REFERENCES

1. Lorde A. *Sister Outsider: Essays and Speeches.* Clarkson Potter/Ten Speed; 2007.
2. Asian American Journalists Association. *AAJA Handbook to Covering Asian America.* 3rd ed. 2015. Accessed May 12, 2025. http://www1.lasalle.edu/~beatty/310/ACES_CD/reference/reference_and_resources/AAJAhandbook.pdf
3. HR 4238, 114th Cong, 2nd Sess (2016). To amend the Department of Energy Organization Act and the Local Public Works Capital Development and Investment Act of 1976 to modernize terms relating to minorities. Accessed May 12, 2025. https://www.congress.gov/bill/114th-congress/house-bill/4238
4. Kambhampaty AP. In 1968, these activists coined the term 'Asian American'—and helped shape decades of advocacy. *TIME.* May 22, 2020. Accessed May 12, 2025. https://time.com/5837805/asian-american-history
5. Mabute-Louie B. *Unassimilable: An Asian Diasporic Manifesto for the Twenty-First Century.* HarperCollins; 2025.
6. Lambert R. "There is nothing minor about us": Why *Forbes* won't use the term minority to classify Black and brown people. *Forbes.* October 8, 2020. Accessed May 12, 2025. https://www.forbes.com/sites/rashaadlambert/2020/10/08/there-is-nothing-minor-about-us-why-forbes-wont-use-the-term-minority-to-classify-black-and-brown-people
7. National Equity Atlas. People of color: Nurturing diversity and fostering racial equity are critical to our future prosperity. Accessed May 12, 2025. https://nationalequityatlas.org/indicators/People_of_color
8. Jones CP. "Race," racism, and the practice of epidemiology. *Am J Epidemiol.* 2001;154(4):299–304. doi:10.1093/aje/154.4.299
9. Mukhopadhyay CC, Moses YT. Reestablishing "race" in anthropological discourse. *Am Anthropol.* 1997;99(3):517–533. doi:10.1525/aa.1997.99.3.517
10. Smitherman G. *Talkin and Testifyin: The Language of Black America.* Houghton Mifflin; 1977.
11. Castro-Atwater SA. Colorblindness. In: Neville HA, Gallardo ME, Sue DW, eds. *The Myth of Racial Color Blindness: Manifestations, Dynamics, and Impact.* American Psychological Association; 2016:213–226.
12. Young C. Is this the end for "urban" music? *NPR.* June 15, 2020. Accessed May 12, 2025. https://www.npr.org/2020/06/15/877384808/is-this-the-end-for-urban-music
13. Rowlands DW, Love H. Mapping rural America's diversity and demographic change. *Brookings Institution.* September 28, 2021. Accessed May 12, 2025. https://www.brookings.edu/articles/mapping-rural-americas-diversity-and-demographic-change

14. Bryant E. No person is illegal—the language we use for immigration matters. Vera Institute of Justice. April 4, 2023. Accessed May 12, 2025. https://www.vera.org/news/no-person-is-illegal-the-language-we-use-for-immigration-matters

15. Pfeiffer D, Hu X. Deconstructing racial code words. *Law Soc Rev.* 2024;58(2):294–328. doi:10.1017/lsr.2024.19

16. Alexander M. *The New Jim Crow: Mass Incarceration in the Age of Colorblindness.* Rev ed. New Press; 2020.

17. Macon TA. Language matters: Why we need to stop talking about eliminating health inequities. *Health Affairs Forefront.* October 24, 2022. Accessed May 12, 2025. https://www.healthaffairs.org/content/forefront/language-matters-why-we-need-stop-talking-eliminating-health-inequities

18. Harris M. Is the tone appropriate? Is the mathematics at the right level? Mathematics Without Apologies. June 2, 2018. Accessed July 15, 2025. https://mathematicswithoutapologies.word-press.com/2018/06/02/is-the-tone-appropriate-is-the-mathematics-at-the-right-level

19. World Health Organization. Constitution of the World Health Organization. Accessed July 15, 2025. https://www.who.int/about/governance/constitution

20. Health Equity & Policy Lab. Human flourishing. Accessed May 12, 2025. https://www.healthequityandpolicylab.com/human-flourishing

21. Institute of Medicine Committee for the Study of the Future of Public Health. Summary and recommendations. In: *The Future of Public Health.* National Academies Press; 1988.

22. Hiscock IV. Public health at Yale. *Yale J Biol Med.* 1947;19(4):393.b1–398.

23. Fakunle DO. Storytelling and public health 101. In: *Arts-Focused Approaches to Public Health Communications.* Public Health Communications Collaborative; February 29, 2024. Accessed June 27, 2025. https://www.slideshare.net/slideshow/artsfocused-approaches-to-public-health-communications/266583002#3

24. @AnandWrites. Coronavirus makes clear what has been true all along. Your health is as safe as that of the worst-insured, worst-cared-for person in your society. It will be decided by the height of the floor, not the ceiling. February 27, 2020. Accessed July 15, 2025. https://web.archive.org/web/20200227145707/https://twitter.com/AnandWrites/status/1233041575414050817

25. Leung CW, Kullgren JT, Malani PN, et al. Food insecurity is associated with multiple chronic conditions and physical health status among older US adults. *Prev Med Rep.* 2020;20:101211. doi:10.1016/j.pmedr.2020.101211

26. National Recreation and Park Association. Parks and chronic disease management. 2015. Accessed June 29, 2025. https://www.nrpa.org/our-work/Three-Pillars/health-and-well-being/ParksandHealth/fact-sheets/parks-chronic-disease-management

27. Altman MC, Kattan M, O'Connor GT, et al. Associations between outdoor air pollutants and non-viral asthma exacerbations and airway inflammatory responses in children and adolescents living in urban areas in the USA: A retrospective secondary analysis. *Lancet Planet Health.* 2023;7(1):e33–e44. doi:10.1016/s2542-5196(22)00302-3

28. FrameWorks Institute. Explaining the social determinants of health. May 5, 2023. Accessed May 12, 2025. https://www.frameworksinstitute.org/publication/explaining-the-social-determinants-of-health

29. Jones CP. Systems of power, axes of inequity: Parallels, intersections, braiding the strands. *Med Care.* 2014;52(10 suppl 3):S71–S75. doi:10.1097/MLR.0000000000000216

30. Whitehead M. The concepts and principles of equity and health. *Health Promot Int.* 1991;6(3):217-228. doi:10.1093/heapro/6.3.217

31. Global Health Europe. Inequity and inequality in health. August 24, 2009. Accessed May 13, 2025. https://globalhealtheurope.org/values/inequity-and-inequality-in-health

32. CityHealth. Equity statement. Accessed May 13, 2025. https://www.cityhealth.org/about-us/equity-statement

33. powell ja, Menendian S, Ake W. Targeted universalism: Policy & practice. Othering & Belonging Institute, University of California, Berkeley. December 2022. Accessed May 12, 2025. https://belonging.berkeley.edu/sites/default/files/2022-12/Targeted%20Universalism%20Primer.pdf

34. Katznelson I. *When Affirmative Action Was White: An Untold History of Racial Inequality in Twentieth-Century America.* W. W. Norton & Company; 2005.

35. Turner SE, Bound J. Closing the gap or widening the divide: The effects of the GI Bill and World War II on the educational outcomes of Black Americans. *J Econ Hist.* 2003;63(1):145-177. doi:10.1017/S0022050703001761

36. Clark A. Returning from war, returning to racism. *New York Times Magazine.* July 30, 2020. Accessed May 31, 2025. https://www.nytimes.com/2020/07/30/magazine/black-soldiers-wwii-racism.html

37. Piketty T, Saez E, Zucman G. Distributional national accounts: Methods and estimates for the United States. *Q J Econ.* 2018;133(2):553-609. doi:10.1093/qje/qjx043

38. Congressional Budget Office. The distribution of household income and federal taxes, 2019. Congressional Budget Office. 2022. Accessed May 12, 2025. https://www.cbo.gov/publication/58353

39. New Jersey State Bar Foundation. What is chattel slavery and how did it dehumanize Black people? 2020. Accessed May 13, 2025. https://njsbf.org/wp-content/uploads/2020/10/Theme-One-Background-Info-1.pdf

40. The Baltimore Story. 1662: Racial chattel slavery—permanent and inheritable. Accessed May 16, 2025. https://www.thebaltimorestory.org/history-1/1662-racial-chattel-slavery-permanent-and-inheritable

41. Mohsini M, Lopez A, Msibi K, Haley D, Campos-Melchor P. Introducing community data. Coalition of Communities of Color. 2024. Accessed August 8, 2025. https://www.coalitioncommunitiescolor.org/research-and-publications/introducing-community-data

42. Fakequity. Welcome to the Fakequity blog. August 30, 2015. Accessed May 12, 2025. https://fakequity.com/welcome-to-the-fakequity-blog

43. NAACP. The origins of modern-day policing. Accessed May 12, 2025. https://naacp.org/find-resources/history-explained/origins-modern-day-policing

44. Lepore J. The invention of the police. *The New Yorker.* July 20, 2020. Accessed May 12, 2025. https://www.newyorker.com/magazine/2020/07/20/the-invention-of-the-police

45. Hadden SE. *Slave Patrols: Law and Violence in Virginia and the Carolinas.* Harvard University Press; 2001.

46. Ritchie AJ. *Invisible No More: Police Violence Against Black Women and Women of Color.* Beacon Press; 2017.

47. hooks b. *Feminism Is for Everybody: Passionate Politics.* South End Press; 2000.

48. Krieger N, Birn AE. A Vision of social justice as the foundation of public health: Commemorating 150 years of the spirit of 1848. *Am J Public Health*. 1998;88(11):1603–1606. doi:10.2105/AJPH.88.11.1603

49. Yong E. How public health took part in its own downfall. *The Atlantic*. October 23, 2021. Accessed May 3, 2025. https://www.theatlantic.com/health/archive/2021/10/how-public-health-took-part-its-own-downfall/620457

50. Fairchild AL, Rosner D, Colgrove J, Bayer R, Fried LP. The EXODUS of public health: What history can tell us about the future. *Am J Public Health*. 2010;100(1):54–63. doi:10.2105/AJPH.2009.163956

51. Aly S, Diaby A, Drix J. The five dimensions of inside–outside strategy: A guide for public health and social movements to build powerful partnerships. Health in Partnership. April 29, 2025. Accessed May 19, 2025. https://www.healthinpartnership.org/resources/the-five-dimensions-of-inside-outside-strategy-guide

52. Rowlands DW, Donoghoe M, Perry AM. What the lack of premium grocery stores says about disinvestment in Black neighborhoods. Brookings Institution. April 11, 2023. Accessed May 6, 2025. https://www.brookings.edu/articles/what-the-lack-of-premium-grocery-stores-says-about-disinvestment-in-black-neighborhoods

53. National Academies of Sciences, Engineering, and Medicine; Health and Medicine Division; Board on Population Health and Public Health Practice; Roundtable on the Promotion of Health Equity. Mass incarceration as a public health issue. In: Anderson KM, Olson S, eds. *The Effects of Incarceration and Reentry on Community Health and Well-Being: Proceedings of a Workshop*. National Academies Press; September 18, 2019. Accessed June 16, 2025. https://www.ncbi.nlm.nih.gov/books/NBK555719

54. National Institute for Health Care Management Foundation. Incarceration: A public health crisis. August 29, 2023. Accessed June 26, 2025. https://nihcm.org/publications/incarceration-a-public-health-crisis

55. The Sentencing Project. Growth in mass incarceration. Accessed June 28, 2025. https://www.sentencingproject.org/research

56. American Public Health Association. Advancing public health interventions to address the harms of the carceral system. October 25, 2021. Accessed June 28, 2025. https://www.apha.org/policy-and-advocacy/public-health-policy-briefs/policy-database/2022/01/07/advancing-public-health-interventions-to-address-the-harms-of-the-carceral-system

57. Fines and Fees Justice Center. COVID-19 policy tracker: Reform tracker. Accessed May 31, 2025. https://web.archive.org/web/20250126023851/https://finesandfeesjusticecenter.org/covid-19-policy-tracker/reform-tracker

58. Sun N, Christie E, Cabal L, Amon JJ. Human rights in pandemics: Criminal and punitive approaches to COVID-19. *BMJ Global Health*. 2022;7(2):e008232. doi:10.1136/bmjgh-2021-008232

59. Stanley J, Granick J. The limits of location tracking in an epidemic. American Civil Liberties Union. 2020. Accessed June 26, 2025. https://www.aclu.org/wp-content/uploads/publications/limits_of_location_tracking_in_an_epidemic.pdf

60. Podcast: Facial recognition is quietly being used to control access to housing and social services. *MIT Technology Review*. December 3, 2020. Accessed June 26, 2025. https://www.technologyreview.com/2020/12/02/1012901/no-face-no-service

61. Purewal Boparai S, Dominie W. Corporate wealth vs. community health: How corporate landlords' profit-seeking strategies harm health. Health in Partnership. June 17, 2024. Accessed June 28, 2025. https://www.healthinpartnership.org/resources/corporate-wealth-vs-community-health-how-corporate-landlords-profit-seeking-strategies-harm-health

62. Desmond M. *Evicted*. Crown Publishers; 2016.

63. Centers for Disease Control and Prevention. Safety and effectiveness of syringe services programs. February 8, 2024. Accessed May 13, 2025. https://www.cdc.gov/syringe-services-programs/php/safety-effectiveness.html

64. San Francisco AIDS Foundation. Living our values: A new strategic plan for San Francisco AIDS Foundation. September 8, 2019. Accessed May 13, 2025. https://www.sfaf.org/collections/status/living-our-values-a-new-strategic-plan-for-san-francisco-aids-foundation

65. Harris AP. Anti-colonial pedagogies: "[X] justice" movements in the United States. *Can J Women Law*. 2018;30(3):567–594. doi:10.3138/cjwl.30.3.010

66. Harris AP, Pamukcu A. The civil rights of health: A new approach to challenging structural inequality. *UCLA Law Rev*. 2020;67(6):1254–1282. Accessed May 17, 2025. https://www.uclalawreview.org/the-civil-rights-of-health-a-new-approach-to-challenging-structural-inequality

67. The White House. Ending illegal discrimination and restoring merit-based opportunity [executive order]. January 21, 2025. Accessed May 13, 2025. https://www.whitehouse.gov/presidential-actions/2025/01/ending-illegal-discrimination-and-restoring-merit-based-opportunity

68. The White House. Ending radical and wasteful government DEI programs and preferencing. January 20, 2025. Accessed May 13, 2025. https://www.whitehouse.gov/presidential-actions/2025/01/ending-radical-and-wasteful-government-dei-programs-and-preferencing

69. Murray C, Bohannon M. IBM reportedly walks back diversity policies, citing "inherent tensions": Here are all the companies rolling back DEI programs. *Forbes*. April 11, 2025. Accessed May 13, 2025. https://www.forbes.com/sites/conormurray/2025/04/11/ibm-reportedly-walks-back-diversity-policies-citing-inherent-tensions-here-are-all-the-companies-rolling-back-dei-programs

70. Izaguirre A. DeSantis curtails diversity, equity and inclusion programs in Florida state colleges. *AP News*. May 15, 2023. Accessed May 13, 2025. https://apnews.com/article/desantis-florida-diversity-programs-colleges-cb0402f8194b70a06e9ef970fa08c9d8

71. Coronado A. Texas ban on university diversity efforts provides a glimpse of the future across GOP-led states. *AP News*. January 29, 2024. Accessed June 3, 2025. https://apnews.com/article/texas-university-diversity-ban-dei-46e4b6193abe27b6abbdffcd1945cf38

72. Ray R, Gibbons A. Why are states banning Critical Race Theory? Brookings Institution. November 2021. Accessed June 1, 2025. https://www.brookings.edu/articles/why-are-states-banning-critical-race-theory

73. Miller V, Fernandez F, Hutchens NH. The race to ban race: Legal and critical arguments against state legislation to ban Critical Race Theory in higher education. *Missouri Law Rev.* 2023;88(1):1–76. Accessed June 1, 2025. https://scholarship.law.missouri.edu/mlr/vol88/iss1/6

74. Trump's orders take aim at Critical Race Theory and antisemitism on college campuses. *CBS News.* January 29, 2025. Accessed June 1, 2025. https://www.cbsnews.com/news/trumps-orders-critical-race-theory-college-protests

75. Huo J, Lawrence Q. Here are all the ways people are disappearing from government websites. *NPR.* March 19, 2025. Accessed May 13, 2025. https://www.npr.org/2025/03/19/nx-s1-5317567/federal-websites-lgbtq-diversity-erased

76. Hamilton VE. Reform, retrench, repeat: The campaign against Critical Race Theory, through the lens of Critical Race Theory. *Wm Mary J Race Gend Soc Justice.* 2021;28(1):61–93. Accessed June 1, 2025. https://scholarship.law.wm.edu/wmjowl/vol28/iss1/5

77. Lowery W. *American Whitelash: A Changing Nation and the Cost of Progress.* Mariner Books; 2024.

78. Douglass F. The significance of emancipation in the West Indies: Address delivered in Canandaigua, New York, on 3 August 1857. Frederick Douglass Papers Digital Edition. Accessed May 13, 2025. https://frederickdouglasspapersproject.com/s/digitaledition/item/10509

79. Blackwell AG. The curb-cut effect. *Stanford Social Innovation Review.* Winter 2017. Accessed May 13, 2025. https://ssir.org/articles/entry/the_curb_cut_effect

2

"Race," Racism, and the Struggle for Equity and Justice

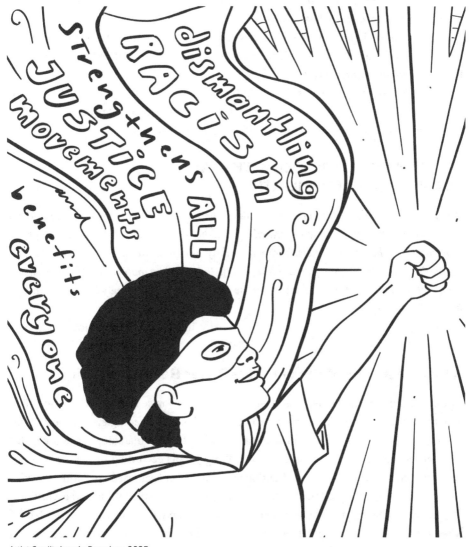

Artist Credit: Jasmin Pamukcu, 2025.
Growing Justice

Gulf-sized race-based gaps exist [in] health, wealth, and well-being. . . . They were created in the distant past but have indisputably been passed down to the present day through the generations. Every moment these gaps persist is a moment in which this great country falls short of actualizing one of its foundational principles—the "self-evident" truth that all of us are created equal.

–Ketanji Brown Jackson, US Supreme Court Justice and author[1(p1)]

Across every area of community health—whether it's diabetes diagnoses, premature births, rates of road traffic deaths, or hospitalizations from infectious diseases—the same frustrating and persistent trend appears: In the United States, people of color disproportionately experience worse health outcomes.

It's so common in our health data that we almost take it for granted. Segmenting data by "race" nearly always reveals higher rates of illness, injury, and premature death in Black and brown communities.

This isn't a new phenomenon. In fact, it far predates even our oldest population datasets. But it's not normal or natural either, which raises an unavoidable question: *Why?*

The answer is both straightforward and complex: racism.

"RACE": A FICTIONAL IDEA WITH REAL CONSEQUENCES FOR HEALTH

What people look like, or rather, the race they've been assigned . . . is the historic flashcard to the public of how they are to be treated . . . whether they will be administered pain relief in a hospital, whether their neighborhood is likely to adjoin a toxic waste site or to have contaminated water flowing from their taps. Whether they are more or less likely to survive childbirth in the most advanced nation in the world. Whether they may be shot by authorities with impunity.

–Isabel Wilkerson, author and journalist[2(p18-19)]

A False Hierarchy of Human Value Drives Health Inequities

At the founding of the United States—and long before—false and opportunistic beliefs about racial superiority were woven into the nation's fabric, shaping every aspect of life, including health. These beliefs formed the bedrock of a dehumanizing racial order that rationalized domination and violence by ranking people according to physical appearance, especially skin color. This fraudulent racial order was used to define the very boundaries of humanity, all in an effort to justify violence, exploitation, and exclusion.

This malignant and deadly racial hierarchy took hold under colonialism (see Box 2-1),[3-12] when 15th-century European settler colonists arrived in what would become the Americas and encountered Indigenous peoples.

Box 2-1. Why the Legacy of Colonialism Matters for Public Health

We are not a 'historically' underserved population. My history is one of ancestors who survived so I could thrive. My history didn't start with 'western civilization.' I am colonially underserved. I am institutionally underserved. And I am historically resilient.

– Abigail Echo-Hawk (Pawnee), public health researcher and data decolonization scholar[3]

Colonialism is both a system and a process through which one nation asserts control over another geographic area and its people through violence, land dispossession, and political domination. A central mechanism of colonialism is **colonization**: the process of establishing foreign control over land and people through displacement and subjugation. Colonization involves taking land through violence and coercion, extracting its resources, and exploiting its people. These terms are often used to describe European expansion beginning in the 15th century, including the invasion and control of lands across the Americas, Australia, and parts of Africa and Asia.[4]

In the United States, colonialism specifically took the form of **settler colonialism**: an ongoing process of taking land, even when clearly inhabited by others. Settler colonialism requires the removal, elimination, and replacement of Indigenous peoples with a permanent settler society.[5] To do this, settler colonists deployed tactics that included genocide, forced relocation, cultural erasure, destruction of systems of governance, and policies designed to break Indigenous peoples' ties to land and community.[6]

Colonialism was integral to the creation of "race"—which was used to justify violence, theft, subjugation, and domination. Colonial powers defined and enforced racial categories that positioned Indigenous peoples as obstacles to be eliminated and Black people as enslaved and exploited labor to make invaded lands profitable. These two racial engines of colonialism—elimination and exploitation—are both are rooted in the pursuit of profit, control, and dominance.

For example, during the Long Walk of the Diné (also referred to as the Navajo Nation or Navajo People[7,8])—a campaign of forced removal from 1863 to 1866—the US military undertook an effort to extinguish the Navajo people and claim their land for white settlers. Soldiers waged a scorched-earth campaign across Diné homelands, burning villages, killing livestock, and destroying water sources to force surrender through starvation and desperation. Thousands of Diné were then marched, at gunpoint, as far as 450 miles to Bosque Redondo, a remote camp under military control.[9]

Puerto Rico, as another example, has functionally remained a US colony since 1898. Its status as a territory has allowed the United States to extract land, labor, and profit from the island without granting full political rights or self-determination to its people.[10] Over generations, this colonial relationship has fueled disinvestment, forced migration, and cycles of economic exploitation. At the same time, colonial narratives claimed the island's Indigenous Taíno people had disappeared—an erasure that continues today through the US government's refusal to formally recognize Taíno identity or sovereignty.[11]

While the destructive impacts of colonialism have fallen most acutely on Indigenous peoples, they do not stop there. The legacy of colonialism continues to ripple across generations and geographies. Native Nations across the United States still face its enduring impacts, including federal policies that undermine Tribal sovereignty and self-determination. Despite treaty obligations, for instance, the US government systematically underfunds the Indian Health Service, leading to chronic gaps in health care access, infrastructure, and life expectancy in Native communities.[12]

Colonialism is a root cause of health inequities. It gave rise to systems that continue to devastate and destabilize communities—from the privatization of public goods, to the criminalization of poverty, to policies that devalue the lives of marginalized people. It lives on today in everything from exclusionary land use policies and environmental racism to mass incarceration and inequitable health care access.

The settler colonists viewed Indigenous people as obstacles to their ambitions of territorial expansion and wealth. This worldview fueled centuries of violence, including massacres, forced removals, cultural erasure, and genocide. Indigenous Nations were violently displaced from their homelands by the US government and confined to reservations—deliberately chosen for their perceived lack of economic value.[13] Indigenous children who survived the violence, disease, and starvation forced on their families and Tribes were often sent to boarding schools designed to erase their cultures, languages, spiritual beliefs, and identities.

During this same period, European settlers kidnapped Africans from their homelands and forced them onto a torturous voyage across the Atlantic. Those who survived were dehumanized as property under a brutal system of chattel slavery in the Americas that lasted nearly 250 years. Enslaved Black people—alongside Indigenous peoples—were placed at the bottom of the false hierarchy of human value.

When slavery was technically abolished in 1865, multiple new systems of racial oppression quickly took its place, including Black Codes,*[6,14,15] Jim Crow laws, racial segregation, redlining, racial terror, state-sanctioned violence, and mass incarceration. These new forms of racial oppression were specifically focused on denying Black people basic human rights—including the right to vote, to live in a safe and desirable home, to travel freely, and to obtain dignified employment. These systems ensured that Black Americans—the descendants of enslaved Africans—would remain oppressed and excluded from the privileges afforded to white people who sat at the top of the hierarchy.

Although this false hierarchy of human value was based on a lie—that a person's worth can be determined by skin color—its consequences are devastatingly real. The systems built on this idea continue to exploit and subjugate Indigenous and Black communities today, resulting in intergenerational poverty, poor health outcomes, and exclusion from resources and opportunity. These harms also ripple outward—to all people of color, other marginalized groups, and even the broader collective—because racism not only targets specific communities but also weakens the health, resilience, and cohesion of our entire social fabric.

The racial health inequities we see today are not random, accidental, or "natural." They are the direct result of systems and structures that were deliberately designed to exclude, exploit, and devalue people based on their position along the false hierarchy of human value that we call "race." To build a healthier future, we must confront this legacy—and dismantle the systems and structures that sustain it.

---

*Black Codes were a series of laws adopted by nearly all Southern states after the Civil War to restrict the rights of Black people, including their labor, voting rights, property ownership, and mobility. Enforced by all-white police and state militia forces, Black Codes were intended to largely restore the system of chattel slavery that existed before the war.

The Origins of "Race"

[R]ace is the child of racism, not the father. And the process of naming "the people" has never been a matter of genealogy and physiognomy so much as one of hierarchy. Difference in hue and hair is old. But the belief in the preeminence of hue and hair, the notion that these factors can correctly organize a society and that they signify deeper attributes, which are indelible—this is the new idea.

—Ta-Nehisi Coates, author and cultural critic[16(p7)]

"Race" is a human-made idea and social construct developed to categorize people solely by their physical appearance.*[18] It forms the basis of the deadly hierarchy of human value that ranks darker skin colors as inferior to lighter, "whiter" skin colors. Despite its pernicious existence in every aspect of our society, "race" has no factual, biological, or genetic basis.

The concept of "race" as we know it dates back to 1795, when German physician Johann Blumenbach published a book featuring a human classification system entirely of his own invention. Blumenbach divided humanity into five groups: "Caucasian," "Mongolian," "Malayan," "Ethiopian," and "American."[19] He assigned white people to the "Caucasian race," claiming that skulls from the Caucasus region of Eastern Europe and Western Asia were the most beautiful and symmetrical.[20]

Blumenbach's categories and their rationale are scientifically baseless. Biologists and geneticists overwhelmingly agree that "race" is not a biological or scientific reality. According to the American Association of Biological Anthropologists,

> the Western concept of race must be understood as a classification system that emerged from, and in support of, European colonialism, oppression, and discrimination. It thus does not have its roots in biological reality, but in policies of discrimination . . . racial classification has long served to justify exploitation, oppression, discrimination, and structural racism.[21]

Racial groups have been socially, politically, and legally engineered over the last five centuries, with racial classifications shifting extensively over time. Because of this, the lens of "race" can obscure and distort people's lived experiences—particularly when individuals are categorized in ways that don't align with how they're perceived or treated in society. The experience of Middle Eastern and North African (MENA) communities illustrates that "race" is not a fixed truth, but an adaptable weapon—reshaped across time by those who benefit from its use (Box 2-2).[22-25]

---

*According to the National Museum of African American History and Culture, a **social construction** or **social construct** is "an idea or collection of ideas that have been created and accepted by the people in a society. These constructs serve as an attempt to organize or explain the world around us." A social construct is not an immutable truth, but rather a creation of human thought and belief.[17]

Box 2-2. Middle Eastern and North African: A Case Study in the Social and Legal Construction of "Race"

Racial categories have never been fixed. They have been shaped, defined, and redefined over time by laws, policies, and institutions. The experience of *Middle Eastern and North-African (MENA)* communities, including Arab Americans, illustrates this evolving dynamic.[a]

The Naturalization Act of 1790 restricted US citizenship to "free white persons," making "whiteness" a legally and socially desirable classification. In the early 20th century, immigrants from the MENA region, particularly Arab people, challenged this restriction in court. Starting with the 1915 Supreme Court case *Dow v United States*, MENA communities eventually won the ability to be legally recognized as "white."[22]

The legal designation of "white" holds real power and benefits, but it also created a paradox: Although legally classified as "white," MENA communities were never truly regarded as such. To this day, they face social exclusion, discrimination, state-sanctioned violence, and government surveillance, particularly during times of heightened nativism and racial prejudice, such as during the post-9/11 era.[23] Although it seemed that whiteness could be granted overnight by a court, the unearned privilege attached to it diverged sharply from MENA individuals' lived experiences.[24]

For decades, this paradox was visible in the fight for a MENA category within the US Census. MENA individuals were categorized as white, erasing their unique racialized[b] experiences and making it difficult to track inequities experienced across daily life. Without accurate data, MENA communities struggled to access resources, gain civil rights protections, and advocate for policies that addressed their communities' specific needs.

In 2024, after years of advocacy and research, the Biden administration announced a long-awaited change: For the first time, the Census and other federal data systems would include a MENA category.[25] This historic shift acknowledged that MENA communities have distinct racialized experiences not endured by white Americans. It was also a crucial step toward ensuring that inequities faced by MENA communities—from housing to health—could be measured, addressed, and remedied through policy change and resource allocation.

Yet progress is never guaranteed. While a MENA category in federal data standards marked a major milestone, its full implementation is vulnerable to shifting political priorities and administration changes. How MENA communities are seen and treated both legally and socially continues to reflect the fact that "race" is not fixed; it is subjectively defined, politically shaped, and continually changing.

[a]While we use the term *MENA* to align with federal data standards and the terminology used by many advocates, we note that some community members prefer SWANA (Southwest Asian and North African) to reject the Eurocentric framing of the "Middle East" and affirm a self-defined regional identity. As advocacy and language evolve, public health practitioners must look to communities themselves to see how people define how they are named, represented, and understood.
[b]The term *racialized* refers to how people are categorized and treated based on the socially constructed idea of "race." In systems shaped by white supremacy, this process has been used to define and devalue people of color by assigning meaning to their perceived "race" and using that assigned meaning to justify unfair treatment. Racialization isn't about individual identity; it's about how systems label people, shape perceptions, and distribute power.

"Race" has been used as a tool for separation and subjugation, shaping policies, systems, and decisions that determine who has access to the resources and opportunities necessary for good health—and who does not. It functions as a "master category" in American society—an enduring organizing principle that shapes institutions, identities, and power relations. Sociologists and critical race theorists Michael Omi and Howard Winant explain that "race" is unique in the United States as a foundational structure that influences everything from political rights to labor markets and cultural belonging.

"Race" is the category that "set[s] the template for other forms of discrimination and oppression."[26(p106)] This framing underscores how "race" not only structures racism but also informs how other health-endangering social hierarchies are constructed and maintained.

Understanding that "race" is a human invention—and not an innate or fixed identity of a person or group—is essential to solving the problem of health inequities.

When we see Black and brown communities suffering disproportionately from disease, poverty, and premature death, we are not witnessing the "natural" outcome of differences between people. We are witnessing the long-term consequences of systems, structures, and policies that have systematically disadvantaged entire groups of people for centuries simply based on the color of their skin.

"Race": A Proxy for Exposure to Racism

In order to get beyond racism, we must first take account of race. There is no other way.
    -Harry Blackmun, US Supreme Court Justice[27]

If "race" is a human invention with no biological basis, why do such stark health inequities between racial groups exist? It's because "race"—the way we categorize and value people based on the color of their skin—functions as a stand-in for people's exposure to racism. It is racism—not "race"—that is a root cause of health inequities.

Epidemiologist and antiracism scholar Camara Jones defines **racism** as a system of structuring opportunity and assigning value based on how people look (their "race") that

• Unfairly disadvantages some individuals and communities;
• Unfairly advantages other individuals and communities; and
• Undermines our realization of the full potential of the whole society through the waste of human resources.[28]

While the financial costs of racism to the US economy are staggering—measured in the trillions each year[29,30]—the deepest, most devastating loss is the theft of human ingenuity and promise. Because of racism, entire populations of people have been denied resources and rights—keeping them from fulfilling their dreams, stifling or negating their contributions, and robbing us all of the collective benefit of everyone meeting their full potential.

Imagine how different our communities would be if colonialism and chattel slavery—which gave rise to "race" and racism as we know it—had never existed. How many lives could have been saved? How many more people could have lived freely, fully, and with dignity? How much deeper would our collective wisdom, culture, and connections be? What possibilities were lost—in terms of scientific discoveries and medical advancements, as well as the everyday contributions, relationships, and dreams that were never allowed to bloom?

Although "race" is a fiction, the consequences of racism are very real. Racism structures opportunity, controls resources, and assigns value to people simply and solely based on how they look. The toll racism takes on health is unmistakable and well-documented, from cancer and chronic disease diagnoses to infant mortality and premature death.[31-33] Racism shapes how people are valued—and, in turn, how they are treated, what resources they can access, the rights and freedoms they are granted, and even how long they live. *It is not possible to understand "race" without understanding racism.*

Racism can take different forms,[34] each of which contributes to health inequities in different ways and on different scales. These are some common examples:

- **Personally mediated racism** refers to interpersonal acts of racial prejudice and discrimination, such as treating someone unfairly because of their perceived "race."
- **Internalized racism** occurs when individuals from racialized groups come to accept negative messages about their own value or the value of people who look like them.
- **Institutional racism** describes how racial inequities are embedded in the policies, practices, and procedures of organizations and institutions, such as hospitals, schools, or employers. It shapes opportunities and outcomes within a system.

Structural racism, however, operates at a broader level and has the most far-reaching impact on population health. Researchers and antiracism scholars Zinzi D Bailey, Nancy Krieger, Madina Agénor, Jasmine Graves, Natalia Linos, and Mary T. Bassett define structural racism as "the totality of ways in which societies foster racial discrimination through mutually reinforcing systems of housing, education, employment, earnings, benefits, credit, media, health care, and the criminal [legal and carceral systems]. These patterns and practices in turn reinforce discriminatory beliefs, values, and distribution of resources."[31(p1453)] Over time, these systems interact, evolve, and reinforce each other to entrench racism and sustain the privileges of "whiteness" and the disadvantages assigned to "color."[35]

Structural racism encompasses institutional racism, but it also goes much further: It describes how institutions, systems, and structures collectively reinforce and amplify racism in ways that shape our lives. As public health practitioners, understanding structural racism is nonnegotiable. It reveals how seemingly isolated health issues are, in fact, deeply interrelated. It allows us to zoom out to see how racism operates across systems and structures that affect our health and longevity, both individually and collectively.

While often used interchangeably with *systemic racism*, this book refers to *structural racism* because of the tangible and powerful nature of structures. The term emphasizes that racism does not exist in the abstract; it is built into the very foundations of our society. The *structures* of racism—laws, practices, institutions, social norms, and culture—affect all aspects of our daily lives. Structural racism is inescapable because it is indeed everywhere. Poet and author Claudia Rankine writes:

[Racism is] in our laws, in our advertisements, in our friendships, in our segregated cities, in our schools, in our Congress, in our scientific experiments, in our language, on the Internet, in our bodies no matter our race, in our communities and, perhaps most devastatingly, in our justice system.[36]

The effects of structural racism are intergenerational. They stretch from the past into the present and future to shape opportunities and outcomes across our lifetimes, and potentially across the lifetimes of our descendants (see Box 2-3).[37-45] Structural racism is ultimately fueled and perpetuated by the ideology and belief system known as *white supremacy*.[46-48c]

Box 2-3. Redlining and the Intergenerational Harms of Structural Racism

Beginning in the 1930s as part of President Franklin D. Roosevelt's New Deal, the federal government launched a national effort to assess the lending "risk" of neighborhoods across the country. The Home Owners' Loan Corporation (HOLC) collaborated with state and local officials, bankers, realtors, and appraisers to create color-coded maps that graded neighborhoods based on their perceived investment potential and used the "race" of residents as a proxy for risk.

Using these maps, they assessed neighborhoods and applied one of four grades: "A" or "Best" (green), "B" or "Still Desirable" (blue), "C" or "Definitely Declining" (yellow), and "D" or "Hazardous" (red). These color-coded maps were used to determine where banks would issue loans, where businesses could invest, and where government resources would be allocated.

These grades were motivated first and foremost by white supremacy and racism, alongside nativism, classism, and anti-Semitism. All-white neighborhoods were deemed the most "desirable." For example, Ladue—a white middle-class suburb in St. Louis, Missouri—was graded "A" and colored green by an HOLC appraiser in 1940 because it had "not a single foreigner or negro."[37(p64)]

Conversely, neighborhoods populated by Black people, immigrants, and other marginalized people were graded "C" and "D" and color-coded yellow and red, respectively. These neighborhoods, which were categorized as "declining" and "hazardous," were considered financial risks and categorically denied public and private loans and investments. This systematic refusal to provide loans and funding to areas colored red came to be known as "redlining."[37,38] A neighborhood in Milwaukee, Wisconsin, for example, was graded "D" and colored red because—according to the HOLC appraiser—it was "the Negro and slum area of Milwaukee. . . . Besides the colored people, a large number of lower type Jews are moving into the section."[39]

Neighborhoods with Black residents were color-coded red and labeled financial risks—regardless of housing quality or economic stability. Even stable, middle-class neighborhoods received the lowest grade solely because Black people lived there.[37]

Redlining codified racial segregation, homeownership denial, and economic exclusion on a national scale. HOLC produced maps for more than 200 cities, covering every metropolitan area in the US. Redlining was reinforced and entrenched by other federal agencies, such as the Federal Housing Administration (FHA), and it remained federal policy for more than three decades. Although banned by the Fair Housing Act of 1968, the damage was done. The government-sanctioned denial of home loans to Black families and the racist designation of thousands of neighborhoods as "hazardous" produced devastating and lasting effects. It entrenched segregation, fueled disinvestment, blocked opportunities for wealth-building through homeownership, and concentrated environmental hazards and poor health outcomes in redlined areas.

Nearly a century later, the destructive legacy of redlining continues. Many neighborhoods that were redlined in the early 20th century remain among the most disinvested and impoverished.[40] Mounting research links redlining to a host of present-day health inequities, including lower life expectancy, preterm birth, cancer diagnoses, pedestrian fatalities, and firearm violence.[41-45]

WHITE SUPREMACY DRIVES RACISM, COLONIALISM, AND OTHER SYSTEMS OF OPPRESSION

White supremacy is not merely the individual delusion of being superior to Black people. Institutionalized white supremacy does not need individual bigotry in order to function, because it is a universal operating system that relies on entrenched patterns and practices to consistently disadvantage people of color and privilege whites.

–Barbara Smith, feminist author and activist[49]

White supremacy is often portrayed as an extremist ideology confined to hate groups like the Ku Klux Klan and neo-Nazis. In reality, it is more mundane and pervasive—deeply embedded in our structures, institutions, policies, and cultural norms.

White supremacy is a belief system and ideology that centers whiteness and perpetuates the myth of white racial superiority—politically, socially, and economically—while marginalizing and devaluing people of color. It underpins structural racism, transforming individual prejudice into systemic and enduring forms of discrimination and oppression. White supremacy and structural racism permeate daily life, determining who has access to resources, who holds power, and whose lives are valued.[46,47]

The false hierarchy of human value is sustained by positioning whiteness as the default, the standard, and the ideal across all domains of life—including our economic, housing, education, employment, and criminal legal systems.[50] Its core belief—that the "white race" is superior to all other "races"—has shaped US institutions and policies since the nation's founding.[46,47,50]

To fully understand racism, we must understand white supremacy. Without it, there would be no racial hierarchy to enforce. Attempting to understand racism without understanding white supremacy is like trying to understand gravity without recognizing that objects fall. The two are inseparable.

Yet, structural racism and white supremacy do not exist in isolation. They are deeply intertwined with other systems of oppression. **Intersectionality**—a concept rooted in Black feminist thought[51] and named by civil rights advocate and legal scholar Kimberlé Crenshaw[52]—describes how different forms of oppression overlap and interlock to produce compounded effects. It reveals how multiple systems work together to intensify inequities for people with multiple marginalized identities.

One way to picture intersectionality is as a Venn diagram (Figure 2-1). Multiple identities dynamically overlap and intersect to create unique lived experiences. Racism surrounds all identities, including "race," because racism amplifies all other forms of oppression. Racism adversely impacts us, no matter who we are; it is a system through which many other "isms"—such as sexism, classism, ableism, and others—are intensified and upheld.

Rather than treating inequities as the result of singular forces in isolation—such as "race" (racism) *or* gender (sexism)—intersectionality reveals how systems of oppression interact to shape people's experiences, opportunities, and outcomes (see Box 2-4).[53-57]

INTERSECTIONALITY

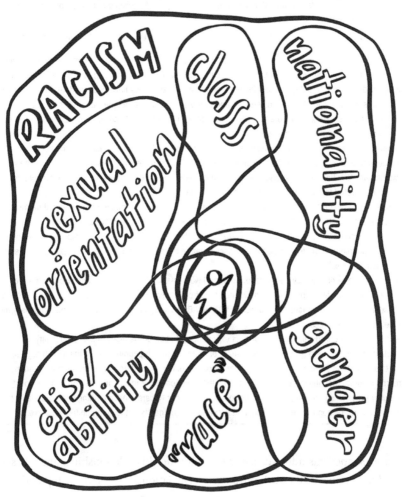

Artist Credit: Jasmin Pamukcu, 2025.
Figure 2-1. Intersectionality

To help illustrate the real-world implications of intersectionality, consider the story of Jose Antonio Vargas, a journalist and filmmaker who was born in the Philippines and made national news in 2011 when he publicly came out as undocumented. Since then, he has become one of the most visible advocates for undocumented immigrants in the United States. Vargas has spoken openly about the mental health toll of navigating life under constant threat of detention and deportation—particularly as a racialized immigrant with limited access to services or protections. He has shared how these

Box 2-4. Seeing the Whole: Lessons From Black, Trans, and Feminist Leadership

> *When you're able to describe exactly what people are experiencing, it makes it that much easier to address it. It's hard to address something that you don't have context for. Giving the experience of misogynoir a name gives us a place to build and organize from.*
>
> —Moya Bailey, Black feminist scholar and author[53]

Different aspects of identity come together in ways that bring the concept of intersectionality to life. The terms *misogynoir, transmisogynoir,* and *transmisogyny* describe specific intersections of oppression and reflect the intellectual and activist leadership of Black, women, and trans thinkers. They have deepened our understanding of how systems of oppression like racism, sexism, and cissexism function in people's daily lives. They do not act independently, but instead compound and intensify one another, creating distinctly different experiences of how we perceive—and are perceived by—those around us.

Misogynoir—a term coined by Black feminist scholar and author Moya Bailey—describes the specific form of discrimination that Black women face at the intersection of racism and sexism.[54] Misogynoir captures the ways Black women are simultaneously hypervisible and devalued—praised for their strength while denied softness, for example, or celebrated for style while dismissed as threatening.[55]

Transmisogyny—first articulated by activist and biologist Julia Serano—names the intersectional harms of *traditional sexism* (which devalues femininity) and *oppositional sexism* (which enforces rigid gender norms and punishes those who defy them). Serano explains that while all trans people experience cissexism, trans women and transfeminine people face an intensified form of discrimination because their identity challenges social hierarchies of both gender and sex.[56]

Building on the work of Bailey and Serano, writer and womanist Trudy introduced **transmisogynoir**, which describes the compounded harm Black trans women face from racism, sexism, and cissexism.[57] Trudy's work has pushed feminist and queer spaces alike to reckon with anti-Blackness, anti-trans prejudice, and transmisogyny within their own communities.

Bailey, Serano, and Trudy highlight the distinct experiences that lie at the heart of intersectionality.

In public health, failing to account for the impact of interventions on people who are uniquely marginalized can result in efforts that are ineffective—or worse, counterproductive. Whether addressing reproductive health inequities, HIV prevention, or mental health access, as public health practitioners we must consider how compounding systems of oppression shape people's exposure to risk and access to care. Understanding intersectionality helps us see more clearly, respond more effectively, and honor the full humanity of the communities we serve.

experiences shaped his adolescence and adulthood, his relationships, and his sense of home and belonging.[58] His work reframes conversations about citizenship and "race" to instead center dignity and shared humanity. Vargas's advocacy is both inseparable from his intersecting identities and powered by them.

Intersectionality helps us understand that identities are not fixed; they shift over time as we encounter changes in our lives, circumstances, and experiences. Intersecting identities can deepen disadvantage or confer advantages depending on the context. A person's disability status, for example, may change over time: Someone may may live without disability at one time and with disability later, or vice versa. These shifts change not only people's daily experiences but also how society treats them, reshaping where they encounter barriers or access advantages.

Our identities are also shaped by how external systems categorize us, sometimes in ways that conflict with how we understand ourselves. Gender identity illustrates this:

Someone who is perceived as fitting binary gender norms may experience unearned privileges—such as easier navigation of health care or legal systems. However, these privileges can disappear if they later come out as queer or present as gender nonconforming, especially in contexts that enforce assigned-at-birth labels.

As these examples show, identity is fluid and socially mediated. They also underscore that public health efforts must be intersectional to address connections between our identities, our health, and systems of oppression. Intersectionality does not suggest that people are defined solely by their demographic categories or the barriers they face. Rather, it helps us see how experiences are shaped by the ways we move through the world. Intersectionality reveals how complex systems can create compounding harms or advantages across different areas of life.

Intersectionality is most often discussed in terms of burdens and barriers, but it also highlights the unique perspectives, strength, and pride people draw from their identities and lived experiences. These vantage points—whether shaped by marginalization, privilege, resistance, or some combination—offer insights that are essential to understanding and transforming the systems around us. By recognizing how "race," gender, disability, and other identities intersect, we gain a deeper understanding of not only people's specific contexts and challenges but also their resilience, adaptability, and agency.

THE CONNECTIONS BETWEEN RACISM, CAPITALISM, AND HEALTH

We live in capitalism, its power seems inescapable—but then, so did the divine right of kings. Any human power can be resisted and changed by human beings.
                                        -Ursula K. Le Guin, novelist and poet[59]

Structural racism and white supremacy—and their centuries-long legacies of subjugation, dispossession, and exclusion—have produced and sustained the **racial wealth gap**: a profound and persistent disparity in assets, income, and intergenerational wealth between white households and households of color.[60] The racial wealth gap reinforces, entrenches, and perpetuates the **racial health gap**—the well-documented pattern in which people of color in the United States tend to live shorter, sicker lives than white people.[61-66] The racial wealth gap and the racial health gap are deeply intertwined and rooted in capitalism, the system that structures our nation's economy.

Capitalism is an economic system in which private individuals and businesses own and control property as well as the *means of production* (such as factories, labor, and land) to generate goods and services. Capitalism relies on markets and competition to determine prices and wages. The underlying assumption is that private self-interest, channeled through markets, leads to benefits for society as a whole.

Supporters of capitalism argue that it contributes to economic growth by driving innovation, rewarding efficiency, and responding dynamically to consumer needs.[67] However, critics point out that these benefits are not equally shared, with gains concentrated at the top and profits prioritized over the well-being of workers, communities, and the environment.[68] For example, in times of crisis like the COVID-19 pandemic, profit incentives undermined equitable access to goods, services, and essential resources.[69,70]

From its inception, capitalism has been racialized.[71] Sociologists and authors Crook et al. explain that capitalism grew in tandem with colonization, slavery, violence, and genocide.[72] In other words, as political scientist and historian Cedric Robinson points out, racism wasn't incidental to capitalism—it was built into it.[73]

The term **racial capitalism** captures this interdependence: It describes the ways in which our economic system is set up to extract value from the exploitation of racialized people.[74] Capitalism structures economic opportunity and labor along racial lines, relying on land dispossession, resource extraction, labor exploitation, and the enforcement of a racial hierarchy to generate wealth for the few at the expense of the many.

We see racial capitalism at work in the colonialist goals that drove the violent seizure of lands from Indigenous communities—laying the groundwork for land ownership structures in the United States today. We see it in how economic disinvestment and residential racial segregation produce communities that concentrate disadvantage—places with fewer assets like grocery stores and libraries, higher pollution, and underfunded schools. We see it in persistent racial inequities in wages, employment opportunities, and access to wealth-building resources. And we see it in how public health crises—like the COVID-19 pandemic and climate-related disasters—disproportionately harm those who have been denied economic security.

As public health practitioners, we cannot ignore racial capitalism because it fundamentally structures the conditions that drive health inequities.[75] These outcomes are not inevitable; they are engineered by policies designed to protect wealth and power for the few at the expense of health and dignity for all. To improve health, we must name and confront the systems that endanger it.

SCIENTIFIC RACISM IN PUBLIC HEALTH

Since enslaved people were first brought to this country, promoters of anti-Black racism and white supremacy have co-opted the authority of science to justify racial inequality.

                                                              -Harvard University Library[76]

Across public health and medicine, differences in health outcomes between white people and people of color have long been documented. But rather than blaming the true root causes of health inequities—systems of oppression like white supremacy and structural racism—many in these fields have invoked unscientific claims of racial inferiority connected to biology and genetics. These ideas are rooted in **scientific racism**—the co-optation, abuse, and distortion of science to uphold a false hierarchy of human value and legitimize the myth of white racial superiority.

Scientific racism has been repeatedly deployed throughout our nation's history. Often, these beliefs emerged *after* widespread acts of subjugation and exploitation, retroactively justifying violence against racialized people. As discussed earlier in this chapter, Indigenous people were displaced and killed to clear land for settler colonists, and Africans were enslaved so that their forced labor could sustain plantation-based economies. Only later were false claims of Indigenous and Black people's "nonhuman"[77] and "savage natures"[78] promoted to legitimize genocide, enslavement, and land theft. These malevolent narratives have proven both persistent and effective: Scientific racism has been called "one of the most effective tactics" for justifying racism and white supremacy.[76]

Scientific racism has long shaped public health tools and methods. *Eugenics*— the unfounded and pseudoscientific theory that selective breeding can "improve" human populations—was championed by prominent statisticians like Karl Pearson and Ronald Fisher.[79] Pearson, Fisher, and other eugenicists weaponized statistics to rationalize their racist and anti-Semitic worldviews.[80] The statistical tools they developed to advance these beliefs—including the Pearson chi-square test, the Fisher exact test, and the Fisher analysis of variance test (ANOVA)—remain widely used by biostatisticians, public health students, and practitioners today. As a field, we are taught to rely on these tools without reckoning with the inhumane ideologies behind their origins.

Scientific racism continues to permeate public health (see Box 2-5) and medicine (see Box 2-6) today.[81-91]

Box 2-5. The Problem With Controlling for "Race" in Epidemiology

Today, epidemiologists still treat "race" as a confounding variable, "adjusting" for it as though it were an innate and permanent biological trait that affects health outcomes. But "race" is not a biological reality—it is an unscientific categorization and human-made construct that functions as a proxy for exposure to racism.

This baseless and unnecessary statistical adjustment obscures and distorts the role that systems of oppression play in driving racial health inequities. For example, if researchers are studying the link between air pollution and asthma rates and they "control for 'race,'" they actually conceal facts and critical context relevant to their research. For instance, Black and Latine communities are more likely to live near sources of pollution precisely because of racist policies like redlining, exclusionary zoning, and community disinvestment.

By "adjusting for 'race'," even well-intentioned researchers will erroneously conclude that "race" explains asthma disparities rather than recognizing that racism—through environmental injustice—is the root cause.

If we fail to conduct analyses that properly account for systemic and contextual forces, we risk misdiagnosing problems, drawing faulty conclusions, and reinforcing the very inequities we aim to expose and eliminate.

Box 2-6. Reckoning With Medical Racism

False beliefs that different "races" are biologically distinct or "abnormal" continue to taint public health and medicine. These myths form the foundation of *scientific racism*, which has long been used to legitimize a false racial hierarchy under the guise of scientific objectivity. Scientific racism, in turn, underpins medical racism, with each reinforcing and justifying the other.

Medical racism refers to the ways in which racial discrimination—whether conscious or not—is embedded in the medical system, including medical training, clinical guidelines, diagnostic tools, and patient care. It shows up in how pain is assessed, how symptoms are interpreted, who receives care, and how medical research is conducted and applied. These patterns of racial discrimination not only drive persistent health inequities but also perpetuate ongoing harm, neglect, and mistrust.[81] Medical racism has a long history in the United States, with many examples:

- **Gynecology's foundation in chattel slavery:** J. Marion Sims, who has been called the "father of modern gynecology," developed surgical techniques by performing repeated, unanesthetized, and cruel procedures on enslaved Black women in the 1840s. He and others justified his inhumane actions using the racist belief that Black women experience less pain than white women—a myth that continues to influence medical treatment today.
- **Forced medical examinations at Angel Island:** Between 1910 and 1940, Asian immigrants arriving at Angel Island in San Francisco Bay were subjected to invasive and discriminatory medical inspections not required of European arrivals.[82] Under the pretense of public health and medical necessity, US authorities carried out dehumanizing examinations in prison-like conditions, particularly targeting single women as "moral risks" and "likely public charges." They were deemed by officials to be an "economic burden" to the United States.[83,84] These practices reinforced false and racist beliefs about Asian bodies and disease, using medicine as a guise to justify immigration restriction.
- **The exploitation of Henrietta Lacks and use of her cells without consent:** In 1951, Henrietta Lacks, a Black woman and mother of five, sought treatment for cervical cancer at Johns Hopkins Hospital. While there, physicians removed cell samples from her body without her knowledge or consent. Her cells—commonly known as *HeLa cells*—became the first immortal human cell line[85] and are the most widely used human cells in scientific research. HeLa cells have been central to decades of medical advancements, including the development of the polio vaccine, the identification of HIV, and the discovery of the COVID-19 vaccines. Nearly 100 pharmaceutical companies have profited from HeLa cells,[86] yet Lacks's family went uncompensated for decades.[87] Her story exposes how racism and exploitation have shaped the medical system and perpetuated unethical research practices that violate Black patients' bodily autonomy and dignity, use Black bodies to fuel scientific progress and profits, and exclude Black people from sharing in the benefits of medical research.
- **Tuskegee Syphilis Study (1932-1972):** In this government-sponsored study, 600 Black men in Alabama—399 of whom were known to have syphilis—were observed for decades and deliberately denied treatment so researchers could study the progression of the disease. The men were lied to and cruelly denied care, even after penicillin became widely available and the standard treatment for syphilis. The study continued for 40 years before it was exposed, causing needless death and suffering and spreading infection to wives and children, who were neither informed nor treated.

Sadly, many contemporary examples of medical racism exist today:

- **Refusal to properly treat pain in clinical settings:** Many clinicians have been formally—and wrongly—taught the racist idea that Black people don't feel pain as acutely as white people. This is based on the false claim that "Black bodies have fewer nerve endings than white bodies." Medical treatment based on this racist idea often results in Black and darker-skinned patients—both adults and children—being systematically undertreated for pain.[88]

(Continued)

Box 2-6. (Continued)

- **Unscientific "race"-based kidney calculation:** For years, a clinical equation used to assess kidney function (eGFR) included a "'race' correction" for Black patients, based on the unsubstantiated and racist belief that Black people had greater muscle mass that affected their kidney function compared with people of other "races."[89] This "adjustment" delayed referrals for specialist care and negated transplant eligibility for many Black patients. After years of advocacy, many medical institutions have discontinued the "race" adjustment, but the practice has not yet been fully abandoned.
- **False attributions of COVID-19 infections to "race":** During the pandemic, so-called research studies—amplified by media reports—attributed higher rates of COVID-19 infection and death among people of color to alleged "biological racial differences."[90] Yet the studies never provided evidence to support these false claims. In reality, these disparities stemmed from the consequences of structural racism and racial capitalism, including economic injustice, unequal access to health care, and chronic stress from discrimination.[91]

There are many commonplace examples of scientific racism:

- **Misattribution of "race" as a risk factor for chronic disease:** Myriad studies incorrectly claim that "race" is related to diseases like asthma and hyperlipidemia (high cholesterol). Even the Centers for Disease Control and Prevention lists being Black, Latine, or Indigenous as a "risk factor" for a chronic disease like type 2 diabetes.[92] But "race" is a human-made fiction—it is a social construct with no factual, biological, or genetic basis. This means that "race" cannot be a risk factor—but racism is. When public health institutions present "race" as a legitimate variable that puts people at risk for disease or injury, they distort and distract from the truth: Systems of oppression like structural racism, white supremacy, and colonialism are the root causes of health inequities—not the color of someone's skin.
- **Misuse of body mass index (BMI):** BMI, a widely used measure of health, was never designed for medical purposes. It was developed in the 19th century by a Belgian mathematician who based it entirely on the bodies of white European men[93] and who never intended it to account for the natural diversity in body types that exists across different people. Yet BMI became central to public health campaigns in the United States and globally in the 20th century. Sociologist and Black Studies scholar Sabrina Strings has documented how thinness was racialized in the 19th century, when fatness was framed as oppositional to white European ideals of self-discipline and moral superiority.[94] Today, using BMI as a clinical tool is dangerous and discriminatory. BMI fails to account for differences in age, muscle mass, bone density, and overall health—inappropriately labeling individuals as "overweight" or "obese."[95] People who are classified as having a high BMI are subjected to prejudice and stigma, alongside economic harms like lower wages and insurance penalties.[96-98]
- **Myth of "genetic predisposition" to disease:** For decades, Indigenous people were told the lie that they were genetically predisposed to alcoholism. This "firewater myth"—as it was later called—claimed that Indigenous people were biologically

incapable of processing alcohol and that intoxication made them unusually violent and aggressive.[99] In addition to being scientifically baseless, this myth conceals the true causes of alcohol-related harm in many Indigenous communities: the long-standing devastation of colonization, genocide, land theft, family separation, forced assimilation, and state-sanctioned violence. These intergenerational traumas created conditions where alcohol misuse became a coping mechanism, not a genetic condition. The issue was never genes.[100] It was—and continues to be—racism, colonialism, and their enduring legacies.

Despite overwhelming evidence that social and environmental factors are primarily responsible for determining health outcomes, unsupported claims about genetics continue to distract from systems of oppression. For example, a study cited hundreds of times incorrectly claimed that 30% of premature deaths in the United States could be explained by "genetic predisposition," while only 20% were attributed to social and environmental conditions.[101] These conclusions are false. Your zip code—your surrounding environments, infrastructure, policies, and socioeconomic conditions—is a far stronger predictor of health and longevity than your genetic code.[102]

Genetic ancestry and "race" are distinctly different. **Genetic ancestry** refers to paths through which genetic material has been inherited. People are born with a genetic ancestry; they are socially assigned a "race."[18] Despite clear evidence that systems of oppression like racism, white supremacy, and classism drive poor health outcomes, public health and medical practitioners wrongly, but persistently, suggest that racial health inequities are rooted in biology.[103]

The problem is not, and never has been, the bodies of racialized and marginalized people; the problem lies in unjust policies and systems steeped in racism. As sociologist and author Troy Duster notes, the impact of "race" on disease is not biological in *origin*, but it is biological in *effect*.[104,105] Although "race" is not a genetic reality, it is a social reality because of racism, leading to real biological and physiological damage.[106]

The repeated stress of enduring racism and other forms of oppression can take a physical toll through *weathering*—a term coined by public health scholar Arline Geronimus. **Weathering** describes how chronic exposure to structural racism, social marginalization, and economic hardship wears down the body over time, accelerating aging and increasing the risk of chronic illness and early death.[107-110]

Scientific racism isn't just a wrong rooted in the past; it continues to distort our understanding of health and undermines public health and medicine today. When false biological and genetic explanations for racial inequities are accepted as "fact," they mask the real drivers of these inequities: systems of oppression. If left unchallenged, scientific racism will continue to generate invalid and dangerous research, harmful clinical decisions, and lost opportunities for improving health.

Advancing equity and justice requires confronting and rejecting racist ideas and narratives. Identifying and dismantling structural racism must be a priority for all of us. We must be dynamic and adaptable in our approaches, particularly given the many ways that racism changes and evolves over time.

THE EVOLVING NATURE OF RACISM

When we think of racism we think of Governor Wallace of Alabama blocking the schoolhouse door . . . water hoses, lynchings, racial epithets, and "whites only" signs. These images make it easy to forget that many wonderful, goodhearted white people . . . nevertheless went to the polls and voted for racial segregation. . . . Our understanding of racism is therefore shaped by the most extreme expressions of individual bigotry, not by the way in which it functions naturally, almost invisibly . . . when it is embedded in the structure of a social system.

–Michelle Alexander, civil rights attorney and legal scholar[111(p183-184)]

Racism is not a relic of the past. It thrives in new forms that produce racist outcomes without explicitly using or referring to the term "race." This evolution makes racism more deeply entrenched in our institutions and policies, while simultaneously making it harder to identify and address.

An instructive example of how racism has adapted over time is the "Southern Strategy." This political tactic was initially deployed in the 1960s following the passage of the Civil Rights Act of 1964 and the Voting Rights Act of 1965—policies that aimed to end racial segregation and protect voting rights for Black Americans. White Southern voters who opposed civil rights became a key political constituency that could be mobilized by "using race as a wedge issue."[112] Politicians found that they could tap into this bloc of white voters' anger and resentment about desegregation, the expansion of voting rights to Black people, and other racial justice reforms.

Over time, the Southern Strategy evolved. It matured, spreading nationally and ultimately exemplifying a form of "dog-whistle politics." Like a dog whistle, these political messages were pitched at a "frequency" that only certain audiences could "hear" or accurately decode. These coded messages signaled racist and white supremacist ideas to receptive voters, while remaining inaudible—or at least plausibly deniable—to the general public.

The Southern Strategy helped racism reenter the mainstream, but it had a cost for everyone—not just people of color but for white people, too (see Box 2-7).[113,114] The architects of the Southern Strategy understood that racism could be used to divide potential cross-racial movements for economic justice, keeping elites in power. Historians and political leaders of the time acknowledged this reality. President Lyndon Baines Johnson described it bluntly, noting the political power of racism to divide working people and distract them from shared economic interests: "If you can convince the lowest white man he's better than the best colored man, he won't notice you're picking his pocket. Hell, give him somebody to look down on, and he'll empty his pockets for you."[115]

Box 2-7. Racism Costs Us All: The Cautionary Tale of Our Nation's Drained Public Pools

In the early 20th century, many US cities boasted large public pools that were a symbol of national pride. Despite being funded by taxpayers of all racial backgrounds, only white people were allowed to use these pools. The desire to maintain segregation was so strong that, when ordered to integrate the pools, white communities instead chose to drain and close them entirely so that no one could enjoy them. In some areas, white communities decided to defund and close their parks and recreation departments entirely to avoid sharing amenities with Black people.

These actions deprived everyone, including Black and white people, access to a valuable community asset. This willingness to destroy public goods, rather than share them—to essentially burn down the house rather than open the door—is a sentiment that continues to shape policy decisions across the United States today.

Author and attorney Heather McGhee uses the story of America's drained public pools as a metaphor for how racism harms everyone, including white people. McGhee explains that the refusal to share resources, even when it clearly damages society as a whole, reflects a deep societal divide rooted in racism.[113] Consider these examples:

- **Failure of Medicaid expansion in all states:** The Affordable Care Act, which was adopted in 2010, expanded the eligibility criteria for Medicaid—a joint federal and state program that provides health care coverage for low-income people. The law would have provided federal funding to cover 90% of costs for all states well into the future. But because Medicaid was perceived as helping Black people and others that powerful constituencies considered "undeserving," many states refused to accept the additional funding, which would have benefited millions of people, particularly white people—the largest share of Americans who would have received health care coverage under Medicaid.

- **Home foreclosures during the Great Recession:** In the 1990s and 2000s, unscrupulous lenders targeted Black and Latine communities with predatory subprime mortgages, even when borrowers qualified for better terms. These loans, laden with excessive fees, unreasonable interest rates, and penalties made default likely and set the stage for mass foreclosures. When the housing market collapsed in 2007, triggering the Great Recession, millions lost their homes. Black and Latine families faced disproportionately higher foreclosure rates and suffered the greatest relative losses in wealth, but ultimately, the majority of foreclosed homes belonged to white people.

- **Environmental injustice and shared harm:** Although segregated communities of color are more likely to be located next to landfills or in areas with high degrees of air contamination, the pollutants do not stay confined—they inevitably travel to neighboring communities, including white ones. Research shows that white residents living near racially segregated, pollution-burdened neighborhoods often assume that environmental hazards stay within communities of color. As a result, white residents are less likely to use their political power to advocate for environmental justice, ultimately allowing the pollution to persist and spread and endangering their neighborhoods as well.[114]

Denying everyone access to needed resources and sabotaging public goods in order to preserve power and privilege is a persistent pattern in our nation. McGhee writes: "When the people with power in a society see a portion of the populace as inferior and undeserving . . . they'll tear apart the web that supports everyone, including them."[113(p30)]

The story of the drained public pool also reflects a broader truth: Structural racism and white supremacy prioritize exclusion and inequity over collective prosperity. Racism robs us of health, well-being, and quality of life—not only for people of color, but for *everyone*.

Johnson's observation highlights how racism has been strategically wielded and weaponized to fracture potential coalitions for economic justice, protecting wealthy and powerful interests while leaving most people of all "races" worse off.

Although it was originally devised more than six decades ago, the Southern Strategy continues to define political discourse, elections, and government actions to this day.[116] The Southern Strategy continues to drive the adoption of policies and laws that weaken civil rights protections, deny people rights and resources, and defund essential government programs—including public health services. To this day, dog-whistle politics allow politicians to subtly communicate racist messages in plain sight. Seemingly innocuous terms like "fiscal conservatism," "tax cuts," "welfare," and "states' rights" have all been used as code for racist ideas.[117]

Racism's adaptability is not limited to politics. Across public health and many other spaces, we must reckon with **cultural racism**: defining white cultural norms as the standard or ideal, while portraying the traditions and behaviors of people of color as abnormal, inferior, or even pathological.[71]

Cultural racism operates by allowing people to avoid explicit references to "race" by blaming seemingly "colorblind" proxies—such as language, religion, immigration status, or participation in social safety net programs—as "problems" to be fixed, ultimately ensuring racist ideas can persist.[118] Sociologist and critical race theorist Eduardo Bonilla-Silva describes this dynamic as "racism without racists,"[119] where overt discrimination shifts to deceptively "race-neutral" explanations that blame marginalized communities for the conditions created by systems of oppression.

Culturally racist ideas are often invoked to "explain" health inequities. Like attempts to "control for race" in research, this framing obscures the root causes—racism and other systems of oppression—that lead to shorter and sicker lives for many. There are multiple examples:

- **The racist trope of Black criminality** has been deployed for decades to racially profile Black people as suspects in crimes[120] and to justify the disproportionate use of violence, incarceration, and force.[121] This racist narrative fuels heightened surveillance and policing of Black communities, leading to trauma, chronic stress, and poor health,[122] as well as unjust and disproportionate imprisonment of Black people.
- **The diets of Black, Latine, and Indigenous people have been vilified,** with false claims that these communities make worse lifestyle choices and eat unhealthier foods. This culturally racist idea has been used to "explain" the higher prevalence of diabetes and cardiovascular diseases in these communities, ignoring systemic factors like *food apartheid** and economic injustice.[124]
- **The "model minority myth"** portrays Asian Americans as more intelligent, high-achieving, hardworking, and deferential to authority compared with other racialized groups.[125] The insidiousness of this expression of cultural racism lies in its disguise as a "compliment." In reality, the stereotype functions to "divide and conquer" communities of color as well as obscure the numerous challenges to health and well-being that many Asian Americans communities face, such as mental health struggles and barriers to health care access.

***Food apartheid** is a term coined by organizer and food justice advocate Karen Washington that refers to the ways in which food is segregated so that "healthy, fresh food is accessible in wealthy neighborhoods while unhealthy food abounds in poor neighborhoods"—an injustice resulting from decades of policy and planning decisions that have perpetuated segregation and disinvestment, like Jim Crow and redlining.[123]

Cultural racism does not just distort how we explain inequities, it actively sustains them. By framing inequity as a product of cultural "deficiencies" rather than systemic oppression, public health interventions risk perpetuating harms rather than addressing their root causes.

Racism exists across all domains of society, shaping institutions, systems, and daily life. It is insidious and highly adaptable, often evolving to take new forms even as old ones are challenged or dismantled. As public health practitioners, we must be vigilant to actively address the ways in which racism evolves. We have an essential role in preventing racist ideas from operating in discreet ways that continue to drive unjust health disparities, poor quality of life, and premature death.

CONCLUSION

Structural racism has strong and deep roots in the United States that were planted long before the nation existed. It is a root cause of health inequities and a fundamental barrier to fulfilling the mission of public health. Too often, as public health practitioners, we simply document inequities—measuring differences in health outcomes across racial groups—without confronting why these differences exist, why they persist, and what we must do to eliminate them. As clinicians and interdisciplinary scholars Elle Lett, Emmanuella Asabor, Sourik Beltrán, Ashley Michelle Cannon, and Onyebuchi A. Arah explain,

> The scientific record is saturated with research demonstrating differences in health outcomes between racial and ethnic groups. Where these studies often fall short is in linking racial health disparities to the precise mechanisms that produce them, such as manifestations of racism, including poverty and state violence . . . [W]e suggest understanding race as a proxy measure for exposure to experiences of structural and individual racism. It is through this conceptualization that *racial disparity*, or difference in health outcomes across racialized groups, can be understood as *racial inequity*, a lack of health justice.[103]

Dismantling structural racism must be core to our work as public health practitioners. Its powerful and pernicious influence demonstrates several lessons:

- **Systems built to control one group inevitably expand to control others.** The carceral structures of surveillance and punishment developed under chattel slavery and settler colonialism evolved to target others—such as Latine and MENA communities—through militarized borders and immigration detention, students of color through school policing and harsh disciplinary policies, and many others through criminalization, austerity, and neglect.
- **Systems that devalue some lives ultimately devalue all lives.** Systems built on anti-Blackness and anti-Indigeneity have failed not only those most directly targeted but also other communities, such as Asian Americans, undocumented immigrants, unhoused people, and low-income white populations. Racist attacks on Black mothers

in politicized debates about welfare, for example, helped dismantle a social safety net that benefited everyone and distracted from the ways in which economic injustice suppresses opportunity for all.

- **When systems are built to exclude, they eventually fail everyone.** Racial scapegoating has justified disinvestment in health care, housing, education, and climate resilience—leaving crumbling infrastructure that puts us all at risk. Racialized opposition to Medicaid expansion, for example, blocked access to care for millions of people across all racial groups.

By challenging the systems, policies, institutions, and ideologies that uphold structural racism, we create opportunities to disrupt multiple forms of oppression and promote health and well-being for all. As Bailey et al. note, addressing structural racism provides us with a "concrete, feasible, and promising approach towards advancing health equity and improving population health."[32]

Racism has been a primary mechanism for justifying inequity and legitimizing white supremacy. By addressing its structural roots, we create pathways for systemic transformation that benefit everyone.

KEY TAKEAWAYS

 A false hierarchy of human value is the foundation of "race" and racism. The origins of the United States are inseparable from its violent history of ranking and valuing people according to their appearance. This deadly human hierarchy was invented to uphold colonialism and justify chattel slavery, positioning those categorized as "white" at the top and people with darker skin at the bottom. This is a lie on a colossal scale. All people are equally worthy of dignity and rights. Though this racial hierarchy has no scientific or moral basis, its consequences are real, far-reaching, and deeply embedded in the systems that shape our daily lives—including our health.

 "Race" is invented, not biological—it's racism that drives health inequities. "Race" is not a fixed or immutable characteristic. It is a constantly evolving social construct used to justify unfair treatment of groups of people. The stark disparities in health outcomes across racialized groups are not natural or inevitable. They are the result of racist policies, environments, and systems. From disproportionately high rates of pregnancy-related deaths among Black and Indigenous people to elevated exposure to environmental toxins in communities of color, racism must be understood as a root cause of sickened and shortened lives.

 Scientific racism co-opts and distorts science to legitimize white supremacy. For centuries, science has been weaponized to advance myths of racial superiority and inferiority. This is known as *scientific racism*. It has justified the exploitation, exclusion, and dehumanization of racialized groups. Scientifically racist ideas persist today across medicine and public health, from the continued misuse of "race" as a risk factor to statistical tools with origins in eugenics. These practices perpetuate dangerous narratives that certain bodies are inherently flawed, when in fact, racism—not biology—is what produces patterns of disease and early death.

 Racial capitalism fuels and entrenches inequities. Racism is economic as well as social, shaping how power and resources are distributed. *Racial capitalism* describes how our economic system generates profits through racialized land, labor, and resource exploitation to create wealth for the few at the expense of the many. Public policy has consistently reinforced and bolstered racial capitalism. While communities of color are most directly targeted, racial capitalism ultimately harms everyone—deepening inequality, suppressing wages, and eroding public goods for all but the wealthiest few. Naming this helps expose how racism is used to justify exploitation and prevent solidarity across "race" and class lines. This system shapes whose lives are devalued, whose labor is exploited, and whose communities are underfunded.

Racism is adaptive and amplifies other systems of oppression. Racism is not static; it has evolved to survive social, legal, cultural, and political change. Dog-whistle politics, like the Southern Strategy, show how racist ideas are repackaged over time to hide their true nature and to maintain mainstream acceptance. Even when its most explicit forms are outlawed or disavowed, racism can adapt to preserve white supremacy. It also intensifies other systems of oppression, including cissexism, ableism, classism, and nativism. This is the core insight of *intersectionality*: that multiple forms of marginalization compound harm for those who live at their intersections. Racism is used to justify gender-based violence, deny rights to disabled people, and entrench economic exclusion—making it a central force for sustaining multiple systems of oppression and ultimately suppressing health and prosperity for all.

REFERENCES

1. *Students for Fair Admissions Inc v President and Fellows of Harvard College*, 600 US 181 (2023). Accessed May 13, 2025. https://www.supremecourt.gov/opinions/22pdf/20-1199_hgdj.pdf
2. Wilkerson I. *Caste: The Origins of Our Discontents*. Random House; 2020.
3. @echohawkd3. We are not a "historically" underserved population [post]. X (formerly Twitter). September 7, 2019. Accessed June 1, 2025. https://x.com/echohawkd3/status/117037160 8894046208
4. Stanford Encyclopedia of Philosophy. Colonialism. January 17, 2023. Accessed May 16, 2025. https://plato.stanford.edu/entries/colonialism

5. Dartmouth College Library. Indigenous people & settler colonialism. Accessed July 24, 2025. https://www.library.dartmouth.edu/slavery-project/indigenous-people-settler-colonialism

6. Batra Kashyap M. US settler colonialism, white supremacy, and the racially disparate impacts of COVID-19. *Calif Law Rev Online*. 2020;11:517–529. Accessed May 16, 2025. https://digitalcommons.law.seattleu.edu/cgi/viewcontent.cgi?article=1832&context=faculty

7. Navajo Nation Department of Information Technology. Introduction. Accessed July 7, 2025. https://www.navajo-nsn.gov/history

8. Navajo People - The Diné. Accessed July 7, 2025. https://navajopeople.org

9. Iverson P. *Diné: A History of the Navajos*. University of New Mexico Press; 2002.

10. Ayala CJ, Bernabe R. *Puerto Rico in the American Century: A History Since 1898*. University of North Carolina Press; 2007.

11. Batista-Kunhardt G. Beyond paper genocide: Taíno recognition in Puerto Rico. *Brown Political Review*. February 17, 2022. Accessed June 3, 2025. https://brownpoliticalreview.org/beyond-paper-genocide

12. Warne D, Frizzell LB. American Indian health policy: Historical trends and contemporary issues. *Am J Public Health*. 2014;104(suppl 3):S263–S267. doi:10.2105/AJPH.2013.301682

13. Institute for Government Research. *The Problem of Indian Administration*. Johns Hopkins Press; 1928.

14. National Constitution Center. Mississippi & South Carolina Black Codes, 1865. Accessed May 16, 2025. https://constitutioncenter.org/the-constitution/historic-document-library/detail/mississippi-south-carolina-black-codes-1865

15. HISTORY.com editors. Black codes. History. February 27, 2025. Accessed May 16, 2025. https://www.history.com/topics/black-history/black-codes

16. Coates T-N. *Between the World and Me*. Spiegel & Grau; 2015.

17. National Museum of African American History and Culture. Historical foundations of race. May 31, 2020. Accessed June 1, 2025. https://web.archive.org/web/20240929122221/https://nmaahc.si.edu/learn/talking-about-race/topics/historical-foundations-race

18. Jones CP, Truman BI, Elam-Evans LD, et al. Using "socially assigned race" to probe White advantages in health status. *Ethn Dis*. 2008;18(4):496–504. Accessed June 1, 2025. https://www.ethndis.org/archive/files/ethn-18-04-496.pdf

19. Saini A. *Superior: The Return of Race Science*. Beacon Press; 2019.

20. Rambachan A. Overcoming the racial hierarchy: The history and medical consequences of "Caucasian." *J Racial Ethn Health Disparities*. 2018;5(5):907–912. doi:10.1007/s40615-017-0458-6

21. American Association of Biological Anthropologists. AABA statement on race & racism. March 2023. Accessed May 13, 2025. https://bioanth.org/about/aaba-statement-on-race-racism

22. Tehranian J. *Whitewashed: America's Invisible Middle Eastern Minority*. Vol 46. NYU Press; 2009.

23. Cainkar LA. *Homeland Insecurity: The Arab American and Muslim American Experience After 9/11*. Russell Sage Foundation; 2009.

24. Maghbouleh N, Schachter A, Flores RD. Middle Eastern and North African Americans may not be perceived, nor perceive themselves, to be white. *Proc Natl Acad Sci U S A*. 2022;119(7):e2117940119. doi:10.1073/pnas.2117940119

25. Wang HL. Next US census will have new boxes for "Middle Eastern or North African," "Latino." *NPR*. March 28, 2024. Accessed June 3, 2025. https://www.npr.org/2024/03/28/1237218459/census-race-categories-ethnicity-middle-east-north-africa

26. Omi M, Winant H. *Racial Formation in the United States.* 3rd ed. Routledge; 2014.
27. *Regents of the University of California v Bakke,* 438 US 265 (1978).
28. Jones CP. Confronting institutionalized racism. *Phylon.* 2002;50(1-2):7-22.
29. Peterson DM, Mann CL. *Closing the Racial Inequality Gaps: The Economic Cost of Black Inequality in the US.* Citi GPS: Global Perspectives & Solutions. Citigroup; September 2020. Accessed June 3, 2025. https://www.citigroup.com/global/insights/closing-the-racial-inequality-gaps-20200922
30. Buckman SR, Choi LY, Daly MC, Seitelman LM. The economic gains from equity. Federal Reserve Bank of San Francisco Working Paper 2021-11. doi:10.24148/wp2021-11
31. Bailey ZD, Krieger N, Agénor M, Graves J, Linos N, Bassett MT. Structural racism and health inequities in the USA: Evidence and interventions. *Lancet.* 2017;389(10077):1453-1463. doi:10.1016/S0140-6736(17)30569-X
32. Williams DR, Lawrence JA, Davis BA. Racism and health: Evidence and needed research. *Annu Rev Public Health.* 2019;40:105-125. doi:10.1146/annurev-publhealth-040218-043750
33. Ford CL, Griffith DM, Bruce MA, Gilbert KL, eds. *Racism: Science & Tools for the Public Health Professional.* American Public Health Association; 2019.
34. Jones CP. Levels of racism: A theoretic framework and a gardener's tale. *Am J Public Health.* 2000;90(8):1212-1215. doi:10.2105/AJPH.90.8.1212
35. Lawrence K, Sutton S, Kubisch A, Susi G, Fulbright-Anderson K, Aspen Institute Roundtable on Community Change. *Structural Racism and Community Building.* The Aspen Institute; 2004. Accessed May 13, 2025. https://www.aspeninstitute.org/wp-content/uploads/files/content/docs/rcc/aspen_structural_racism2.pdf
36. Rankine C. The condition of Black life is one of mourning. *New York Times Magazine.* June 22, 2015. Accessed May 13, 2025. https://www.nytimes.com/2015/06/22/magazine/the-condition-of-black-life-is-one-of-mourning.html
37. Rothstein R. *The Color of Law: A Forgotten History of How Our Government Segregated America.* W. W. Norton & Company; 2017.
38. Nardone A, Chiang J, Corburn J. Historic redlining and urban health today in US cities. *Environ Justice.* 2020;13(4):109-118. doi:10.1089/env.2020.0011
39. Nelson RK, Winling L, et al. Mapping inequality: Redlining in New Deal America. American Panorama. Accessed June 23, 2025. https://dsl.richmond.edu/panorama/redlining
40. Jan T. Redlining was banned 50 years ago. It's still hurting minorities today. *Washington Post.* March 28, 2018. Accessed May 13, 2025. https://www.washingtonpost.com/news/wonk/wp/2018/03/28/redlining-was-banned-50-years-ago-its-still-hurting-minorities-today
41. Graetz N, Esposito M. Historical redlining and contemporary racial disparities in neighborhood life expectancy. *Soc Forces.* 2023;102(1):1-22. doi:10.1093/sf/soac114
42. Krieger N, Van Wye G, Huynh M, et al. Structural racism, historical redlining, and risk of preterm birth in New York City, 2013-2017. *Am J Public Health.* 2020;110(7):1046-1053. doi:10.2105/AJPH.2020.305656
43. Krieger N, Kim R, Feldman J, Waterman PD. Cancer stage at diagnosis, historical redlining, and current neighborhood characteristics. *Am J Epidemiol.* 2020;189(10):1065-1075. doi:10.1093/aje/kwaa045

44. Taylor NL, Porter JM, Bryan S, Harmon KJ, Sandt LS. Structural racism and pedestrian safety: Measuring the association between historical redlining and contemporary pedestrian fatalities across the United States, 2010-2019. *Am J Public Health.* 2023;113(4):420-428. doi:10.2105/AJPH.2022.307192

45. Mehranbod CA, Gobaud AN, Jacoby SF, et al. Historical redlining and the epidemiology of present-day firearm violence in the United States: A multi-city analysis. *Prev Med.* 2022;165(Pt A):107207. doi:10.1016/j.ypmed.2022.107207

46. National Museum of African American History and Culture. Whiteness. Accessed July 23, 2025. https://web.archive.org/web/20240817141305/https://nmaahc.si.edu/learn/talking-about-race/topics/whiteness

47. Gillborn D. Rethinking white supremacy: Who counts in "WhiteWorld." *Ethnicities.* 2006;6(3):318-340. Accessed May 13, 2025. https://www.ssoar.info/ssoar/bitstream/handle/document/23036/ssoar-ethnicities-2006-3-gillborn-rethinking_white_supremacy.pdf

48. Bush ME. Race, ethnicity and whiteness. *SAGE Race Relations Abstracts.* 2004;29(3-4):5-48.

48a. Delgado R, Stefancic J, eds. *Critical White Studies.* Temple University Press; 1997.

48b. Bush ME, Bush RD. Twilight time: White supremacy, US hegemony, and historical capitalism. Presented at: 102nd Annual Meeting of the American Sociological Association, August 11-14, 2007, New York, NY.

48c. Cross KJ. Racism is the manifestation of white supremacy and antiracism is the answer. *J Eng Educ.* 2020;109(4):625-628. doi:10.1002/jee.20362

49. Smith B. The problem is white supremacy. *The Boston Globe.* June 29, 2020. Accessed May 13, 2025. https://www.bostonglobe.com/2020/06/29/opinion/problem-is-white-supremacy

50. Cheema Z. White supremacy: Whiteness and power. Antiracist Praxis subject guide. American University. Accessed May 13, 2025. https://subjectguides.library.american.edu/c.php?g=1025915&p=7749719

51. Combahee River Collective. The Combahee River Collective statement. 1977. Accessed June 21, 2025. https://americanstudies.yale.edu/sites/default/files/files/Keyword%20Coalition_Readings.pdf

52. Crenshaw KW. Demarginalizing the intersection of race and sex: A Black feminist critique of antidiscrimination doctrine, feminist theory, and antiracist politics. *University of Chicago Legal Forum.* 1989;1989(1):139-167. Accessed June 1, 2025. https://chicagounbound.uchicago.edu/uclf/vol1989/iss1/8

53. Babineau D. Chatting with . . . Moya Bailey. *Northwestern Magazine.* Fall 2023. Accessed June 28, 2025. https://magazine.northwestern.edu/voices/moya-bailey-misogynoir-racism-misogyny-merriam-webster-digital-apothecary

54. Bailey M. They aren't talking about me . . . March 14, 2010. Crunk Feminist Collective. Accessed July 24, 2025. https://www.crunkfeministcollective.com/2010/03/14/they-arent-talking-about-me

55. Bailey M. *Misogynoir Transformed: Black Women's Digital Resistance.* New York University Press; 2021.

56. Serano J. What is transmisogyny? *Medium.* 2022. Accessed May 16, 2025. https://juliaserano.medium.com/what-is-transmisogyny-4de92002caf6

57. Bailey M, Trudy. On misogynoir: citation, erasure, and plagiarism. *Fem Media Stud.* 2018;18(4):762-768. doi:10.1080/14680777.2018.1447395

58. Vargas JA. *Dear America: Notes of an Undocumented Citizen.* Dey Street Books; 2018.

59. Le Guin UK. National Book Foundation Medal for Distinguished Contribution to American Letters. Accessed May 16, 2025. https://www.ursulakleguin.com/nbf-medal

60. Kuhn M, Schularick M, Steins UI. *Income and Wealth Inequality in America, 1949-2016.* Opportunity & Inclusive Growth Institute Working Paper 9. Federal Reserve Bank of Minneapolis; June 14, 2018. doi:10.21034/iwp.9

61. Himmelstein KEW, Lawrence JA, Jahn JL, et al. Association between racial wealth inequities and racial disparities in longevity among US adults and role of reparations payments, 1992-2018. *JAMA Netw Open.* 2022;5(11):e2240519. doi:10.1001/jamanetworkopen.2022.40519

62. Johnson CO, Boon-Dooley AS, DeCleene NK, et al. Life expectancy for white, Black, and Hispanic race/ethnicity in US states: Trends and disparities, 1990-2019. *Ann Intern Med.* 2022;175(8):1057-1064. doi:10.7326/M21-3956

63. Moss E, McIntosh K, Edelberg W, Broady KE. The Black-white wealth gap left Black households more vulnerable. The Hamilton Project, Brookings Institution. December 8, 2020. Accessed May 13, 2025. https://www.hamiltonproject.org/publication/paper/the-black-white-wealth-gap-left-black-households-more-vulnerable

64. McKay LC. How the racial wealth gap has evolved—and why it persists. Federal Reserve Bank of Minneapolis. October 3, 2022. Accessed May 13, 2025. https://www.minneapolisfed.org/article/2022/how-the-racial-wealth-gap-has-evolved-and-why-it-persists

65. Mineo L. Racial wealth gap may be a key to other inequities. *Harvard Gazette.* June 3, 2021. Accessed May 13, 2025. https://news.harvard.edu/gazette/story/2021/06/racial-wealth-gap-may-be-a-key-to-other-inequities

66. Grutman A. The racial wealth gap is a racial health gap. *Kentucky Law J.* 2021;110:723-737. Accessed June 3, 2025. https://www.academia.edu/65139569/The_Racial_Wealth_Gap_is_a_Racial_Health_Gap

67. Jahan S, Mahmud AS. What is capitalism? *Finance Dev.* 2015;52(2):44-45. Accessed June 3, 2025. https://www.imf.org/en/Publications/fandd/issues/Series/Back-to-Basics/Capitalism

68. Surowiecki J. John Cassidy: The author on capitalism's critics, why everyone is so unhappy with the system, and what may come next. *The Yale Review.* May 27, 2025. Accessed July 28, 2025. https://yalereview.org/article/john-cassidy-capitalism-critics-interview

69. Cohen J. COVID-19 capitalism: The profit motive versus public health. *Public Health Ethics.* 2020;13(2):176–178. doi:10.1093/phe/phaa025

70. Paremoer L, Nandi S, Serag H, Baum F. Covid-19 pandemic and the social determinants of health. *BMJ.* 2021;372:n129. doi:10.1136/bmj.n129

71. Kendi IX. *How to Be an Antiracist.* One World; 2019.

72. Crook M, Short D, South N. Ecocide, genocide, capitalism and colonialism: Consequences for indigenous peoples and glocal ecosystems environments. *Theor Criminol.* 2018;22(3):298-317. doi:10.1177/1362480618787176.

73. Kelley RDG. What did Cedric Robinson mean by racial capitalism? *Boston Review.* January 12, 2017. Accessed May 13, 2025. https://www.bostonreview.net/articles/robin-d-g-kelley-introduction-race-capitalism-justice

74. Robinson CE. *Black Marxism: The Making of the Black Radical Tradition.* 3rd ed. University of North Carolina Press; 2022.

75. Pirtle WN Laster. Racial capitalism: A fundamental cause of novel coronavirus (COVID-19) pandemic inequities in the United States. *Health Educ Behav.* 2020;47(4):504–508. doi:10.1177/1090198120922942

76. Harvard Library. Scientific racism. Harvard University. Accessed January 17, 2025. https://web. archive.org/web/20250117041023/https://library.harvard.edu/confronting-anti-black-racism/ scientific-racism

77. Smith A. Indigeneity, settler colonialism, white supremacy. In: HoSang DM, LaBennett O, Pulido L, eds. *Racial Formation in the Twenty-First Century.* University of California Press; 2012:66–90. doi:10.1525/9780520953765-006

78. Sirmans ME. The legal status of the slave in South Carolina, 1670–1740. *J South Hist.* 1962;28(4):462–473. doi:10.2307/2205410

79. Kennedy-Shaffer L. Teaching the difficult past of statistics to improve the future. *J Stat Data Sci Educ.* 2023;32:108–119. doi:10.1080/26939169.2023.2224407

80. Clayton A. How eugenics shaped statistics. *Nautilus.* October 27, 2020. Accessed May 13, 2025. https://nautil.us/how-eugenics-shaped-statistics-238014

81. Bronson E. What is medical racism? *YWCA Firesteel* (blog). July 21, 2020. Accessed May 12, 2025. https://www.ywcaworks.org/blogs/firesteel/tue-07212020-0947/what-medical-racism

82. Angel Island Immigration Station Foundation. History of Angel Island Immigration Station. 2008. Accessed June 28, 2025. https://www.aiisf.org/history

83. Angel Island Immigration Station Foundation. Angel Island Immigration Museum under the microscope. Accessed June 28, 2025. https://www.aiisf.org/aiimicroscope

84. Yung J. "A Bowlful of Tears" revisited: The full story of Lee Puey You's immigration experience at Angel Island. *Frontiers.* 2004;25(1):1–22. Accessed June 28, 2025. http://www.jstor.org/stable/3347251

85. Skloot R. *The Immortal Life of Henrietta Lacks.* Crown Publishers; 2010.

86. Prudente T. Family of Henrietta Lacks hires civil rights attorney to seek funds over famous cells. *Washington Post.* July 31, 2021. Accessed June 3, 2025. https://www.washingtonpost.com/local/ henrietta-lacks-cells-family-compensation/2021/07/31/63935928-f16c-11eb-bf80-e3877d9c5f06_story.html

87. Skene L, Brumfield S. Henrietta Lacks' family settles lawsuit with a biotech company that used her cells without consent. *Associated Press.* August 1, 2023. Accessed July 30, 2025. https:// apnews.com/article/henrietta-lacks-hela-cells-thermo-fisher-scientific-bfba4a6c10396efa34c9 b79a544f0729

88. Dutchen S. Field correction: Race-based medicine, deeply embedded in clinical decision making, is being scrutinized and challenged. *Harvard Medicine Magazine.* Winter 2021. Accessed May 13, 2025. https://magazine.hms.harvard.edu/articles/field-correction

89. Brooks K. Filtering bias out of kidney testing: Q&A with Nwamaka Eneanya, MD, MPH, on advancing health equity and removing race from assessment of renal function. *Penn Medicine Magazine.* March 16, 2021. Accessed May 13, 2025. https://web.archive.org/web/20250307171904/ https://www.pennmedicine.org/news/publications-and-special-projects/penn-medicine-magazine/winter-2021/filtering-bias-out-of-kidney-testing

90. Xue W, White A. COVID-19 and the rebiologisation of racial difference. *Lancet.* 2021;398(10310):1479-1480. doi:10.1016/S0140-6736(21)02241-8

91. Khazanchi R, Evans CT, Marcelin JR. Racism, not race, drives inequity across the COVID-19 continuum. *JAMA Netw Open.* 2020;3(9):e2019933. doi:10.1001/jamanetworkopen.2020.19933

92. Centers for Disease Control and Prevention. Type 2 diabetes. May 15, 2024. Accessed May 13, 2025. https://www.cdc.gov/diabetes/about/about-type-2-diabetes.html

93. Stern C. Why BMI is a flawed health standard, especially for people of color. *Washington Post.* May 5, 2021. Accessed May 13, 2025. https://www.washingtonpost.com/lifestyle/wellness/healthy-bmi-obesity-race/2021/05/04/655390f0-ad0d-11eb-acd3-24b44a57093a_story.html

94. Strings S. *Fearing the Black Body: The Racial Origins of Fat Phobia.* New York University Press; 2019.

95. Office of Minority Health. Obesity and Hispanic Americans. Accessed May 13, 2025. https://minorityhealth.hhs.gov/obesity-and-hispanic-americans

96. Landry M, Song X, Wolfson C, et al. Gender differences in care-seeking and hospitalization for COVID-19 in Ontario, Canada: A population-based cohort study. *J Epidemiol Community Health.* 2023;77(4):233-240. doi:10.1136/jech-2022-219078

97. Mensah GA, Mokdad AH, Ford ES, Greenlund KJ, Croft JB. State of disparities in cardiovascular health in the United States. *Circulation.* 2005;111(10):1233-1241. doi:10.1161/01.CIR.0000158136.76824.04

98. Cromwell L. High BMI can mean penalties for benefits. *The Ledger.* September 10, 2007. Accessed June 3, 2025. https://www.theledger.com/story/news/2007/09/10/high-bmi-can-mean-penalties-for-benefits/25790129007

99. Golding CW. A prairie Polyphemus: The firewater myth in a Canadian legal context. *Sask Law Rev.* 2023;86(1). Accessed May 12, 2025. https://www.canlii.org/en/commentary/doc/2023CanLIIDocs1200

100. Szalavitz M. No, Native Americans aren't genetically more susceptible to alcoholism. *The Verge.* October 2, 2015. Accessed June 3, 2025. https://www.theverge.com/2015/10/2/9428659/firewater-racist-myth-alcoholism-native-americans

101. Schroeder SA. Shattuck Lecture. We can do better—improving the health of the American people. *N Engl J Med.* 2007;357(12):1221-1228. doi:10.1056/NEJMsa073350

102. Ross RK, Iton A. Understanding how health happens: Your zip code is more important than your genetic code. In: Callahan RF, Bhattacharya D, eds. *Public Health Leadership: Strategies for Innovation in Population Health and Social Determinants.* Routledge; 2022:67-80.

103. Lett E, Asabor E, Beltrán S, Cannon AM, Arah OA. Conceptualizing, contextualizing, and operationalizing race in quantitative health sciences research. *Ann Fam Med.* 2022;20(2):157-163. doi:10.1370/afm.2792

104. Smedley B, Jeffries M, Adelman L, Cheng J. Race, racial inequality and health inequities: Separating myth from fact. Briefing paper. Unnatural Causes; 2008. Accessed May 16, 2025. https://unnaturalcauses.org/assets/uploads/file/Race_Racial_Inequality_Health.pdf

105. Duster T. Medicine and people of color: Unlikely mix—race, biology and drugs. SFGate. March 17, 2003. Accessed May 16, 2025. https://www.sfgate.com/opinion/openforum/article/MEDICINE-AND-PEOPLE-OF-COLOR-Unlikely-mix-2628151.php

106. American Sociological Association. Troy Duster. October 23, 2024. Accessed June 3, 2025. https://www.asanet.org/troy-duster

107. Geronimus AT. *Weathering: The Extraordinary Stress of Ordinary Life in an Unjust Society*. Little Brown Spark; 2023.

108. Forde AT, Crookes DM, Suglia SF, Demmer RT. The weathering hypothesis as an explanation for racial disparities in health: A systematic review. *Ann Epidemiol*. 2019;33:1-18.e3. doi:10.1016/j.annepidem.2019.02.011

109. Millstine D. Weathering the storm of chronic racism and oppression [podcast]. *Mayo Clinic Press*. April 12, 2023. Accessed May 13, 2025. https://mcpress.mayoclinic.org/women-health/weathering-the-storm-of-chronic-racism-and-oppression

110. Simons RL, Lei M-K, Klopack E, et al. The effects of social adversity, discrimination, and health-risk behaviors on the accelerated aging of African Americans: Further support for the weathering hypothesis. *Soc Sci Med*. 2021;282:113169. doi:10.1016/j.socscimed.2020.113169

111. Alexander M. *The New Jim Crow: Mass Incarceration in the Age of Colorblindness*. Rev ed. The New Press; 2020.

112. Buck K. The Southern Strategy: The GOP has a history of using racism to its political advantage. *Baltimore Sun*. Accessed May 13, 2025. https://web.archive.org/web/20250416034222/https://digitaledition.baltimoresun.com/tribune/article_popover.aspx?guid=90fa275f-7eca-4fdd-8120-8ba0fd1e8474.

113. McGhee H. *The Sum of Us: What Racism Costs Everyone and How We Can Prosper Together*. One World; 2021.

114. Ash M, Boyce JK, Chang G, Scharber H. Is environmental justice good for white folks? Industrial air toxics and exposure in urban America. *Soc Sci Q*. 2013;94(3):616–636. doi:10.1111/j.1540-6237.2012.00874.x

115. Moyers BD. What a real president was like. *Washington Post*. November 13, 1988. Accessed August 1, 2025. https://www.washingtonpost.com/archive/opinions/1988/11/13/what-a-real-president-was-like/d483c1be-d0da-43b7-bde6-04e10106ff6c

116. Stanley J. We are witnessing the rise of a new Republican "Southern Strategy." *The Guardian*. February 10, 2025. Accessed May 13, 2025. https://www.theguardian.com/us-news/2025/feb/10/we-are-witnessing-the-rise-of-a-new-republican-southern-strategy

117. Perlstein R. Exclusive: Lee Atwater's infamous 1981 interview on the Southern Strategy. *The Nation*. November 13, 2012. Accessed May 13, 2025. https://www.thenation.com/article/archive/exclusive-lee-atwaters-infamous-1981-interview-southern-strategy

118. Chua R. Cultural racism. In: *The Wiley Encyclopedia of Social Theory*. Wiley; 2017. doi:10.1002/9781118430873.est0079

119. Bonilla-Silva E. *Racism Without Racists: Color-Blind Racism and the Persistence of Racial Inequality in America*. 6th ed. Rowman & Littlefield; 2022.

120. Levin S. California police show severe racial bias in stops and searches, data finds. *The Guardian*. January 3, 2024. Accessed May 13, 2025. https://www.theguardian.com/us-news/2024/jan/03/california-police-stops-racial-bias

121. Najdowski CJ. How the "Black criminal" stereotype shapes Black people's psychological experience of policing: Evidence of stereotype threat and remaining questions. *Am Psychol.* 2023;78(5):695–713. doi:10.1037/amp0001159

122. Alang S, Haile R, Hardeman R, Judson J. Mechanisms connecting police brutality, intersectionality, and women's health over the life course. *Am J Public Health.* 2023;113(suppl 1):S29–S36. doi:10.2105/AJPH.2022.307064

123. Walker J. 'Food desert' vs. 'food apartheid': Which term best describes disparities in food access? University of Michigan School for Environment and Sustainability. November 29, 2023. Accessed May 12, 2025. https://seas.umich.edu/news/food-desert-vs-food-apartheid-which-term-best-describes-disparities-food-access

124. Hirsch JS. The racial transformation of diabetes. *Clin Diabetes.* 2022;40(4):511–512. doi:10.2337/cd22-0064

125. Ruiz NG, Im C, Tian Z. Asian Americans and the "model minority" stereotype. Pew Research Center. November 30, 2023. Accessed May 13, 2025. https://www.pewresearch.org/race-and-ethnicity/2023/11/30/asian-americans-and-the-model-minority-stereotype

The Root Causes of Health Inequities

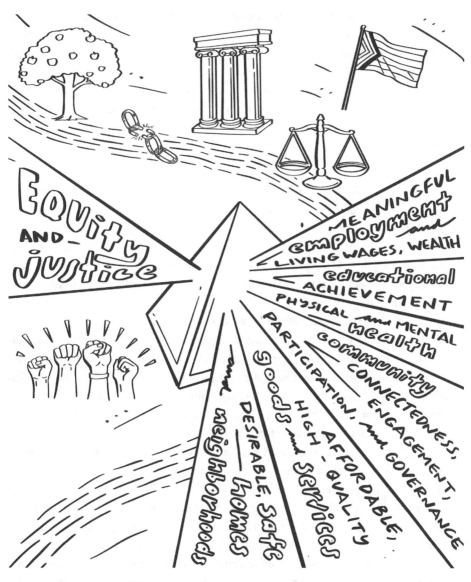

Artist Credit: Jasmin Pamukcu, 2025.

A Prism of Possibility

A primary goal of public health is to address the root causes of social injustice: widening gaps between rich and poor, the unequal distribution of resources within our society, discrimination, and the disenfranchisement of individuals and groups from the political process.
        –Marian Wright Edelman, civil rights activist and children's advocate[1(pviii)]

Health is often described as a personal responsibility—determined by lifestyle choices, genetics, and access to medical care—but this description of health is both inaccurate and incomplete. In reality, the forces that shape our health are much more fundamental—what those of us in the field of public health call the **social determinants of health.** As discussed in Chapter 1, these are a complex and often invisible web of conditions and contexts that shape not only our health but also our options, our opportunities, and the structure of our daily lives. The social determinants of health—and the systems and structures that give rise to them—have far more influence on our well-being than our personal choices or the medical treatment we receive, and these influences are numerous:

Economics shape health: Across and within countries, income is highly correlated with health, as measured by life expectancy and multiple other health indicators.[2] Wealthier children tend to be healthier, and adults with higher incomes tend to live longer.[3] Countries with lower income inequality tend to have better population health outcomes: They have lower rates of chronic disease, mental health disorders, and preventable deaths.[4] Even small changes in economic policy can make a big difference: for example, increasing the minimum wage by just one dollar can potentially prevent thousands of suicides.[5] Economic policies are public health policies—with consequences that can be life-or-death. Moreover, a **guaranteed income**—recurring cash payments that are distributed to members of a community, with no strings attached—can create an income floor beneath which no one can fall.[6] This offers not only financial stability but also a foundation for better health: A guaranteed income has been shown to improve health outcomes, particularly those related to adult physical and mental health and maternal and child well-being.[7]

Education shapes health: Higher educational attainment is closely linked to longer, healthier lives. Adults with more years of education tend to live longer and have better health outcomes than those with less education.[8] The relationship between education and health in the United States is particularly strong because of the way health insurance is structured: Insurance coverage is generally tied to employment. In the United States, those with more education are more likely to secure jobs that include health insurance benefits,[9] which is, in turn, associated with better health outcomes.[10] In general, higher levels of education typically lead to more stable, higher-paying jobs. In turn, higher-paying jobs contribute to greater social status[11]

and improved access to health-promoting resources—such as safe and stable housing, nutritious food, and time for rest and recovery. Compared with other high-income countries, the United States has one of the largest gaps in life expectancy
between people with high and low levels of education.[12]

 Housing shapes health: Housing is foundational to well-being. Lack-
ing it can be deadly: People experiencing homelessness face a significantly higher risk of death compared with people who have stable
housing.[13,14] And simply having shelter is the bare minimum. Unstable
housing increases the risk of illness, stress, lost income, school disruption, and even early death—harming not just individuals but entire families and communities.[15] By contrast, affordable housing improves health by reducing stress,
preventing disease, enhancing environmental safety, and enabling people of all ages
and abilities to live with stability and dignity.[16] Unsurprisingly, then, homeownership
in the United States is generally associated with longevity.[17] However, the powerful
health benefits of housing are not available to everyone. This is due in large part to the
way we as a nation treat housing as a commodity—something to be bought, owned,
and sold—not a right to which everyone is entitled. It's also because of racist policies
like redlining and "urban renewal,"* which forced Black people and other marginalized communities into segregated neighborhoods that were cut off from lending,
investment, and other resources. For decades, these neighborhoods have been subjected to substandard housing, fewer resources, poor neighborhood infrastructure,
and greater exposure to environmental toxins.[19]

 Transportation shapes health: The way our communities are designed
governs how safe it is to travel through them.[20] When policies ensure
roads are built to prioritize people over cars, thousands of lives can be
saved[21]—particularly among those who are walking, biking, and using
wheelchairs to travel throughout communities. A well-designed public
transit system is a public health intervention that can reduce traffic crashes, improve
air pollution, and enhance access to jobs, goods, services, and social spaces.[22] Yet
transportation infrastructure in the United States has long reflected and reinforced
racial and economic inequities. Communities that were redlined nearly a century ago

---

*From the late 1940s through the 1970s, the federal government funded a nationwide "urban renewal" pro-
gram. Its stated goals were to "revitalize American cities, create a decent home for every family, improve transportation, and accommodate suburban sprawl."[18] In reality, these efforts targeted low-income and communities
of color under the guise of eliminating "blight" and promoting public health. Across the country, thousands of
neighborhoods were razed and nearly a million people were uprooted to make way for highways, corporate
development, and gentrification—with little to no replacement housing and no deference to the people and
communities being displaced and destroyed. "Urban renewal" efforts caused the irreversible loss of diverse and
vibrant neighborhoods, as well as the people and cultures that defined them. Backed by federal funding and
support, "urban renewal" became yet another tool for state-sanctioned violence against Black, low-income, and
other marginalized communities.

continue to experience higher rates of pedestrian deaths to this day.[23] And in a nation where mobility is often dependent on car ownership, low-income individuals and communities of color are disproportionately burdened by transportation inequities.

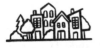 **Social and physical features of neighborhoods shape health:** The physical and social environment of a neighborhood has a profound effect on well-being. Living in a safe, walkable area with access to parks, grocery stores, and strong social networks supports both physical and mental health.[24-26] Conversely, neighborhoods contribute to chronic stress and poor health when they have high-speed roads running through them, inadequate pedestrian safety infrastructure, high levels of pollution, little to no green space, and limited access to fresh food. Climate change is exacerbating these inequities. Today, communities of color disproportionately bear the brunt of dangerous environmental hazards like extreme heat, wildfires, hurricanes, flooding, and disruptions to food and energy systems.[27] For example, neighborhoods without green space and tree canopies are more likely to become *heat islands*—places with significantly higher temperatures than their surroundings—which can create dangerous and extreme heat waves and increase the risk of heat-related illnesses.[28,29]

The influences on our health go far deeper than we may realize. When we talk about the social determinants of health, we're describing symptoms we can see, but not the root causes that give rise to them. Powerful forces are at work below the surface of what we can see.

Housing, education, employment, health care, and other social determinants of health are all shaped by the root causes of health inequities: **systems of oppression**—the entrenched social, economic, and political structures that distribute power and resources unfairly, creating advantages for some groups while marginalizing and disadvantaging others. These systems of oppression include white supremacy, structural racism, colonialism, racial capitalism, and more—all of which produce conditions and contexts that govern how well and how long we live.

These underlying systems of oppression ultimately determine who flourishes and who is left behind. Take housing, for example: In the United States, housing is considered a commodity. It is bought, sold, rented, and withheld rather than being guaranteed and equitably allocated as a public good and human right. This commodification reflects and reinforces deeper systems at play: Racial capitalism has distorted and restricted access to stable housing and wealth-building opportunities by tying them to inherited money and resources that have been systematically denied to many. Simultaneously, structural racism and colonialism have historically denied Indigenous and Black people access to land, quality mortgages, and health-promoting neighborhoods. The end result is a housing system that allows some to build stability and intergenerational wealth while leaving others—disproportionately low-income households and communities of color—precarious, segregated, and exposed to damaging conditions that cut years off their lives.

To advance equity and justice and create long-term, meaningful change, we must directly confront systems of oppression. But first, we must understand the powerful connections that exist between the root causes of health inequities and the many other forces that shape our daily lives.

This chapter introduces the *Root Causes Roadmap*—a multilayered framework that illustrates how and where these connections exist, identifies intervention points to disrupt systems of oppression, and lays out tools to promote community health and well-being.

THE ROOT CAUSES ROADMAP

There is no such thing as a single-issue struggle because we do not live single-issue lives.
                                        –Audre Lorde, poet and feminist scholar[30(p138)]

The Root Causes Roadmap*[31] allows us to zoom out and see the dynamic interrelationships between the systems, structures, tools, and outcomes connected to community health. These include *systems of oppression, structural inequities, tools for systems change*, the *social determinants of health*, and *outcomes for healthy and flourishing communities* (Figure 3-1).

This chapter will unpack the Root Causes Roadmap layer by layer, starting at the bottom with the root causes—systems of oppression and structural inequities—then returning to the top to walk through the social determinants of health and outcomes for healthy and flourishing communities. Given their dynamic impact across all of the layers, the tools for systems change will be discussed last.

ROOT CAUSES: SYSTEMS OF OPPRESSION AND STRUCTURAL INEQUITIES

[S]ystems, as it turns out, change all the time, and systemic change can be dangerous if it doesn't center both equity and power.
                                        –Farhad Ebrahimi, organizer and philanthropic strategist[35]

At the base of the Root Causes Roadmap are the root causes of health inequities: *systems of oppression*. These are white supremacy, structural racism, racial capitalism, colonialism, sexism, ableism, classism, and more. These forces are deeply interconnected and operate across every level of society—shaping policies, institutions, and social norms in ways that determine who has access to resources and opportunities and who does not. As discussed in Chapter 2, the inequities these systems produce not only harm marginalized communities but also weaken the health and well-being of society as a whole.

---

*The Root Causes Roadmap was adapted from a framework published by Porter et al.[31] The framework from Porter et al. was informed and inspired by works published by Jones,[32] Yearby,[33] and ChangeLab Solutions.[34]

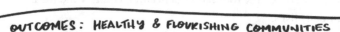

ROOT CAUSES Roadmap

OUTCOMES: HEALTHY & FLOURISHING COMMUNITIES

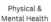

Physical & Mental Health	Meaningful Employment, Living Wages, & Wealth	Safe, Stable, & Desirable Homes & Neighborhoods	Educational Achievement	Affordable, High-Quality Goods & Services	Community Connectedness & Civic Participation

SOCIAL DETERMINANTS of HEALTH

Economic Stability & Security	Education	Neighborhoods, Housing & Built Environment	Public Heath & Health Care	Resources, Goods, & Services	Social & Community Contexts

TOOLS for SYSTEMS CHANGE

Laws & Public Policies	Organizational Policies	Practices	Budgets	Collaborative Governance or Co-Governance	Data & Research

STRUCTURAL INEQUITIES

Structural Discrimination	Inequities in Income & Wealth	Inequities in Opportunity	Inequities in Political Power	Governance that Limits Meaningful Participation

ROOT CAUSES: SYSTEMS of OPPRESSION

WHITE SUPREMACY   STRUCTURAL RACISM   COLONIALISM   RACIAL CAPITALISM

CLASSISM   SEXISM   ABLEISM   NATIVISM   AGEISM   HETEROSEXISM   CISSEXISM   & MORE

Source: Porter et al.[31] Adapted with permission from Wolters Kluwer Health.
Artist Credit: Jasmin Pamukcu, 2025.

Figure 3-1. The Root Causes Roadmap

ROOT CAUSES: SYSTEMS of OPPRESSION

WHITE SUPREMACY   STRUCTURAL RACISM   COLONIALISM   RACIAL CAPITALISM

CLASSISM   SEXISM   ABLEISM   NATIVISM   AGEISM   HETEROSEXISM   CISSEXISM   & MORE

Systems of oppression are built on destructive and exclusionary ideas about who is valuable, who gets to make decisions, and who is allowed to flourish. Because these ideas are deeply woven into the fabric of our nation, they can often be hard to name or even notice. But the effects of systems of oppression are visible and real. They produce and reinforce **structural inequities**—large-scale, patterned, and entrenched disadvantages that shape people's everyday lives.

STRUCTURAL INEQUITIES

| Structural Discrimination | Inequities in Income & Wealth | Inequities in Opportunity | Inequities in Political Power | Governance that Limits Meaningful Participation |

The impacts of systems of oppression are often easier to see in their outcomes than in their underlying mechanisms. Even if we don't always talk about structural racism, for example, we see its impact in the racial wealth gap that leaves people of color with a fraction of the generational assets held by white households; the underrepresentation of people of color in leadership roles across society; and in voter suppression laws that intentionally target and undermine the political power of communities of color. We may not see colonialism directly, but its legacy is visible in public health datasets that erase Indigenous people's experiences and in the daily lives of people living in territories like Puerto Rico, where communities have been denied essential resources and self-determination for centuries. Sexism shows up in wage gaps, disproportionate caregiving burdens, and the erosion of reproductive rights. Ableism manifests in inaccessible infrastructure, discriminatory health care practices, and exclusion from educational and employment opportunities. The list goes on.

When people are shut out of decision-making, denied access to opportunities and resources, and excluded from the political process, it's not a coincidence; it's the result of systems that were built to intentionally benefit some at the expense of others. These oppressive systems fuel multiple structural inequities:

Structural discrimination. Interlocking and unjust laws, policies, practices, and societal norms systematically disadvantage marginalized people. They deny some groups fair access to power, resources, and opportunities while upholding advantages and privileges for others. Together, these forms of injustice reinforce one another, embedding inequities into daily life and across generations. Even policies designed to protect marginalized groups can perpetuate injustice if they are implemented in a "colorblind" or one-size-fits-all manner that ignores the specific barriers that different people face. Dismantling structural discrimination requires an intentional focus on justice and redress.

Inequities in income and wealth. Economic inequities refer to sustained, systemic, and unfair disparities in earnings, asset ownership, and wealth-building opportunities between different groups. These inequities limit most people's ability to attain economic stability, invest in their futures, and build generational wealth—especially if they hold marginalized identities. While wealth is increasingly concentrated among the already-wealthy, others face persistent barriers to obtaining dignified employment, fair wages, and access to high-quality financial services. These conditions create fertile ground for economic exploitation and exacerbate other forms of oppression—such as environmental injustice caused by corporate profit seeking and government inaction.

Inequities in opportunity. Meeting basic needs, pursuing personal goals, and leading fulfilling lives are all essential for health and flourishing. But unfair and systemic differences in access to opportunities—especially in education, economic mobility, and social support—create profound barriers to our health and longevity. These inequities not only restrict access to health-promoting resources but also contribute to harms like chronic stress, poor living conditions, and the inability to afford essential services. Inequities in opportunity block paths to upward mobility and widen racial health and wealth gaps, fueling cycles of poverty and marginalization that follow families across generations.

Inequities in political power. Political power—the ability to vote, organize, influence policy, and shape civic life—is directly connected to health and well-being.[36] Yet marginalized communities face significant barriers to participating in the democratic process. This is because of policies and practices—past and present—that deliberately suppress their ability to influence decisions that shape their lives. Antidemocratic tactics like voter ID laws, gerrymandering, voter roll purges, winner-take-all elections,[37] and the disenfranchisement of formerly incarcerated individuals are all intentionally deployed to negate the political power of communities of color, low-income communities, and other historically excluded groups. Meanwhile, communities with concentrated political power are better positioned to shape laws and policies, direct public resources, and maintain systems that benefit them. Unfair differences in access and resources between communities further entrench inequities in power and opportunity.

 Governance that limits meaningful participation. Governance refers to processes by which communities make collective decisions and distribute power and resources. Ideally, governance structures— such as state legislatures, city councils, school boards, and county commissions, as well as community-led structures like land trusts, neighborhood associations, and participatory budgeting assemblies—reflect broad consensus and serve the needs of all community members. But in communities where civic and democratic participation is suppressed—through barriers to voting, inaccessible decision-making spaces, and the silencing of marginalized voices—governance structures often fail to address the priorities and desires of all communities. When people are excluded from shaping the decisions that impact their lives, their priorities are ignored, their influence is diminished, and policies and decisions perpetuate inequity rather than prevent it.

The Root Causes Roadmap presents each structural inequity as distinct for the sake of clarity and understanding. In reality, these forces are deeply intertwined and frequently overlap. From inequities in opportunity to governance that limits meaningful participation, each structural inequity interacts with and intensifies the others—operating within broader systems of oppression to collectively form a dense web of systemic harm. When these forces converge, they compound disadvantage and create conditions that make it extraordinarily difficult—if not impossible—for marginalized people to break free from cycles of exclusion, subjugation, and exploitation.

SOCIAL DETERMINANTS OF HEALTH

[Change] looks like everybody having an economic floor and not having to worry about making sure their necessities are met: shelter, health care, food, just the bare necessities needed to function in a civilized society. We will . . . see more of a healthy community . . . We will also see civic engagement, engagement with the community at large increasing, and I think you will see people happier.

–Michael Tubbs, political leader and anti-poverty advocate[38]

Toward the top of the Roadmap are the social determinants of health—a set of interconnected conditions and contexts that shape our health by influencing the opportunities, resources, and choices available to us in our daily lives.

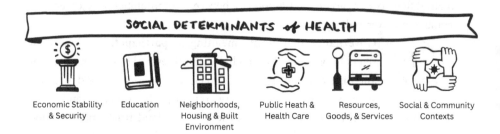

SOCIAL DETERMINANTS of HEALTH

| Economic Stability & Security | Education | Neighborhoods, Housing & Built Environment | Public Heath & Health Care | Resources, Goods, & Services | Social & Community Contexts |

The social determinants of health are essential building blocks for health and flourishing. These determinants include economic stability; education; neighborhoods, housing, and the built environment; public health and health care; resources, goods, and services; and social and community contexts.

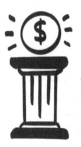

Economic stability goes beyond income to encompass all the resources and opportunities that open the door to financial security and well-being, both now and across generations. Economic stability is influenced by a variety of interdependent systems, including employment structures, financial institutions, credit networks, public assistance programs, nonprofit initiatives, stock markets and investment systems, and support from community and family. Policies set the stage for whether people will experience job security, earn a living wage, build wealth, and access important financial resources. In the long term, these systems dictate whether or not someone has a path to prosperity—and whether they can grow and maintain that prosperity for future generations.

Education is the process of gaining knowledge, skills, and opportunities through structured learning systems. It encompasses a broad network of institutions and organizations, including early childhood programs, K–12 school systems, school boards, parent–teacher associations, colleges and universities, technical and vocational schools, apprenticeships, continuing education programs, professional associations, and student loan institutions. Policies heavily shape these systems—and in turn, those systems determine who can access educational opportunity, what kind of education they receive, how they can apply their training, and the resources available to support them. Access to a quality education—and the professional network that often accompanies it—directly influences future job prospects, earning potential, wealth building, and long-term health outcomes.

Neighborhoods, housing, and the built environment refer to the human-made surroundings that provide the setting for daily life—where people live, work, and interact. This includes buildings, roads, sidewalks, and parks, as well as infrastructure systems like water and energy networks. The built environment plays a major role in shaping our opportunities, social participation, and well-being. Policies governing housing, zoning, transportation, and urban planning deeply influence how these spaces function. Well-designed, safe, affordable, and desirable neighborhoods promote health and provide easy access to destinations and essential resources. By contrast, health is endangered by poorly planned neighborhoods, such as those characterized by sprawl, high-speed roads, limited green space and shade, and unsafe or abandoned infrastructure.

 Public health and health care encompass the systems entrusted with safeguarding people's health—individually and collectively. These systems include hospitals, medical offices, clinics, government agencies like health departments, pharmacies, mental health services, community-based organizations, and professional associations. As discussed in Chapter 1, public health focuses on protecting and improving the health of entire populations, while health care delivery systems are concerned with diagnosing, treating, and supporting the health of individual patients. Some health care and public health programs—like Medicare, Medicaid, and vaccination campaigns funded by government agencies or supported by nonprofit organizations—are publicly supported, helping specific groups access low- or no-cost services. But the broader health care system functions as a for-profit, market-based environment where access is determined by people's ability to pay. In the United States, health care is more about transaction than treatment. Low-income and marginalized communities face steep barriers to quality care—especially when access to publicly supported programs is deeply restricted or these programs are cut entirely.

 Resources, goods, and services refer to the necessities of life, including affordable and nutritious food, utilities like power and water, dependable and affordable childcare, and essential services—from public transportation and libraries to sanitation services and fire stations. The availability of these resources is shaped not only by geography but also by decisions about which parts of daily life are treated as public goods—funded and governed collectively—and which are left to the private market to manage and sell.[39] Policy choices dictate whether daily necessities are universally available or if they are privatized, to be purchased by those who can afford them. In marginalized communities, chronic disinvestment leads to fragmented or absent necessities, resulting in dire consequences like food insecurity, unreliable or nonexistent public transportation systems, and utility shortages that compound economic hardship and reinforce health inequities.

Social and community contexts refer to the relationships, institutions, structures, and places that shape civic participation and social connection. These include voting and democratic processes, civic engagement opportunities, gathering spaces, and community-based organizations. When functioning well, these systems can foster a sense of belonging, access to decision-making power, and the ability to collectively advocate for shared goals and priorities—all of which are critical to health and well-being. In marginalized communities, these social structures and relationships have been fractured and suppressed by past and present policies that isolate residents physically, socially, and economically. As a result, communities are left with fewer tools and resources to advocate for their needs, build social capital, and flourish.

OUTCOMES: HEALTHY AND FLOURISHING COMMUNITIES

By and large, the poor do not want some small life. They don't want to game the system or eke out an existence; they want to thrive and contribute.
                                        –Matthew Desmond, sociologist and author[40(p310)]

At the top of the Root Causes Roadmap is our north star: flourishing communities, rich in opportunity, where everyone lives a full and meaningful life. In truly healthy communities, people aren't forced to make impossible tradeoffs—like having to choose between paying rent, purchasing medication, or putting food on the table. Instead, people have what they need to flourish: dignified and desirable housing, quality education, good jobs, clean air and water, affordable goods and services, and opportunities for connection, rest, and joy.

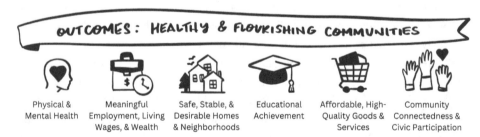

| Physical & Mental Health | Meaningful Employment, Living Wages, & Wealth | Safe, Stable, & Desirable Homes & Neighborhoods | Educational Achievement | Affordable, High-Quality Goods & Services | Community Connectedness & Civic Participation |

Flourishing communities are supported by a shared set of **health and quality-of-life outcomes***—overarching and culminating effects that reflect levels of physical, mental, emotional, and social well-being. These outcomes are not static; they change dynamically

---

Quality of life (QOL) is defined by the World Health Organization as "an individual's perception of their position in life in the context of the culture and value systems in which they live and in relation to their goals, expectations, standards and concerns."[41] QOL is connected to *health-related quality of life*, defined by the Centers for Disease Control and Prevention as "an individual's or group's perceived physical and mental health over time."[42]

over time based on the conditions, systems, and environments that impact people's lives. Communities are much more likely to be healthy and flourishing when people feel safe, respected, included, and fulfilled. When people have power over decisions that shape their lives—and when the environments and contexts that surround them make it possible to live with dignity and purpose—surviving can give way to thriving.

Collectively, these outcomes describe communities that are adaptable, powerful, and connected. They include physical and mental health; meaningful employment, livable wages, and wealth; dignified and desirable homes and opportunity-rich neighborhoods; educational achievement; access to affordable and high-quality goods and services; and community connectedness and civic participation:

Physical and mental health. Healthy and flourishing communities prioritize the well-being of every individual, and people have what they need to thrive physically, mentally, and emotionally. Health care, mental health support, wellness programs, and public health services are high-quality and universally available. Health is not narrowly viewed as the absence of disease or disability; it includes joy, connection, and adaptability. This holistic and collective approach to health honors the full humanity of people navigating chronic conditions and disabilities, ensuring they have the resources and support needed to lead connected, meaningful, and self-determined lives. Community services are inclusive, respectful, and tailored to meet the needs of all people. Health is seen as a shared responsibility and a benefit to the community at large, so everyone has access to the resources they need to live well. This community chooses care over control, creating the fertile ground for health, dignity, and abundance—now and for generations to come.

Meaningful employment, livable wages, and wealth. Every person can secure dignified work that offers more than a paycheck: It provides purpose and opportunities to positively contribute to their surrounding community. People earn livable wages, allowing them to provide for their families and invest in their futures. Economic opportunities are abundant, and systems are in place to ensure that wealth is built ethically and equitably. Opportunities for wealth are plentiful and shared across generations, creating a foundation of financial security for families and communities for years to come.

Dignified and desirable homes and opportunity-rich neighborhoods. Every community is anchored by safe and stable housing for all, with homes that are affordable, appealing, and a source of fulfillment and comfort. Neighborhoods are thoughtfully designed to be vibrant, resilient, and interconnected. They provide easy access to resources and services that support the social, economic, and emotional well-being of all residents.

These neighborhoods are rich in opportunity: All children are cherished and supported, adults experience belonging and purpose, and seniors find connection and fulfillment. Neighborhoods are welcoming and well-connected places, with ample green space, climate-resilient infrastructure, and seamless transit and mobility options that link people across regions.

Educational achievement. Education is universally accessible, inclusive and enriching, and a powerful gateway to opportunity. From early childhood through lifelong learning, everyone receives the support and resources they need to explore their interests, achieve their goals, and grow into thoughtful and civically engaged people. Schools and training centers are vibrant places of learning, where everyone—from young children to older adults—gains knowledge and expands their practical skills, critical thinking, creativity, and personal growth. Students are not just prepared for the workforce—they are primed to become empathetic and effective leaders who positively shape the future of their communities.

Affordable and high-quality goods and services. Every neighborhood is fully equipped to provide the necessities of daily life: affordable and well-stocked grocery stores, reliable public transit systems, environmentally responsible utilities, and access to other high-quality goods and services. These resources are not just available—they are abundant, sustainable, and intentionally designed to support the well-being of all residents. They also fuel the local economy—creating good jobs, supporting small businesses, fostering environmental sustainability, and keeping wealth circulating within the community.

Community connectedness and civic participation. Every person has a voice that deserves to be heard when it comes to decisions that shape their lives. In a healthy and flourishing community, civic engagement is a protected right as well as a way of life. Community members are actively involved in governance, from voting and participating in decision-making processes to leading initiatives that impact local policies, budgets, and programs. Governance is transparent, just, and rooted in the collective wisdom of the community, ensuring decisions reflect the diverse needs and aspirations of all.

TOOLS FOR SYSTEMS CHANGE

We need more than justice in the moment—we need an overhaul of our systems. This is our opportunity as a people and world citizens to address the root of the larger issues that affect all our communities and the injustices that we deal with.

–Ras Baraka, poet and political leader[43]

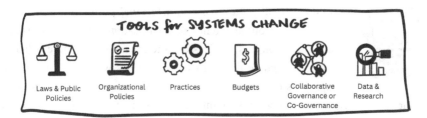

At the center of the Root Causes Roadmap are **tools for systems change**—powerful levers and mechanisms that can directly influence every layer of the Roadmap. The tools for systems change include law and public policy, organizational policy, practice, budgets, collaborative governance or co-governance, and data and research:

Law and public policy. Laws are codified and enforceable rules established by governments to regulate behavior, allocate power and resources, protect rights, resolve disputes, and set the terms for how government authority is used—including when it can compel or coerce. Although law is often portrayed as neutral and fair, in practice, it has long served to protect those in power, enforce social hierarchies, and authorize state-sanctioned force—deciding when and how that force is deemed "legitimate." While modern legal systems operate on the assumption that coercion and control are necessary features, we reject that premise. Instead, we envision a legal and political order rooted in care, consent, and collective accountability—where justice is cultivated not through domination but through relationships of mutual responsibility and repair.

Laws can take various forms: ordinances and statutes passed by legislative bodies, regulations issued by administrative agencies, case law established through judicial decisions, and executive orders issued by presidents, governors, or other executive officials.[44,45] All laws are policies, but not all policies are laws.[34] **Public policy** refers to governments' decisions and priorities to address societal issues. This can be expressed through laws, as well as through funding allocations, program design, and administrative actions.

Together, laws and public policies create a formal framework that structures societal behavior in ways that can protect or undermine rights and the collective good. For instance, antidiscrimination laws are vital for protecting marginalized groups and ensuring equitable access to important resources such as health care, education, and housing. Laws also influence societal norms and drive systems change. During the *Civil Rights Movement*, for example, landmark legislation and court rulings upended de jure racial segregation and expanded civil and voting rights.

Both laws and public policies either institutionalize justice or entrench oppression, depending on how they are designed, implemented, and assured (see Chapter 6 for more on assurance).

Organizational policy. An **organizational policy** is a written statement that sets out an agency or organization's position, decision, or course of action on specific issues and procedures.[34] These policies are designed to guide decisions and behaviors within an organization, shaping its operations, culture, and actions. Organizational policies define how an organization engages with internal constituents (such as employees and members) and external constituents (such as clients, communities, and the public).

Organizational policies influence a wide range of practices—from programmatic activities and ethical stewardship to operational processes and strategic planning. They shape how services and functions are carried out and for what purpose. For example, in the 1930s, federal housing institutions enacted policies that firmly embedded racial discrimination into lending on a national scale. The Federal Housing Administration codified redlining through underwriting guidelines that discouraged loans in neighborhoods where Black people and other marginalized people resided. Meanwhile, the Home Owners' Loan Corporation implemented a policy of producing neighborhood maps that institutionalized racial prejudice and shaped broader lending and development practices. These organizational policies have held entire communities back from homeownership and wealth-building opportunities for generations. (See Chapter 2 for more on redlining, structural racism, and intergenerational harm.)

Practice. A **practice** refers to an informal or customary procedure or norm that shapes how things are done within an organization or community. Unlike formal policies, practices are not always written down or legally mandated. They evolve over time and often reflect shared habits, expectations, and cultural norms. Practices influence everyday behaviors and responses across all domains of society.

Practices are powerful tools that either promote or hinder equity and justice. They may align with formal policies or, in some cases, contradict them. For example, even though many police departments have policies prohibiting racial profiling, the informal practice of "stop-and-frisk" has disproportionately targeted Black and Latine people.[46] Between 2004 and 2012, more than 4 million stops were conducted by the New York City Police Department, with more than 80% involving Black or Latine individuals, despite these groups making up less than half the city's population.[47]

On the other hand, practices can go above and beyond what a policy requires. For example, an epidemiology team might go beyond health department requirements by partnering with community organizations to utilize *community data* that reflect residents' realities and lived experiences, going beyond reporting narrowly-defined agency metrics. (See Chapter 6 for more on community data.) Over time, practices can influence the creation of formal policies, as they become institutionalized and widely adopted.

Budgets. A **budget** is a plan for managing funds, setting levels of spending, and financing expenditures. Budgets are aligned with policy decisions and direct how resources are allocated. The budget process is the primary means by which organizations and agencies select among competing demands for the allocation of resources.[48]

Budgets reflect our values: They show where attention and effort will be directed—and what will be neglected. Budgets can even serve as policy statements in themselves, reflecting the values and priorities of communities and institutions.

Budgets are powerful tools for shaping how the social determinants of health are distributed across communities. For example, if a city allocates a larger share of its budget to policing and incarceration and a smaller share to health-affirming solutions that help prevent social problems—like dignified housing and mental health support—it signals a commitment to punitive approaches rather than prevention. (See Chapter 6 for more on budgets.) As another example, a city could choose to invest in safe, accessible, and sustainable public transit instead of expanding highways, showing a commitment to community well-being and environmental justice. In these ways, budgets either perpetuate inequities or advance equity by reorienting resources toward prevention and care.

 Collaborative governance or co-governance. Co-governance refers to a shared decision-making approach in which government agencies and community members—especially those who have been historically excluded and oppressed—work together to shape and implement public policies, programs, and the allocation of resources.[49] (See Chapter 5 for more on co-governance and power.) In authentic co-governance processes, communities are not merely consulted—they hold real authority and leadership. Governments act as partners and implementers of the community's will.

When practiced with integrity, co-governance enhances democratic participation, centers community members' voices, and ensures that policies are aligned with the lived experiences of all people—especially the most marginalized. It can also lead to more transparent and accountable decision-making processes, increasing trust and communication between governments and communities. Participatory budgeting, for example, is a co-governance process through which communities formally decide how public funds are allocated, helping transform civic engagement into tangible outcomes.[50]

 Data and research. Data are facts, statistics, and other basic units of information about people, places, communities, conditions, and systems. They are the building blocks that elected officials, policymakers, organizers, advocates, and the public use to draw conclusions about how a community functions and the realities of people living within them. Data are collected all the time, often without our conscious awareness. On their own, data are raw information. They become meaningful when analyzed, interpreted, and placed in context—often by combining different data points or connecting them to a broader story.[51,52] **Research** refers to creating new knowledge and the innovative use of existing knowledge to generate new concepts, methodologies, and insights.[53] It involves the analysis, synthesis, and interpretation of data to produce actionable learnings and to guide informed decision-making.

Reliable research and data can help identify the root causes of problems, measure progress and impact, and predict future needs.[54] In public health, data-driven decisions can help address unjust health disparities, evaluate the effectiveness of interventions, and shape more equitable and just policies. Research across the social determinants of health can be particularly powerful in driving policy reforms. For instance, research that affirms connections between housing instability and poor health has led agencies to invest in evidence-based and dignity-centered solutions like *Housing First*—a strategy that provides permanent housing without preconditions and requirements,[55] rather than criminalizing people who are experiencing homelessness.

In the Root Causes Roadmap, tools for systems change—laws, policies, practices, budgets, governance, and data—interact dynamically with every layer. Double-sided arrows show this two-way relationship. Most arrows in the Roadmap point upward—illustrating the need to confront systems of oppression to achieve collective health and flourishing. However, the arrows flanking the tools for systems change point in both directions. These double-sided arrows indicate that the tools shape structural inequities and systems of oppression and are also shaped by them.

We see this two-way relationship in action every day. Structural inequities—such as unjust disparities in wealth, opportunity, and political power—are directly shaped by how tools for systems change are designed and deployed. For example, when communities are denied political power or the ability to meaningfully participate in governance, they are more likely to be the targets of oppressive laws and policies. Voter suppression laws,[56] cuts to critical public health and medical services,[57] and efforts to undermine birthright citizenship[58] show how inequities in governance deepen harm for already marginalized communities.

Tools for systems change are pivotal to our experience of health. They have the power to influence—and be influenced by—all other layers of the Root Causes Roadmap: systems of oppression, structural inequities, social determinants of health, and outcomes for health and flourishing. What makes these tools especially powerful is that they sit within our collective locus of control. They are the primary means through which we can change the status quo—or reinforce it. Like any tool, their impact depends on who wields them and for what purpose.

Tools for systems change can never be used neutrally. They either promote equity and justice, or they entrench oppression and widen unjust disparities. For instance,

- **Budgets can either fund or undermine justice.** Since 2011, New York City has implemented participatory budgeting in several districts, allowing residents to directly decide how to allocate portions of public funds to community projects. This approach has helped communities to turn ideas into funded projects and to distribute resources in ways that prioritize local needs.[50] Yet at the same time, New York City's fiscal year 2024 budget allocated an additional $42 million to the New York City Police Department's Domain Awareness System—a vast surveillance project that raises serious concerns about privacy and racial profiling, while simultaneously expanding punitive enforcement strategies at the expense of community health.[59]

- **Data and research can either guide equitable solutions or perpetuate harm.** During the early months of the COVID-19 pandemic, federal and state agencies failed to accurately collect "race" and ethnicity data on infections and deaths— irreparably damaging efforts to understand and address the virus's disproportionate impact on people of color. These failures were further compounded by so-called research that attributed higher rates of COVID-19 infections and deaths among people of color to false "biological racial differences"[60] rather than confronting the real root causes: systems of oppression such as white supremacy, structural racism, colonialism, and racial capitalism.

- **Co-governance can either shift power to communities or reinforce power imbalances.** In Milwaukee, Wisconsin's public school system, Black students were disproportionately referred to police. In response, students, youth organizers, and the nonprofit Leaders Igniting Transformation led co-governance efforts that resulted in the school board unanimously voting to end all police contracts for school resource officers. The school board also passed a resolution requiring school administrators to work with an advisory council to collaboratively create a plan for reallocating funds formerly budgeted for police.[61] Yet in 2025, police officers were reinstated in Milwaukee public schools as part of a deal that city officials struck with the Wisconsin state legislature.[62] This backlash underscores the need for ongoing community power building and grassroots advocacy efforts. Constant pressure is necessary to resist threats to progress and fortify wins for equity and justice. (See Chapter 5 for more on community power building.)

Tools for systems change can either dismantle or reinforce structural inequities— depending on whether they are applied with intentional focus on equity and justice. The next section delves deeper into policy—a powerful tool for systems change that can similarly be used to perpetuate or rectify structural inequities. Policies directly shape the structures in our lives. They determine our access to resources and opportunities that can bring us closer to health and flourishing or take us—and our descendants—farther from it. Recognizing this dual nature of policy is essential—not only to confront historical injustices but also to harness its power for transformative change.

THE OUTSIZED ROLE OF POLICY IN SUSTAINING INJUSTICE

We now must put a face on this crisis of possibility. It is a crime in a rich nation for people to receive starvation wages . . . [Poverty is] human-made because of policy. It is the result of policy and the interlocking injustices of systemic racism, ecological devastation, the denial of health care, the defunding of our children's possibilities through public education, militarism and the war economy, and the distorted moral narrative of religious nationalism . . . It is wrong.

–William J. Barber II, pastor and social justice leader[63]

Policies—including laws, executive orders, and organizational rules—are among the most powerful tools for systems change in public health. They determine how resources are allocated, what actions are taken, and who ultimately benefits. Policy is a tool that is used by all levels of government and institutions: from federal sentencing laws to city-level parking enforcement rules, from mayoral executive orders to internal public health department protocols.

At their best, policies shape conditions, environments, and systems in ways that produce lasting improvements in health and well-being. Fortunately, there are many positive examples. In Florida, a Complete Streets state law helped save the lives of nearly 4,000 pedestrians over four decades by requiring that roadways be designed for all users—particularly people who are walking, bicycling, and using public transit.[21] The state of California implemented a regulatory tool called CalEnviroScreen that guides investments and interventions in environmentally burdened communities[64]—demonstrating how rulemaking can institutionalize equity in agency decisions. And in moments of crisis, governors and mayors have used executive authority to direct resources or waive potentially burdensome regulations, as seen in emergency actions—such as eviction moratoria—taken during the COVID-19 pandemic and during housing crises.

At their worst, harmful policies—or the failure to enact, implement, and fund necessary policies—can devastate families and communities for generations. In the United States, countless local, state, and federal policies have produced ripple effects that touch every aspect of life, from housing to health care. These policies have reinforced the false hierarchy of human value described in Chapter 2 and contributed directly to the unjust health disparities we see today.

Appendix 3A highlights influential policies—many overtly and intentionally oppressive, others harmful in implementation or shaped by racist ideologies, flawed evidence, shortsightedness, and political opportunism. Together, they have profoundly shaped life in what we now know as the United States. These policies have repeatedly slammed the door shut on opportunity and well-being—particularly for people of color—denying access to education, housing, intergenerational wealth, and political power.

Collectively, these policies paint a damning picture of the vast scope and scale by which white supremacy, structural racism, and other systems of oppression have been codified into the very foundations of US law. They work cumulatively to reinforce "race" and racism, concentrate wealth and power in the hands of a few, and drive vast inequities in health, well-being, and life expectancy.

While some of the most explicitly racist laws from our past—such as Jim Crow laws (Box 3-1)[65-76] and redlining—have been prohibited, their consequences remain deeply entrenched. Many unjust health disparities that people experience today—including higher rates of aggressive breast cancer,[73] premature death,[74] pedestrian fatalities,[23] and preterm births[77]—are linked to laws that were adopted and implemented decades ago.

Meanwhile, contemporary policies continue to compound and worsen these inequities. For example, while redlining is no longer legal, modern banking and real estate practices still create significant barriers to homeownership for people of color, reinforcing the racial wealth gap. While explicit racial segregation in schools is no longer law, regressive tax policies that govern how schools are funded and punitive discipline measures that are used against students continue to perpetuate inequitable educational outcomes among students of color.[78] These policies undermine young people's educational attainment, opportunities, and life expectancy.[79-81]

Polices can worsen structural inequities in several ways:

- **Direct negative impacts.** Some policies directly cause harm by codifying and entrenching structural racism and inequity. For example, Jim Crow laws made racial segregation the law of the land and systematically denied Black people access to voting, education, housing, employment, and more. Similarly, redlining policies intentionally denied people of color and other marginalized communities access to homeownership and wealth-building opportunities by marking certain neighborhoods as "hazardous" for investment.
- **Harmful and discriminatory implementation.** Even policies intended to help can cause harm without proper implementation. For instance, the Federal Highway Act of 1956 was meant to create a national interstate system, but its implementation was disproportionately detrimental to communities of color. Highways were routinely constructed through Black communities, destroying entire neighborhoods, displacing residents, and irreparably damaging the social fabric and economic stability of whole areas without ever providing compensation or support to the people and families who were harmed.
- **Inaction in the face of systemic injustice.** A lack of necessary policies—or the failure to implement them—can also devastate marginalized communities. Preventing the adoption of a living wage policy, undermining voting rights, underfunding public transit, denying resources to public schools, and cutting nutrition assistance programs are all examples of **policy violence**—making unjust policy choices in the face of abject need. This includes policy decisions that actively harm people by denying them resources and rights, as well as a failure or outright refusal to adopt essential

Box 3-1. Jim Crow Laws

Named for a minstrel show character that caricatured and dehumanized Black people,[65,66] **Jim Crow laws** were a system of state and local laws that legalized racial segregation and racial discrimination against Black people in the United States. Enacted after the end of Reconstruction in 1877, these laws formalized white supremacy and entrenched structural racism, codifying the "systematic subordination" of Black people across all aspects of daily life.[67(p2)]

Jim Crow laws restricted Black people's access to and movement within all public spaces—including schools, public transit, restaurants, retail stores, parks, beaches, and hospitals—and barred interaction between Black and white people. These laws denied Black people public services as well as the right to vote, obtain employment, earn an education, purchase homes and land, and participate fully in society. Jim Crow laws made racial terror both commonplace and legal, with state-sanctioned violence, surveillance, and intimidation all deployed to keep Black people "in their place."[68(p220-221)] The US judicial system—from local courts to the Supreme Court—widely upheld Jim Crow laws.[69] Black people and others who were accused of violating them faced arrest, beatings, imprisonment, and death at the hands of law enforcement and white civilians.

Jim Crow laws remained on the books for nearly a century. No single law ever overturned them. Instead, decades of organizing and advocacy—led by civil rights and human rights leaders, many of whom remain unnamed in history—forced a gradual dismantling of Jim Crow through court rulings and federal legislation. This intergenerational activism, advocacy, and policy change is now known as the *Civil Rights Movement*. This movement catalyzed a number of landmark laws and cases, including these examples:

- *Brown v Board of Education* (1954): The Supreme Court unanimously struck down racial segregation in public schools, ruling that "separate but equal" educational facilities were inherently unequal and in violation of the Equal Protection Clause of the 14th Amendment.
- Civil Rights Act of 1964: This sweeping federal legislation outlawed segregation in public places and banned discrimination in employment based on "race," color, religion, sex, and national origin. Title VII of the act established the Equal Employment Opportunity Commission to enforce these protections.
- Voting Rights Act of 1965: This federal law prohibited racial discrimination in voting. It was especially impactful for Black people, who had long been systematically disenfranchised through racist tactics like literacy tests, poll taxes, intimidation and violence, and *"grandfather clauses"*—provisions within Jim Crow laws that allowed people to bypass voting restrictions if they or their ancestors had voted before 1867. Grandfather clauses effectively prohibited Black people from voting but ensured that poor white men—who likely would have failed literacy tests or been unable to afford poll taxes—could still vote.[70,a] The Voting Rights Act also introduced *preclearance*, which required certain jurisdictions with histories of discrimination to obtain federal approval before changing voting laws.
- *Loving v Virginia* (1967): The Supreme Court struck down state laws banning marriage between individuals of different "races." The case challenged Virginia's Racial Integrity Act of 1924, a law emblematic of white supremacist and eugenicist policies common across many states, which sought to preserve "racial purity" by criminalizing interracial marriages.[71]
- Fair Housing Act of 1968: Passed as Title VIII of the Civil Rights Act of 1968, this law prohibited discrimination in housing based on "race," color, national origin, religion, and sex (and later, disability and family status).[72,b]

Although the system of Jim Crow may seem like a relic of the past, its devastating legacy is very much alive. The harms it inflicted—racial segregation, discrimination, violence, and systemic exclusion—continue to shape our society. Today, many Black families remain concentrated in racially segregated neighborhoods and are still excluded from the opportunities of homeownership and intergenerational wealth that were also denied to their ancestors. Jim Crow laws have also been linked to numerous unjust health disparities, from Black women's increased likelihood of developing aggressive forms of breast cancer[73] to premature mortality among Black people.[74]

(Continued)

Box 3-1. (Continued)

> Jim Crow never fully disappeared—instead, it has evolved over time to replicate injustice against other marginalized groups. Latine communities, for instance, have experienced what journalist and human rights activist Roberto Lovato has called *Juan Crow*—a system of laws, policies, and practices that systematically criminalize, exploit, and exclude Latine people in the United States.[75] From workplace immigration raids and family separations to anti-immigrant laws, English-only ordinances, and voter ID restrictions, Juan Crow reflects Jim Crow in its intent: to oppress and exploit racialized people through legal, economic, and social mechanisms of control.
>
> Today, Jim Crow looms large over the United States, especially because those who survived the era know it not as history but as their own lived experience. Millions of Black people in the United States were subjected to the horror of these laws, and continue to live with the traumatic, intergenerational consequences.[76]

Note: ID = identification.
[a]The phrase "grandfathered in"—often used to describe allowing people or organizations to continue under old rules after new ones are introduced—originates from racist "grandfather clauses" in Jim Crow laws. Like many seemingly neutral expressions, it has roots in structural racism and white supremacy. "Grandfathered in" is one of many examples of how systems of oppression have shaped everyday language. Understanding the history behind the words we use (several of which are discussed in this book) is part of an ongoing learning journey that can help us evolve our language in ways that reflect equity and justice.
[b]As noted by public policy scholar and author Richard Rothstein, housing discrimination had already been technically outlawed by the 1866 Civil Rights Act, which declared that housing discrimination was "a residue of slave status that the 13th Amendment empowered Congress to eliminate."[72(pk)] However, the 1866 law gave the government no powers to enforce it. The law had little practical effect until the Supreme Court's 1968 decision in *Jones v Mayer*, which gave new legal force to the 1866 Civil Rights Act, finally making it a usable tool for civil rights advocates and complementing the newly enacted 1968 Fair Housing Act.

policies in the face of clear need.* Policy violence is an effective means of perpetuating and reinforcing systems of oppression.

- **Action and inaction that compound harm.** The interaction of multiple policies—or the absence of corrective action—can come together to create unjust outcomes. For example, many undocumented young people in California are caught in a policy bind: They are excluded from DACA (Deferred Action for Childhood Arrivals) protections because of its strict age requirements.[†84] Then, in a blow to California's Health4All campaign, undocumented adults face a proposed freeze on new enrollment in Medi-Cal (California's Medicaid program), while those currently enrolled may face new and potentially cost-prohibitive premiums.[85] Meanwhile, undocumented students without federal work authorization—including those without DACA—remain barred from on-campus work–study jobs at University of California campuses due to the Regents' refusal to adopt a hiring policy—an approach recently found to violate state civil rights law.[86] Although no single policy is responsible, this combination of political inaction and exclusionary policies is a form of policy violence. It leaves young undocumented people unable to work legally, without health

---

*According to the Center for the Study of Social Policy, "The term 'policy violence' was first used in the 1960s by the original Poor People's Campaign. More recently, the revived Poor People's Campaign[82] has used the term to change the narrative around poverty, positioning it as the consequence of immoral public policy choices that promote and sustain structural racism and [inequity]."[83]

†To qualify for DACA, applicants must have arrived in the United States before age 16 and have been under age 31 as of June 15, 2012. Many young undocumented people do not fall within these age restrictions.

care, and vulnerable to deportation—further marginalizing them through policy fragmentation and systemic neglect.

Given the profound role that policy has played in cementing racism and oppression into the foundations of our country, it must now play an equally transformative role in disman-tling those structures. We cannot rely on small, incremental changes alone—we need bold shifts that directly address the harms created by past and present policies. This means fundamentally rethinking how policies are written, implemented, and assured. (See Chapter 6 for more on assurance.) We must be at least as intentional about using policy to rectify injustices as those who used policy to create and uphold injustice in the first place.

GOING BEYOND INTENT: THE DISPARATE IMPACT OF UNJUST POLICIES

[T]he law isn't about the school. It's about the mind. The heart. About understanding what the law intends as much as reading beneath what it says. Knowing how to find one's way to the truth.

—Stacey Abrams, political leader and voting rights attorney[87(p12)]

Jim Crow laws and redlining were tools for systems change explicitly used to advantage white people and to disadvantage and punish Black people. Laws like the Civil Rights Act of 1964, the Voting Rights Act of 1965, and the Fair Housing Act of 1968 were adopted to address these injustices. Yet even the groundbreaking policy victories of the Civil Rights Movement fell short of dismantling the deep-rooted inequities embedded in systems throughout the United States. This reveals a sobering truth: No single tool, law, or reform is a substitute for sustained, structural transformation centered on equity and justice.

One reason progress stalls is that racism is often and incorrectly framed as a problem of individual prejudice. As a result, solutions tend to focus too narrowly on changing hearts and minds through education, dialogue, and personal reflection. While a person's efforts to grow, change, and gain awareness are important, they are not enough.

We cannot personally reflect or self-actualize our way out of structural injustice. Equity and justice require a shift in focus—from intent to impact, from personal inten-tions to structural outcomes. Author and historian Ibram X. Kendi explains that we must be *outcome-centered*,[88] meaning that we must look beyond what may be intended by a policy or process and instead focus on what actually happens because of it. Kendi reminds us that intent is not the measure of justice—outcomes are: "If a policy is leading to racial injustice, it doesn't really matter if the policymaker intended for that policy to lead to racial injustice."[88]

This distinction between *intent* and *outcome* is critical when it comes to law and policy—two of the primary tools we use to organize our society. Even policies that appear "neutral" on paper can reinforce inequity if they disproportionately harm specific groups, such as poor people and people of color. Recognizing how racism operates through systems—not just individuals—is essential for our efforts to advance equity and justice.

Even with its limitations (see Box 3-2[89,90]), civil rights law remains an incredibly powerful tool that offers two ways of understanding and challenging systems of oppression: the doctrines of *disparate treatment* and *disparate impact*. These legal frameworks have been instrumental in shifting the focus beyond individual intent and toward structural outcomes. They can help us assess how injustice persists in policy, even without having overt discrimination written into policy language.

Disparate treatment occurs when individuals or groups are intentionally treated differently based on their "race" or another legally protected identity, such as religion, gender identity, or disability status. A real estate agent's overt refusal to sell a home to a family because they are Muslim or a company's denial of an employee's promotion because of their gender are both examples of disparate treatment.

Disparate impact, by contrast, addresses policies that may appear "neutral" on paper but result in disproportionate harm to specific protected groups. Crucially, proving disparate impact does not require evidence of discriminatory intent—the emphasis is on effects, not motives. This shift has been key to advancing civil rights protections in areas like housing, employment, and education—particularly where discrimination is woven into systems and policies rather than openly expressed.

Exclusionary zoning policies provide a powerful example of the everyday ways in which disparate impact shows up in our lives. These regulations, which are still widely used today, limit or outright prevent the construction of affordable housing. While the official text of these policies rarely states discriminatory intent outright, the aims, structure, and implementation of these policies accomplish exactly that.[91] They include onerous requirements—such as mandating that people purchase large and expensive lots for single-family homes, limiting the number of homes that can be built in an area, or banning multifamily housing like apartments and townhomes. Functionally, they exclude low-income people and people of color from living in specific places,[92] barring entry into well-resourced, majority-white neighborhoods and instead concentrating these communities in places burdened by pollution, environmental hazards, and chronic disinvestment.[93-95] In this way, seemingly "neutral" policies—policies that do not discriminate in word but discriminate in effect—have well-documented health consequences, such as increased rates of cancer, heart disease, and chronic illness,[96] as well as inequitable access to education,[97] transportation,[98] and economic opportunities.

As scholars and historians have documented, these outcomes reflect the true aims of exclusionary zoning policies. Public policy scholar and author Richard Rothstein[72] and urban planning researcher and educator Rolf Pendall[99] have explained how exclusionary zoning policies were not merely tools of economic planning but strategies of racial and economic segregation. Global development scholar and urban theorist Ananya Roy also

Box 3-2. Civil Rights, Human Rights, and the Future of Public Health

The fight for equity and justice in the United States has often been framed through the lens of civil rights—legal protections against discrimination and the right to participate fully in civic life. This framing has delivered landmark victories, from the Civil Rights Act (1964), which outlawed segregation and discrimination, to the ADA (1990), which extended protections to people with disabilities across public and private life. It has enabled social movements to challenge exclusion and assert the fundamental principle that every person deserves equal treatment under the law.

Yet civil rights alone are not enough. While they serve the important function of protecting individuals from certain forms of exclusion and unequal treatment, they do not guarantee the material conditions required to live a dignified, healthy life—such as housing, clean air and water, education, and health care. As human rights attorney and public health scholar Alicia Ely Yamin observes, "the great power of applying a human rights framework to health lies in denaturalizing the inequalities that pervade our societies and our world, and in establishing that all people—by virtue of being human—have both a claim for redress when they are treated unfairly and a right to participate in determining what equity and equality require in a given context."[89(p1)]

Civil rights and human rights offer complementary—but distinct—understandings of what justice requires. A *civil rights frame* asks whether individuals are being treated fairly and have equal access within existing systems. It is essential for identifying and remedying discrimination and exclusion. A *human rights frame* expands the focus: it asks whether those systems themselves are designed to provide the fundamental conditions necessary for health and dignity—and what must be transformed when they fall short.

Human rights are rooted in the belief that every person is entitled to the basic conditions that support health and well-being—not because they are citizens, or belong to a protected class, or have met certain conditions, but because they are human. This insight has long been part of the Black radical tradition. Human rights activist and Black liberation leader Malcolm X, for instance, argued that the plight of Black people in the United States "is not a problem of civil rights, it is a problem of human rights"[90]—highlighting that US law alone could not address the full scope of racial injustice. The same conviction drove the 1968 *Poor People's Campaign* and Indigenous sovereignty movements, as well as contemporary demands for reproductive justice, housing justice, and environmental justice.

Yet in the United States, human rights frameworks rarely shape domestic law or policy. While the global community widely recognizes human rights as a foundation for dignity, equity, and material well-being, the United States has historically emphasized civil rights—a comparatively narrower legal lens centered around individual protections against discrimination and government interference. This reflects a deeply rooted constitutional emphasis on *negative rights*, such as freedom of speech and due process, rather than *positive rights* to basic conditions for health and well-being. As a result, civil rights have become the dominant lens for justice in the United States. But this limited scope has constrained our political imagination, making it harder to assert rights to basic necessities like housing, health care, education, and livable wages.

All struggles for justice are connected. Embracing a human rights frame allows us to learn from global movements for liberation and to ground public health in an ethos of shared obligation and transnational solidarity. To advance equity and justice in public health, we must build on the powerful foundation of civil rights while expanding our scope. We must recognize that flourishing is not a personal responsibility or a privilege of the few. It is a collective good. Making flourishing our goal invites us to not only ask, *Are civil rights being violated?* but also, *What systems are failing to meet people's needs—and what must we do to transform them?*

For public health practitioners, this means aligning our work not just with antidiscrimination efforts but with movements for economic, racial, climate, gender, and global justice. It means expanding beyond the US- and law-centered framework of civil rights—which often focuses on meeting minimum legal requirements—toward the broader, more global framework: one that affirms every person's entitlement to dignity and the conditions necessary to thrive, regardless of whether their country's laws uphold them. Embracing this framework means making a commitment to build systems that ensure the material conditions necessary for health and dignity for all.

Ultimately, no single framework or field—whether civil rights, human rights, or beyond—offers a perfect path to liberation. But each brings tools, insights, and histories that can strengthen our collective efforts. To achieve health and flourishing, we must honor their contributions, learn from their strengths, and apply them strategically to advance equity and justice.

Note: ADA = Americans With Disabilities Act.

emphasizes that zoning, planning, and land use are not neutral or technical processes; they are shaped by power—often used to marginalize and displace communities of color—a process she calls *racial banishment*.[100]

Exclusion was not a side effect—it was the purpose. Even after explicitly racist zoning laws were declared unconstitutional, jurisdictions adopted policies cloaked in "race-neutral" language that achieved the same results. In fact, many of our current zoning policies and practices nationwide are still fulfilling their original, discriminatory purposes.

The disparate impact doctrine helps illuminate yet another way structural racism operates and evolves. A policy may lack explicitly discriminatory language yet still produce deeply inequitable outcomes. Sometimes these outcomes are intended: Elected officials and other decision-makers may craft laws with a discriminatory purpose while disguising that intent through seemingly "neutral" language. In other cases, people may unknowingly uphold unjust systems they've inherited, unaware of the cumulative harms those systems perpetuate. Either way, focusing only on intent misses the broader reality: Laws and policies that appear "neutral" can reinforce racial hierarchies and produce devastating and dangerous consequences.

Disparate impact explains why, even if individual prejudice was eliminated today, we would still have to contend with systems of oppression and structural inequities that influence all of the social determinants—from housing policies to economic systems. Without bold, deliberate, and transformative policy interventions, these oppressive systems and structures will continue to generate injustices that will endure for generations to come.

CONCLUSION

Powerful, overlapping systems shape how well and how long we live. Because health is influenced by every aspect of our lives—and because the systems of oppression that undermine health are structural, not individual—public health efforts must be at least equally structural, expansive, and transformative.

The social determinants of health—contexts that shape economic mobility, education, housing, transportation, and neighborhood conditions—are governed by the enduring legacies of systems of oppression, such as white supremacy, structural racism, racial capitalism, and colonialism. Powerful tools for systems change have cemented inequity into our daily lives and institutions. We now have an opportunity and a moral imperative to use those same tools—laws, policies, practices, budgets, and more—to demolish the foundations of injustice and build new structures rooted in equity, justice, and liberation.

The Root Causes Roadmap helps us visualize the dynamic relationships that exist between the systems, structures, tools, and determinants that influence health and flourishing. We can use it as a strategic guide to understand how complex forces interact, and how we can intervene—no matter our sector or role—to create meaningful change.

From health department staff and academic researchers to urban planners, transportation engineers, loan officers, business owners, and policymakers, we all have a role to play as community health champions. When we understand the root causes, we can begin to address them, no matter our role or vantage point. And when we act together, we can build communities where everyone has the opportunity to flourish.

KEY TAKEAWAYS

 The *social determinants of health* are shaped by *systems of oppression—* the root causes of health inequities. As public health practitioners, we seek to look beyond individual behaviors to the broader systems that influence well-being. We understand that the choices people make are shaped by the choices they're given. Social determinants like housing, education, employment, and transportation do not exist in a vacuum—they are driven by underlying *systems of oppression*, including white supremacy, structural racism, racial capitalism, and colonialism. These forces determine how resources and opportunities are distributed, leading to predictable and preventable health inequities. To meaningfully improve community health, we must confront root causes directly.

Systems of oppression have deep historical roots and continue to evolve. The prejudice of the past haunts the present. Forces embedded at the nation's founding—white supremacy, racial capitalism, and colonialism—continue to shape the air we breathe, the schools we attend, the homes we live in, and the futures we're able to imagine. Widespread injustices like redlining, Jim Crow, and "urban renewal" carried the weight of state authority as they destroyed communities and built lasting barriers to opportunity. That's why, even when laws change, the harm remains—felt in neighborhoods, homes, and bodies through generations. The health inequities we see today are the cumulative result of systemic and policy violence— from the stress of survival to the unequal distribution of care, safety, and dignity.

The *Root Causes Roadmap* helps us connect the dots between powerful forces and tools that influence community health. The Roadmap illustrates how health outcomes are influenced by interacting layers: root causes (like white supremacy and racial capitalism), *structural inequities* (like structural discrimination and inequities in opportunity), social determinants of health (like economic stability and education), and *outcomes for healthy, flourishing communities*. The Roadmap helps us simultaneously see the big picture and identify where we can intervene to advance community health.

Tools for systems change are never neutral—they either reinforce or reject injustice. Whether we're talking about policies, budgets, or data— each tool for systems change reflects the priorities and values of those who wield it. Policy, in particular, is one of the most influential tools for shaping health and well-being. Even when written in seemingly "neutral" language, policies like zoning laws, tax codes, school funding formulas, and public health guidance can produce inequitable outcomes. What matters most is not what a policy promises on paper, but what it delivers in practice. Policies with *disparate impact*—those that disproportionately harm specific groups—can uphold systemic oppression, even without explicit intent to discriminate. Advancing equity and justice requires examining these tools for their real-world effects. It requires us to ask: *Who benefits? Who is burdened? And does this shift power toward—or away from—equity and justice?*

 Healthy systems produce healthy communities. Flourishing communities are the result of systems that are supportive, caring, and inclusive. These systems ensure that everyone has the necessities of life as well as honor self-determination by placing community members at the center of decision-making and supporting everyone's ability to live with dignity and purpose. When systems are built on justice and shared well-being—not extraction and exclusion—entire communities can truly thrive, and the benefits ripple outward to all of society.

REFERENCES

1. Levy BS, Sidel VW. *Social Injustice and Public Health*. Oxford University Press; 2009.
2. Weil DN. Health and economic growth. In: Aghion P, Durlauf SN, eds. *Handbook of Economic Growth*. Vol 2. Elsevier; 2014:623–682.
3. Frakt AB. How the economy affects health. *JAMA*. 2018;319(12):1187–1188. doi:10.1001/jama.2018.1739
4. Pickett KE, Wilkinson RG. Income inequality and health: A causal review. *Soc Sci Med*. 2015;128:316–326. doi:10.1016/j.socscimed.2014.12.031
5. Dangor G. Raising the minimum wage by $1 may prevent thousands of suicides, study shows. *NPR*. January 8, 2020. Accessed May 13, 2025. https://www.npr.org/sections/health-shots/2020/01/08/794568118/raising-the-minimum-wage-by-1-may-prevent-thousands-of-suicides-study-shows
6. Kline S. Guaranteed income: A primer for funders. Asset Funders Network, Center for High Impact Philanthropy, Economic Security Project, Springboard to Opportunities. May 2022. Accessed August 5, 2025. https://assetfunders.org/resource/guaranteed-income-a-primer-for-funders
7. Nishimura HM, Snguon S, Moen M, Dean LT. Guaranteed income and health in the United States and Canada: A scoping review. *Epidemiol Rev*. 2025;47(1):mxaf003. doi:10.1093/epirev/mxaf003
8. Zajacova A, Lawrence EM. The relationship between education and health: Reducing disparities through a contextual approach. *Annu Rev Public Health*. 2018;39:273–289. doi:10.1146/annurev-publhealth-031816-044628

9. Institute of Medicine, Committee on the Consequences of Uninsurance. Effects of health insurance on health. In: *Care Without Coverage: Too Little, Too Late*. National Academies Press; 2002.

10. Hummer RA, Hernandez EM. The effect of educational attainment on adult mortality in the United States. *Popul Bull*. 2013;68(1):1–16. Accessed May 13 2025. https://pmc.ncbi.nlm.nih.gov/articles/PMC4435622

11. Mirowsky J, Ross CE. *Education, Social Status, and Health*. Routledge; 2017.

12. Lübker C, Murtin F. Changes in longevity inequality by education among OECD countries before the COVID-19 pandemic. *BMC Public Health*. 2023;23:1646. doi:10.1186/s12889-023-16492-z

13. Auerswald CL, Lin JS, Parriott A. Six-year mortality in a street-recruited cohort of homeless youth in San Francisco, California. *PeerJ*. 2016;4:e1909. doi:10.7717/peerj.1909

14. Minnesota Department of Health. People who experience homelessness face earlier and greater risk of death, report finds. January 26, 2023. Accessed May 13, 2025. https://www.health.state.mn.us/news/pressrel/2023/homelessness0102623.html

15. Network for Public Health Law. The public health implications of housing instability, eviction, and homelessness. April 2021. Accessed August 5, 2025. https://www.networkforphl.org/wp-content/uploads/2025/01/The-Public-Health-Implications-of-Housing-Instability-Eviction-and-Homelessness.pdf

16. Maqbool N, Viveiros J, Ault M. The impacts of affordable housing on health: A research summary. Center for Housing Policy. 2015. Accessed August 5, 2025. https://www.melkinginstitute.org/resources/reports/impacts-affordable-housing-health-research-summary

17. Breen TR. The longevity benefits of homeownership: Evidence from early twentieth-century US male birth cohorts. *Demography*. 2024;61(6):1731–1757. doi:10.1215/00703370-11680975

18. University of Louisville. Urban renewal. Uncovering Racial Logics: Louisville's History of Racial Oppression and Activism. May 13, 2025. Accessed August 6, 2025. https://library.louisville.edu/archives/racial-logics/urban-renewal

19. Bailey ZD, Krieger N, Agénor M, Graves J, Linos N, Bassett MT. Structural racism and health inequities in the USA: Evidence and interventions. *Lancet*. 2017;389(10077):1453–1463. doi:10.1016/S0140-6736(17)30569-X

20. Smart Growth America; National Complete Streets Coalition. Dangerous by Design 2024. May 30, 2024. Accessed July 27, 2025. https://wordpress.smartgrowthamerica.org/wp-content/uploads/2024/08/Dangerous-By-Design-2024_5.30.pdf

21. Porter JM, Rathbun SL, Bryan SJ, et al. Law accommodating nonmotorized road users and pedestrian fatalities in Florida, 1975 to 2013. *Am J Public Health*. 2018;108(4):525–531. doi:10.2105/AJPH.2017.304259

22. Heaps W, Abramsohn E, Skillen EL. Public transportation in the US: A driver of health and equity. *Health Affairs Health Policy Brief*. July 29, 2021. doi:10.1377/hpb20210630.810356

23. Taylor NL, Porter JM, Bryan S, Harmon KJ, Sandt LS. Structural racism and pedestrian safety: Measuring the association between historical redlining and contemporary pedestrian fatalities across the United States, 2010–2019. *Am J Public Health*. 2023;113(4):420–428. doi:10.2105/AJPH.2022.307192

24. House JS, Landis KR, Umberson D. Social relationships and health. *Science*. 1988;241(4865):540–545. doi:10.1126/science.3399889

25. Office of the Surgeon General. Our epidemic of loneliness and isolation: The US Surgeon General's advisory on the healing effects of social connection and community. US Dept of Health and Human Services. 2023. Accessed May 16, 2025. https://www.hhs.gov/sites/default/files/surgeon-general-social-connection-advisory.pdf

26. Sallis JF, Floyd MF, Rodríguez DA, Saelens BE. Role of built environments in physical activity, obesity, and cardiovascular disease. *Circulation.* 2012;125(5):729–737. doi:10.1161/CIRCULATIONAHA.110.969022

27. Haines A, Ebi K. The imperative for climate action to protect health. *N Engl J Med.* 2019;380(3):263–273. doi:10.1056/NEJMra1807873

28. Knight T, Price S, Bowler D, et al. How effective is 'greening' of urban areas in reducing human exposure to ground-level ozone concentrations, UV exposure and the 'urban heat island effect'? An updated systematic review. *Environ Evid.* 2021;10:12. doi:10.1186/s13750-021-00226-y

29. Tong S, Prior J, McGregor G, Shi X, Kinney P. Urban heat: An increasing threat to global health. *BMJ.* 2021;375:n2467. doi:10.1136/bmj.n2467

30. Lorde A. *Sister Outsider: Essays and Speeches.* Crossing Press; 2007.

31. Porter JM, Giles-Cantrell B, Schaffer K, Dutta EA, Castrucci BC. Awareness of and confidence to address equity-related concepts across the US governmental public health workforce. *J Public Health Manag Pract.* 2023;29(suppl 1):S87–S97. doi:10.1097/PHH.0000000000001647

32. Jones CP. Systems of power, axes of inequity: Parallels, intersections, braiding the strands. *Med Care.* 2014;52(10 suppl 3):S71–S75. doi:10.1097/MLR.0000000000000216

33. Yearby R. Structural racism and health disparities: Reconfiguring the social determinants of health framework to include the root cause. *J Law Med Ethics.* 2020;48(3):518–526. doi:10.1177/1073110520958876.

34. ChangeLab Solutions. A blueprint for change makers: Achieving health equity through law & policy. March 27, 2019. Accessed June 4, 2025. https://www.changelabsolutions.org/product/blueprint-changemakers

35. Ebrahimi F. How we got here. *Stanford Social Innovation Review.* Winter 2024. Accessed May 16, 2025. https://ssir.org/articles/entry/how_we_got_here

36. Institute for Responsive Government. Health & Democracy Index. Accessed June 6, 2025. https://democracyindex.responsivegov.org

37. Freelander A. Why US elections only give you two choices. *Vox.* March 6, 2024. Accessed June 6, 2025. https://www.vox.com/videos/24091275/why-us-elections-only-give-you-two-choices.

38. Shapiro TM, Loya R. Michael Tubbs on universal basic income: The issue with poverty is a lack of cash. *The Guardian.* March 21, 2019. Accessed June 6, 2025. https://www.theguardian.com/commentisfree/2019/mar/21/michael-tubbs-on-universal-basic-income-the-issue-with-poverty-is-a-lack-of-cash

39. Pamukcu A, Harris AP. Using anti-racist policy to promote the good governance of necessities. *Bill of Health.* October 20, 2020. Accessed May 16, 2025. https://petrieflom.law.harvard.edu/2020/10/20/anti-racist-policy-health

40. Desmond M. *Evicted: Poverty and Profit in the American City.* Crown Publishers; 2016.

41. World Health Organization. WHOQOL: Measuring quality of life. Accessed May 16, 2025. https://www.who.int/tools/whoqol

42. Centers for Disease Control and Prevention. HRQOL concepts. September 12, 2018. Accessed May 16, 2025. https://archive.cdc.gov/#/details?url=https://www.cdc.gov/hrqol/concept.htm

43. Martoccio A. Mayor Ras Baraka drops timely spoken word video, "What We Want." *Rolling Stone.* June 4, 2020. Accessed May 16, 2025. https://www.rollingstone.com/music/music-news/mayor-ras-baraka-what-we-want-video-1009917

44. Hearne S, Pollack Porter KM, Forrest KS. *Policy Engagement.* American Public Health Association; 2023.

45. Pollack Porter KM, Rutkow L, McGinty EE. The importance of policy change for addressing public health problems. *Public Health Rep.* 2018;133(suppl 1):9S–14S. doi:10.1177/0033354918788880

46. Alexander M. *The New Jim Crow: Mass Incarceration in the Age of Colorblindness.* Rev ed. New Press; 2020.

47. Ridgeway G. Analysis of racial disparities in the New York police department's stop, question, and frisk practices. RAND Corporation. 2007. Accessed August 5, 2025. https://www.rand.org/pubs/technical_reports/TR534.html

48. US Government Accountability Office. A glossary of terms used in the federal budget process. 5th ed. Report No. GAO-05-734SP. 2005. Accessed May 16, 2025. https://www.gao.gov/assets/gao-05-734sp.pdf

49. Ansell C, Gash A. Collaborative governance in theory and practice. *J Public Adm Res Theory.* 2008;18(4):543–571. doi:10.1093/jopart/mum032

50. New York City Council. Participatory budgeting. Accessed May 16, 2025. https://council.nyc.gov/pb

51. Black Beyond Data Reading Group. St. Francis Neighborhood Center. Accessed June 30, 2025. https://www.stfranciscenter.org/what_we_do/programs/bbd-sfnc.html

52. US General Services Administration. Data vs. information. Accessed June 30, 2025. https://resources.data.gov/glossary/data-vs.-information

53. Western Sydney University. Definition of research. September 11, 2024. Accessed May 16, 2025. https://www.westernsydney.edu.au/research/researchers/preparing_a_grant_application/dest_definition_of_research

54. Pew Charitable Trusts. How states use data to inform decisions: A national review of the use of administrative data to improve state decision-making. February 21, 2018. Accessed May 16, 2025. https://www.pewtrusts.org/en/research-and-analysis/reports/2018/02/how-states-use-data-to-inform-decisions

55. National Alliance to End Homelessness. Housing First. March 20, 2022. Accessed August 8, 2025. https://endhomelessness.org/resources/toolkits-and-training-materials/housing-first

56. Shelton S. At least 11 states have enacted restrictive voting laws this year, new report finds. *CNN.* June 14, 2023. Accessed August 3, 2025. https://www.cnn.com/2023/06/14/politics/restrictive-voting-laws-brennan-report

57. Elisabeth Rosenthal. How Trump aims to slash federal support for research, public health, and Medicaid. *KFF Health News.* May 20, 2025. Accessed August 3, 2025. https://kffhealthnews.org/news/article/health-care-spending-cuts-research-trump-administration-tariffs-public-health

58. Barclay ML. What's the latest on birthright citizenship? What Trump's order means for immigrant families. *The 19th.* July 10, 2025. Accessed August 3, 2025. https://19thnews.org/2025/07/birthright-citizenship-questions-legal-status-families

59. Kotowski O. Report on the Fiscal 2025 Preliminary Plan and the fiscal 2024 preliminary Mayor's management report for the police department. New York City Council Finance Division. March 20, 2024. Accessed June 9, 2025. https://council.nyc.gov/budget/wp-content/uploads/sites/54/2024/03/056-NYPD.pdf

60. Xue W, White A. COVID-19 and the rebiologisation of racial difference. *Lancet.* 2021;398(10310):1479–1480. doi:10.1016/S0140-6736(21)02241-8

61. Local Progress: Dare to Reimagine. Youth Power Agenda: Milwaukee Public Schools, WI. Accessed June 9, 2025. https://www.daretoreimagine.org/case-studies/milwaukee-youth-power-agenda

62. Rommel N. Milwaukee puts officers in schools, ends dispute. Wisconsin Public Radio. March 17, 2025. Accessed September 6, 2025. https://www.wpr.org/news/milwaukee-officers-schools-dispute-sros-mps

63. Barber W II. Talk for the 2021 Elie Wiesel Memorial Lecture Series. Boston University, Arts and Sciences, Elie Wiesel Center for Jewish Studies. October 27, 2021. Accessed June 5, 2025. https://www.bu.edu/jewishstudies/transcript-of-reverend-dr-william-barber-iis-talk-for-the-2021-elie-wiesel-memorial-lecture-series

64. State of California. CalEnviroScreen. Accessed June 28, 2025. https://oehha.ca.gov/calenviroscreen

65. Pilgrim D. Who was Jim Crow? Jim Crow Museum. Accessed July 27, 2025. https://jimcrowmuseum.ferris.edu/who/index.htm

66. Holloway J. The history of minstrel shows and Jim Crow. MacMillan Center for International and Area Studies at Yale, Gilder Lehrman Center for the Study of Slavery, Resistance, and Abolition. Accessed August 16, 2025. https://macmillan.yale.edu/glc/history-minstrel-shows-and-jim-crow

67. Brundage WF. Introduction. In: Cole S, Ring NJ, eds. *The Folly of Jim Crow.* University of Texas at Arlington; 2012:1–17.

68. Cohen W. *At Freedom's Edge: Black Mobility and the Southern White Quest for Racial Control, 1861–1915.* Louisiana State University Press; 1991.

69. *Plessy v Ferguson,* 163 US 537 (1896).

70. Greenblatt A. The racial history of the 'grandfather clause.' *NPR Code Switch.* October 22, 2013. Accessed August 4, 2025. https://www.npr.org/sections/codeswitch/2013/10/21/239081586/the-racial-history-of-the-grandfather-clause

71. Pascoe P. *What Comes Naturally: Miscegenation Law and the Making of Race in America.* Oxford University Press; 2009:83–85.

72. Rothstein R. *The Color of Law: A Forgotten History of How Our Government Segregated America.* Liveright Publishing; 2017.

73. Krieger N, Jahn JL, Waterman PD. Jim Crow and estrogen-receptor–negative breast cancer: US-born Black and white non-Hispanic women, 1992–2012. *Cancer Causes Control.* 2017;28(1):49–59. doi:10.1007/s10552-016-0834-2

74. Krieger N, Chen JT, Coull BA, et al. Jim Crow and premature mortality among the US Black and white population, 1960–2009: An age-period-cohort analysis. *Epidemiology.* 2014;25(4):494–504. doi:10.1097/EDE.0000000000000104

75. Lovato R. *Unforgetting: A Memoir of Family, Migration, Gangs, and Revolution in the Americas.* Harper; 2020.

76. Bump P. Nearly a third of Americans were alive during Jim Crow. *Washington Post.* August 19, 2019. Accessed July 27, 2025. https://www.washingtonpost.com/politics/2019/08/19/nearly-third-americans-were-alive-during-jim-crow

77. Krieger N, Van Wye G, Huynh M, et al. Structural racism, historical redlining, and risk of preterm birth in New York City, 2013–2017. *Am J Public Health.* 2020;110(7):1046–1053. doi:10.2105/AJPH.2020.305656

78. Taylor J, Lindsay R, Ibrahim M, Kye P, Tegeler P. The persistence of school segregation in the United States, its effects on racial disparities in school funding, achievement, and discipline, and the failure of the US government to sufficiently address it. Poverty and Race Research Action Council. July 14, 2022. Accessed August 7, 2025. https://www.prrac.org/the-persistence-of-school-segregation-in-the-united-states-its-effects-on-racial-disparities-in-school-funding-achievement-and-discipline-and-the-failure-of-the-u-s-government-to-sufficiently-add

79. Library Research Service. EdBuild finds a $23 billion funding gap between white and non-white school districts. March 5, 2019. Accessed June 3, 2025. https://www.lrs.org/2019/03/05/edbuild-finds-a-23-billion-funding-gap-between-white-and-nonwhite-school-districts

80. Leung-Gagné M, McCombs J, Scott C, Losen DJ. *Pushed Out: Trends and Disparities in Out-of-School Suspension.* Learning Policy Institute; September 30, 2022. Accessed May 16, 2025. https://learningpolicyinstitute.org/media/3885/download?inline&file=CRDC_School_Suspension_REPORT.pdf

81. Hahn RA. School segregation reduces life expectancy in the US Black population by 9 years. *Health Equity.* 2022;6(1):263–269. doi:10.1089/heq.2021.0121

82. Poor People's Campaign. About the Poor People's Campaign: A National Call for Moral Revival. Accessed August 4, 2025. https://www.poorpeoplescampaign.org/about

83. Center for the Study of Social Policy. A conversation with: Anthony Iton. Accessed August 4, 2025. https://cssp.org/ideas-in-action/our-work/projects/a-conversation-with-anthony-iton

84. US Citizenship and Immigration Services. Consideration of Deferred Action for Childhood Arrivals (DACA). July 15, 2024. Accessed August 6, 2025. https://www.uscis.gov/DACA

85. California Academy of Family Physicians. Governor's 2025–26 May revision proposes major cuts to healthcare and undermines Medi-Cal expansion commitments. May 14, 2025. Accessed August 7, 2025. https://www.familydocs.org/news-governors-2025-26-may-revision-proposes-major-cuts-to-healthcare-and-undermines-medi-cal-expansion-commitments

86. Egelko B. Court orders UC system to rethink policy against hiring undocumented students. *San Francisco Chronicle.* August 5, 2025. Accessed August 7, 2025. https://www.sfchronicle.com/politics/article/university-of-california-hiring-undocumented-20803842.php

87. Abrams S. *While Justice Sleeps.* Doubleday; 2021.

88. Belli B. Kendi: Racism is about power and policy, not people. *Yale News.* December 7, 2020. Accessed May 16, 2025. https://news.yale.edu/2020/12/07/kendi-racism-about-power-and-policy-not-people

89. Yamin AE. Shades of dignity: Exploring the demands of equality in applying human rights frameworks to health. *Health Hum Rights.* 2009;11(2):1–18

90. Malcolm X. Speech to the African Summit Conference; August 21, 1964. ICIT Digital Library. Accessed June 17, 2025. https://www.icit-digital.org/articles/malcolm-x-s-speech-to-the-african-summit-conference-august-21-1964

91. Clingermayer JC. Heresthetics and happenstance: Intentional and unintentional exclusionary impacts of the zoning decision-making process. *Urban Stud.* 2004;41(2):377–388. doi:10.1080/0042098032000165307

92. Rouse C, Bernstein J, Knudsen H, Zhang J. Exclusionary zoning: Its effect on racial discrimination in the housing market. The White House. November 30, 2021. https://bidenwhitehouse.archives. gov/cea/written-materials/2021/06/17/exclusionary-zoning-its-effect-on-racial-discrimination-in-the-housing-market

93. Shertzer A, Twinam T, Walsh RP. Race, ethnicity, and discriminatory zoning. NBER Working Paper No. 20108. National Bureau of Economic Research. May 2014. Accessed August 7, 2025. https://www.nber.org/papers/w20108

94. Mizutani J. In the backyard of segregated neighborhoods: An environmental justice case study of Louisiana. *Georgetown Environ Law Rev.* 2019;31(2):363–390. Accessed August 7, 2025. https://www.law.georgetown.edu/environmental-law-review/wp-content/uploads/sites/18/2019/04/GT-GELR190004.pdf

95. Moore E, Montojo N, Mauri N. Roots, race, & place: A history of racially exclusionary housing in the San Francisco Bay area. Othering & Belonging Institute, University of California, Berkeley. October 2, 2019. Accessed August 7, 2025. https://belonging.berkeley.edu/rootsraceplace

96. Joint Economic Committee, Democratic Staff. Chronic conditions pose growing health, economic and equity challenges. US Congress. July 8, 2022. Accessed August 7, 2025. https://www.jec.senate.gov/public/index.cfm/democrats/2022/7/chronic-conditions-pose-growing-health-economic-and-equity-challenges

97. Speroni S, Winchell Lenhoff S. School transportation and educational equity. *Regulatory Review.* March 30, 2023. Accessed August 7, 2025. https://www.theregreview.org/2023/03/30/speroni-school-transportation-and-educational-equity

98. Sánchez TW, Stolz R, Ma JS. *Moving to Equity: Addressing Inequitable Effects of Transportation Policies on Minorities.* Civil Rights Project, University of California, Los Angeles. June 1, 2003. Accessed August 7, 2025. https://civilrightsproject.ucla.edu/research/metro-and-regional-inequalities/transportation/moving-to-equity-addressing-inequitable-effects-of-transportation-policies-on-minorities

99. Pendall R. Local land use regulation and the chain of exclusion. *Urban Stud.* 2000;37(1):71–92. doi:10.1080/0042098002300021

100. Roy A. Racial banishment. In: Shaw KSV, Garmany J, eds. *Routledge Handbook on Spaces of Urban Politics.* Routledge; 2018:199–209.

Appendix 3A. Examples of Laws and Policies That Endanger Our Health

Think of the law as like the sail of a boat. The sail, or the law, guarantees motion but not direction. Legal work together with political mobilization, by individuals, organizations, and states, is the wind that determines direction. The law is not loyal to any outcome or player, despite its bias towards the most powerful states. The only promise it makes is to change and serve the interests of the most effective actors. In some cases, the sail is set in such a way that it cannot possibly produce a beneficial direction, and the conditions demand either an entirely new sail, or no sail at all. It is this indeterminacy in law and its utility as a means to dominate as well as to fight that makes it at once a site of oppression and of resistance; at once a source of legitimacy and a legitimating veneer for bare violence; and at once the target of protest and a tool for protest.

– Noura Erakat, human rights attorney and legal scholar[1(p11)]

LAWS AND POLICIES THAT HARM THE STRUCTURE AND RESOURCING OF OUR COMMUNITIES

- **National Housing Act (1934–1968):** This federal law created the Federal Housing Administration (FHA) to stabilize the housing market during the Great Depression but instead hardwired segregation into US communities. Using "redlining" maps and racially coded underwriting standards, FHA denied mortgage insurance to Black families and any neighborhood where they lived, cutting off investment and directing resources into white-only areas. Although formally banned by the Fair Housing Act of 1968, these policies left lasting patterns of segregation and disinvestment that continue to shape community structures and resources today.
- **Community disinvestment (1940s–present):** Government at all levels, alongside private actors like banks and businesses, systematically withheld investment from communities of color and other marginalized neighborhoods, guided by redlining maps and austerity policies. Public spending on infrastructure, schools, and services was curtailed, while credit, capital, and economic development were denied. Meanwhile, resources flowed into already well-resourced white communities. This state-sanctioned and market-reinforced disinvestment led to deteriorating schools, unreliable public services, and crumbling or absent infrastructure, ultimately locking communities of color out of opportunity for generations.

- **Housing Act of 1949 (1949–1970s):** This federal law provided federal funding to states and cities to implement large-scale "slum clearance" and redevelopment projects, which targeted low-income and communities of color under the guise of eliminating "blight" and promoting public health.[2] Across the country, thousands of neighborhoods were destroyed and nearly a million people were displaced[3] to make way for highways, corporate development, and gentrification—with little to no replacement housing and no deference to the people uprooted. These actions deepened segregation and housing insecurity. Backed by federal funding and support, "urban renewal" became yet another tool for state-sanctioned violence against Black, low-income, and other marginalized communities.
- **Inequitable reinvestment (1980s–present):** Federal and state tax reforms—such as the Economic Recovery Tax Act of 1981 (ERTA), which offered accelerated depreciation and tax shelters for real estate investors—channeled capital toward high-return projects, typically in wealthier, white-majority, or gentrified areas. ERTA and other policies fueled redevelopment that excluded and displaced long-term residents of color, compounding decades of disinvestment.
- **Gentrification (1980s–present):** Local zoning and land use decisions have driven up costs, taxes, and rents in historically marginalized neighborhoods and communities of color, contributing to the displacement of long-term residents. Redevelopment has too often proceeded without equitable protections or community benefits, turning past exclusion into present-day displacement.

LAWS AND POLICIES THAT UNDERMINE OUR ECONOMIC OPPORTUNITIES

- **Colonialism and land annexation (1400s–present):** European powers and later, the US government, seized Indigenous lands through conquest, forced removal, and settlement. This was rationalized under the 15th-century Doctrine of Discovery, which claimed non-Christian lands could be taken by colonial powers. Colonizers imposed private property regimes in place of Indigenous communal stewardship, converting stolen land into wealth for settler colonists while stripping Indigenous Nations of sovereignty, resources, and ancestral connections.
- **Slave codes (1600s–1865):** Colonial and later US state laws defined enslaved Africans and their descendants as property, codifying chattel slavery as a permanent, inherited condition.[4] These codes legalized brutal control over enslaved people's bodies, labor, and family life, creating vast wealth for white landowners and investors—and their descendants—while producing a multigenerational underclass.
- **Black Codes (1865–1870s):** In the wake of Emancipation, southern states enacted laws to restrict the rights of Black people, including their labor, voting rights, property

ownership, and mobility. Enforced by all-white police and state militia forces, Black Codes trapped newly emancipated Black people into a system of convict leasing and forced labor that was intended to effectively restore chattel slavery under another name.[5-7]

- **Jim Crow (1877–1960s):** After Reconstruction, Jim Crow emerged as a system of racial control that enforced white supremacy across the South and beyond. State and local governments mandated racial segregation and legalized widespread discrimination against Black people in all public spaces, such as schools, public transit, parks, retail areas, and hospitals. The laws forbade interaction between people of different "races" while denying Black people the right to vote, gain employment, obtain an education, and more. People who resisted faced arrest, heavy fines, jail, violence, and death.[8]

- **Broken treaties with Indigenous Nations (1770s–present):** The US government signed hundreds of legally binding treaties with Indigenous Nations, promising resources, protections, and recognition of sovereignty in exchange for land. Nearly all treaties were knowingly violated, enabling mass land theft, resource exploitation, and lasting economic and cultural harm across nearly all Indigenous peoples and Tribes in the United States.

- **Indian Removal Act of 1830 (1830–1907):** This federal law authorized the forced expulsion of tens of thousands of Indigenous peoples from their homelands east of the Mississippi. The resulting death and suffering—infamously remembered in the Trail of Tears endured by the Cherokee Nation—constituted a federally sanctioned act of genocide. These removals opened seized and stolen lands to white settlers and caused massive, intergenerational loss of land, wealth, and sovereignty for Indigenous Nations. Formal campaigns ended by the 1850s, but dispossession continued through later federal policies, culminating in 1907 with the dissolution of Indian Territory and Oklahoma statehood.

- **Homestead Act (1862–1986):** This federal law distributed millions of acres of stolen Indigenous lands almost exclusively to white settler colonists, while people of color were largely excluded from access to free or low-cost property ownership, entrenching racial wealth gaps. The act remained in effect until 1976, with an extension in Alaska until 1986.

- **Exploitation of marginalized labor (1800s–present):** Employment laws and workplace policies and practices systematically exploited and undercompensated women, people of color, and immigrant workers—especially in agriculture, domestic labor, railroad construction, mining, and service industries. Governments and employers profited from their labor while denying fair pay, safety, and rights, fueling long-standing income and wealth gaps.

- **Employment restrictions (1865–present):** Federal and state laws and private hiring practices have long barred people who have been incarcerated from being able to fairly compete for jobs or obtain employment. These restrictions persist today: Formerly incarcerated people are routinely forced to disclose their criminal legal system history on job applications and are discriminated against in hiring practices. These actions have reinforced cycles of poverty and reincarceration.

- **National Housing Act (1934–1968):** This federal law led to the widespread denial of mortgage credit that systematically excluded Black families and other communities of color from the nation's largest wealth-generating program. It entrenched racial wealth gaps and limited access to capital, education, and economic opportunity for generations. Although redlining was outlawed under the Fair Housing Act of 1968, its economic consequences persist through discriminatory lending practices, policy decisions, and the enduring impact of concentrated poverty.

- **Social Security Act of 1935 (1935–1960s):** This federal law excluded farm and domestic workers—jobs largely held by Black and brown people—denying them retirement and unemployment protections. Though coverage expanded by the 1960s, the initial exclusion delayed benefits and deepened racial wealth gaps.

- **Fair Labor Standards Act of 1938 (1938–present):** This federal law excluded certain industries from protections like minimum wage and overtime pay. Excluded industries were predominantly staffed by people of color and immigrant workers. They included agricultural jobs, domestic work, and service jobs that relied on tips. These actions exacerbated racial wealth gaps and perpetuated the continued racialized exploitation of labor.

- **The GI Bill, or Servicemen's Readjustment Act of 1944 (1944–1960s):** This federal law provided benefits for returning World War II veterans, including financial aid for college and vocational education, unemployment insurance, and government-backed home and small business loans. Although "race-neutral" on paper, the law was implemented in a racially discriminatory manner. Black veterans were largely barred from accessing home loans, higher education, and other benefits that were part of the GI Bill, while white veterans were able to build intergenerational wealth due to subsidized homeownership, small business supports, and educational advancement.

- **Rescission Act of 1946 (1946–2009):** This federal law revoked promises of full pay and benefits to more than 200,000 Filipino soldiers who served under US command in World War II, declaring their service "not to be deemed active service" for most veterans' benefits. Partial benefits were restored in 2009, but the decades-long denial caused lasting economic hardship and deepened racialized inequities among veterans.

- **Welfare Reform Act, or the Personal Responsibility and Work Opportunity Reconciliation Act of 1996 (1996–present):** This federal law replaced guaranteed cash aid with Temporary Assistance for Needy Families (TANF)—imposing work requirements, time limits, and capped state funding on access to the benefits. The change cut support to millions—especially women and children—worsening poverty rather than alleviating it.

LAWS AND POLICIES THAT DENY US DIGNIFIED HOUSING

- **Homeownership tax benefits (1913–present):** Federal tax policies—such as the mortgage interest deduction, capital gains exclusions, and property tax write-offs— provide heavy subsidies for homeowners, disproportionately benefiting wealthier, predominantly white households. These policies offer little support to renters or families historically excluded from homeownership, widening racial wealth gaps exacerbated by past decades of housing discrimination.

- **Racially restrictive covenants (1920s–1968):** These widely used clauses in property deeds prevented people of color—especially Black people—from purchasing homes in specific neighborhoods, reinforcing and further entrenching racial segregation. Though the Supreme Court ruled them unenforceable in *Shelley v Kraemer* (1948), they remained widely used until prohibited by the Fair Housing Act of 1968—and many property deeds still contain this racist language today.[9]

- **Exclusionary zoning policies (1930s–present):** These policies include local laws and land use rules that prohibit or limit the construction of affordable housing. They prevent certain groups—specifically lower-income people and people of color—from being able to live in specific neighborhoods and communities.

- **National Housing Act (1934–1968):** This federal law created FHA to stabilize the housing market during the Great Depression. Alongside the Home Owners' Loan Corporation's "Residential Security Maps" (also referred to as "redlining maps"), FHA underwriting manuals codified racial exclusion, denying mortgage insurance based explicitly on "race" and neighborhood composition, entrenching segregation and long-term disinvestment. Though banned under the Fair Housing Act of 1968, housing discrimination persists through comparatively subtler mechanisms like lending disparities and exclusionary zoning.

- **Public housing and Section 8 (1937–present):** The Housing Act of 1937 created federally funded public housing, which was usually segregated and underresourced. To expand housing options, the Section 8 program (1974) provided rental vouchers, which helped millions of low-income families. Yet discrimination, underfunding, and zoning barriers still confine many families—disproportionately Black and brown—to high-poverty neighborhoods.

- **Federal Highway Act of 1956 (1956–present):** This federal law funded massive interstate highway construction that state and local officials intentionally routed through neighborhoods of color to maintain segregation. This destroyed whole communities—including homes, businesses, and community institutions—and displaced residents on a large scale.[10,11] While the construction era tapered off by the early 1990s, its legacy of segregation, displacement, and disinvestment continues to shape communities today.

- **Policies enabling predatory lending (2000s–present):** Major policy decisions— notably the adoption of the Gramm–Leach–Bliley Act (1999) and repeal of Glass–Steagall Act (1933) restrictions—resulted in the deregulation of mortgage lending and allowed high-risk, discriminatory "subprime" loans to flood the housing market. These events led to the 2008 foreclosure crisis and the national Great Recession. Millions of people across all "races" lost their homes: The majority of foreclosed homes belonged to white people, but Black and Latine families faced disproportionately higher foreclosure rates and suffered the greatest relative losses in wealth.[12]

- **Post-2008 "reverse redlining" (2008–present):** In the wake of the foreclosure crisis, predatory investors and financial institutions disproportionately targeted Black and brown neighborhoods. They bought foreclosed homes in bulk, inflated rents, and used exploitative practices like "contract-for-deed" sales.

- **Eviction moratoria and pandemic housing insecurity (2020–2022):** Federal and state eviction bans provided temporary relief from mass displacement during COVID-19. But when the protections expired, many renters—disproportionately households of color—faced limited rental assistance and a surge in evictions.

LAWS AND POLICIES THAT ERODE OUR CIVIC AND POLITICAL POWER

- **Racist census practices (1790s–present):** Early US censuses failed to count enslaved people. Under the dehumanizing Three-Fifths Compromise, delegates to the 1787 Constitutional Convention agreed that each enslaved person would count as "three-fifths" of a person for the purposes of congressional representation, electoral votes, and the census. US censuses have routinely undercounted or misclassified racialized people—including Black, Indigenous, Middle Eastern and North African, multiracial, and immigrant communities—reducing their political representation and access to resources. This practice persists today.

- **Partisan gerrymandering (1812–present):** States have long drawn district boundaries to dilute or negate the voting power of communities of color. These actions—known as *gerrymandering*—are common and continuous. They are routinely used to weaken the political influence of racialized voters despite protections against racial discrimination in voting.

- **Felony disenfranchisement laws (1865–present):** Following the Civil War, states adopted laws stripping voting rights from people with felony convictions—often alongside racially targeted Black Codes. Discriminatory policing and sentencing have since led to the disproportionate incarceration of Black and brown communities. Today, more than 4 million Americans—disproportionately people of color—are disenfranchised.[13]

- **Voter suppression laws (1870s–present):** From "grandfather clauses," literacy tests, and poll taxes to modern barriers like strict voter ID laws, gerrymandering, voter roll purges, and reduced polling access, states have repeatedly erected obstacles intended to disproportionately disenfranchise marginalized communities and communities of color. The endgame is to prevent people in these groups from participating in elections.

- **Disenfranchisement of territories (1898–present):** People living in US territories (Puerto Rico, Guam, American Samoa, the US Virgin Islands, and the Northern Mariana Islands) are US citizens or nationals. However, they are not allowed to vote in presidential elections, and they have no voting representation in Congress. These territories are home to roughly 3.6 million people who are mostly people of color.[14]

- **Election crisis (2000, *Bush v Gore*):** The Supreme Court halted Florida's ballot recount, effectively deciding the 2000 presidential election in favor of George W. Bush. This crisis exposed serious issues in US election administration: Inconsistent vote-counting standards and unfair voter roll purges disproportionately impacted voters of color, marking a pivotal moment in the undermining of voting rights and election integrity.
- **Unlimited corporate spending in elections (2010–present):** The Supreme Court's decision in *Citizens United v Federal Election Commission* allowed unlimited independent political spending by corporations and wealthy donors, amplifying their influence in elections and drowning out ordinary voters.
- **Gutting the Voting Rights Act (2013–present):** In *Shelby v Holder*, the Supreme Court struck down federal preclearance requirements for states with histories of racial discrimination in voting. Justice Ruth Bader Ginsburg dissented, warning that this was "like throwing away your umbrella in a rainstorm because you are not getting wet."[15] Her words foreshadowed the new wave of voter suppression laws adopted by states, which especially harmed Black and brown voters.

LAWS AND POLICIES THAT EXPAND AND INTENSIFY THE HARMS OF THE CRIMINAL LEGAL SYSTEM

- **Criminalization of poverty (1600s–present):** These laws disproportionately targeted Black, Indigenous, and other communities of color, as well as poor and unhoused people, by criminalizing and punishing "idleness," unemployment, and homelessness. Post–Civil War "vagrancy" codes funneled people into forced labor systems like convict leasing. Modern-day "loitering" and "sit-lie" ordinances continue to allow local governments to fine, arrest, and displace people who are unhoused instead of addressing the root causes of poverty.
- **Criminalization of queer people (1600s–present):** Laws targeting queer communities have long been used to police, punish, and exclude—ranging from "anti-sodomy" statutes and bans on "cross-dressing" to police raids, HIV criminalization, and restrictions on LGBTQ+ military service. While many of these have been repealed or struck down, their legacy of stigma and policing continue. Today, queer and especially trans people continue to face criminalization through legislation that restricts access to public spaces, health care, education, and self-expression.
- **13th Amendment loophole (1865–present):** The 13th Amendment abolished slavery but included an exception allowing involuntary servitude "as punishment for crime." This loophole helped lay the groundwork for today's cruel, dehumanizing, and

highly racialized system of mass incarceration, which exploits and profits from imprisoned people's labor.[16,17]

- **Targeted mass detention and institutionalization (1879–present):** State-sanctioned confinement and control of marginalized communities—often beyond traditional prison systems—have been a persistent feature of US history. These practices reflect a long-standing pattern of using incarceration to enforce racial and economic hierarchies. This pattern has taken many forms and continues today in immigration detention centers, surveillance regimes, and carceral systems. These policies offer historical context for how confinement has been repeatedly used to suppress, displace, and dehumanize:
  - In 1879, the federal government opened the first "Indian boarding school," launching a system that forcibly removed Indigenous children from their families and cultures.
  - Early 20th-century eugenics laws led to the mass institutionalization and sterilization of disabled people, a practice upheld by the Supreme Court in *Buck v Bell* (1927).
  - During World War II, Executive Order 9066 (1942) authorized the incarceration of more than 120,000 Japanese American civilians.
  - The Illegal Immigration Reform and Immigrant Responsibility Act of 1996 expanded mandatory detention and deportation, disproportionately impacting immigrants of color—especially Latine immigrants.
  - The PATRIOT Act (2001) and National Security Entry-Exit Registration System (2002) enabled mass detentions and deportations of men from Muslim-majority countries.
- **Qualified immunity laws (1967–present):** These laws shield government officials—especially police—from civil lawsuits, requiring victims to prove a nearly identical past case to succeed. This almost insurmountable legal barrier largely allows violent acts committed by police—many of which result in people's deaths—to escape accountability.
- **Criminalization of homelessness (1980s–present):** Local laws have increasingly banned sleeping, camping, "panhandling," or storing belongings in public spaces—punishing unhoused people instead of providing them with permanent housing solutions. These ordinances—rising after federal housing cuts—displace, penalize, and criminalize people for the act of surviving in public.
- **Anti-Drug Abuse Act of 1986:** This federal law enforced harsh sentencing laws, including mandatory minimums, and drove mass incarceration of Black and Latine individuals for nonviolent drug offenses—all as part of the "War on Drugs." It also drove the militarization of law enforcement, racial profiling, and the criminalization of addiction.
- **1994 Crime Bill, or Violent Crime Control and Law Enforcement Act of 1994 (1994–present):** This federal law expanded prisons, funded tens of thousands of new police officers, and incentivized states to adopt "three-strikes" laws and mandatory minimum sentencing. This crime bill, the largest ever in US history, fueled racialized mass incarceration with no clear evidence of improving long-term public safety. While some

provisions, like the assault weapons ban, expired in 2004, many of its policing and sentencing structures continue to shape the criminal legal system today.

- **"Broken windows" policing (1990s–present):** Institutionalized through local ordinances and police department mandates, "broken windows" policing strategies disproportionately targeted Black, Latine, and unhoused communities without any meaningful or demonstrated public safety benefits. This form of policing prioritized and glorified the aggressive criminalization and enforcement of minor infractions—like loitering and fare evasion—based on the unproven idea that visible "disorder" causes serious crime.

- **"Stop-and-frisk" policies (1990s–present):** Enabled by the Supreme Court's *Terry v Ohio* (1968) decision, police departments in the 1990s adopted and expanded "stop-and-frisk" practices, permitting officers to stop and search individuals based on the legal standard of "reasonable suspicion." In practice, this standard has been applied broadly and disproportionately against Black and brown people, leading to widespread rights violations, unnecessary and unfounded arrests, and scant evidence of crime reduction.

- **Unjust fines and fees (2000s–present):** Building on revenue-driven court practices that expanded in the 1980s and 1990s, the 2000s saw a surge in state and local laws imposing steep fines and fees for minor offenses and routine legal proceedings. Alongside widespread use of cash bail, these policies transformed courts and law enforcement into revenue-generating systems. Failure to pay these fines and fees can result in suspension, loss of voting rights, arrest, and incarceration. These fines and fees disproportionately burden low-income communities of color, trapping many in deepening cycles of debt, incarceration, and poverty. (See Chapter 6 for more on unjust fines and fees.)

LAWS AND POLICIES THAT LIMIT AND UNDERMINE OUR EDUCATIONAL OPPORTUNITIES

- **School funding tied to local taxes (1800s–present):** Public schools have long relied on local property taxes, creating vast resource inequities between wealthy, predominantly white districts and low-income, often racially diverse communities. State-level funding attempts have narrowed but not eliminated these gaps.

- **Racially segregated schools (1870s–present):** For decades following the Civil War, Black students and white students were forbidden from learning together, and Black schools were starved of resources. While *Brown v Board of Education* (1954) ended formal racial segregation in schools, ongoing policies and practices—such as redlining, unfair tax policies, exclusionary zoning, district secessions, and private academies—have kept many schools in communities of color segregated and underfunded.

- **Special education inequities (1975–present):** The Individuals with Disabilities Education Act expanded access to education for students with disabilities. Yet systemic bias has led to students of color being disproportionately underresourced, placed in restrictive settings, and disciplined at higher rates, reflecting ongoing inequities in educational opportunity.

- **English-only education policies (1980s–present):** Multiple federal and state policy decisions have curtailed bilingual education, including the repeal of the Bilingual Education Act (1968) and its replacement under No Child Left Behind (2002) and state laws like California's Proposition 227 (1998) and Arizona's Proposition 203 (2000). These actions have disproportionately harmed English language learners by restricting access to culturally responsive instruction and undermining long-term academic success.

- **Mandatory standardized testing (1990s–present):** Laws like the Improving America's Schools Act (1994) and No Child Left Behind (2001) tied federal funding to test scores. Standardized tests—which have their origins in eugenics and scientific racism—have never been accurate or reliable measures of student learning.[18] Despite disproportionately penalizing students of color and low-income students, they continue to be widely used in schools today.

- **Zero-tolerance discipline policies (1990s–present):** These policies increased the presence of police in schools (referred to as school resource officers, or SROs), resulting in the disproportionate targeting of students of color by police. This has led to higher suspension, expulsion, and arrest rates among students of color compared with white students who engage in the same behaviors.

- **The end of affirmative action in higher education (2023–present):** In *Students for Fair Admissions v Harvard* and *University of North Carolina*, the Supreme Court struck down "race"-based admissions, stating that the use of "race" in college admissions was unconstitutional. This overturned decades of precedent and dismantled the legal basis for affirmative action in higher education. Following this Supreme Court decision, enrollment of students of color—particularly Black students—in colleges and medical schools declined precipitously.[19-21]

LAWS AND POLICIES THAT CONSTRAIN OUR FREEDOM TO IMMIGRATE AND BE LEGALLY RECOGNIZED

- **Chinese Exclusion Act (1882–1943):** This was the first US law to ban immigration based on nationality. The law prohibited Chinese laborers from entering the country and denied Chinese immigrants the ability to become US citizens. This set a precedent for future exclusionary immigration policies based on "race."

- **Immigration Act of 1924 (1924–1965):** This federal law established strict national origin quotas, favoring immigrants from Northern and Western Europe while severely restricting Southern and Eastern Europeans and banning Asian immigration. This law formalized racial hierarchy in US immigration policy for more than four decades. Although it was formally repealed in 1965, the quota system's legacy continues through racialized visa caps, restrictive border enforcement, and immigration rules that discriminate against people from Africa, Latin America, and Asia.

- **Hart–Celler Act, or Immigration and Nationality Act of 1965 (1965–present):** This federal law repealed national origin quotas but created a preference system prioritizing family ties and "skilled labor." This law reshaped migration from Asia and Latin America and functionally excluded many working-class migrants from these regions and others from consideration for immigration.

- **Illegal Immigration Reform and Immigrant Responsibility Act (1996–present):** This federal law dramatically expanded the grounds for deportation, limited access to legal relief, and introduced mandatory detention and expedited removal. This law laid the groundwork for today's mass deportation system and continues to disproportionately impact immigrants of color, as well as Black and brown communities broadly.

- **Federal reentry laws (2000s–present):** These laws—expanded in 1996 and aggressively enforced in the 2000s—criminalize reentry after deportation, making it a felony to return without authorization, even for those originally deported for minor immigration violations. This disproportionately affects and harms Latine immigrant communities.

- **ICE raids (2003–present):** After the creation of Immigration and Customs Enforcement (ICE) in 2003, workplace and neighborhood raids escalated, often with minimal oversight. These military-style operations have torn families apart, instilled fear in immigrant communities, and created chilling effects on access to due process, education, employment, health care, and social services.

- **Federal family separation policies (2018–present):** At their peak, these federal policies legally separated more than 5,000 migrant children from their parents and guardians. Many children were placed in mass shelters, with no documentation to track their locations. As a result, more than 1,000 children remained separated from their families more than six years after the policy was first implemented, resulting in lasting and ongoing harm to families and communities.[22] While the formal "zero tolerance" policy ended in 2021, family separation continues in various forms—through detention, deportation, and systemic failures in reunification.

LAWS AND POLICIES THAT RESTRICT OUR ABILITY TO TRAVEL AND MOVE FREELY

- **Discriminatory ticketing (1900s–present):** Traffic and minor infraction laws—such as so-called jaywalking, loitering, and expired vehicle tags—have been disproportionately enforced against people of color,[23] creating compounding fines, debt, and criminal records that exacerbate the harms of poverty and racism.

- **Disinvestment in road transportation infrastructure (1900s–present):** Low-income, Native, and racially segregated communities have historically been denied investment in basic road transportation infrastructure. Rooted in colonialism, redlining, and other racist policies and systems of oppression, these areas were starved of public investment, leading to hazards like unsafe roads, poor lighting, missing sidewalks, and nonexistent road safety infrastructure. On Tribal lands and in disinvested urban areas, inadequate infrastructure endangers pedestrians and transit users, and limits access to jobs, schools, health care, and emergency services.

- **Underfunded public transit (1900s–present):** Public transit systems in many cities were defunded or left to decline as white riders shifted to cars—spurred by a combination of desegregation orders, suburbanization, white flight, and federal policies that funneled investment into highways. Decades of disinvestment left transit systems with crumbling infrastructure, fare hikes, and service cuts that disproportionately harm Black, brown, and low-income communities. This forced a reliance on cars—which were often unaffordable—and limited mobility for those without them.

- **Exclusion from transit jobs (1930s–1970s):** Federal infrastructure programs often excluded people of color—especially Black and Indigenous workers—through discriminatory hiring and unfair union-related practices. These programs created tens of thousands of stable, well-paying jobs, but Black people and other people of color were excluded from consideration for them. These racist hiring practices not only denied people economic opportunity but also limited people of color's influence over how transportation systems were designed and who benefited from them.

- **Transportation-related pollution (1950s–present):** Decades of planning decisions have prioritized commerce and cars over health. Highways, airports, and freight corridors expose nearby communities—especially Black, brown, and low-income neighborhoods—to elevated levels of environmental and noise pollution. These conditions discourage outdoor activity, increase health risks like asthma and heart disease, and limit safe access to parks, sidewalks, and green spaces.

- **Federal Highway Act of 1956 (1956–present):** This federal law funded nationwide highway construction that federal, state, and local officials often routed through communities of color to reinforce segregation. In addition to razing neighborhoods and uprooting residents, the resulting infrastructure prioritized car travel for suburban commuters while physically isolating urban communities of color from public transit, walkable routes, and access to jobs, schools, and services. By fragmenting neighborhoods and embedding barriers into the built environment, the policy restricted mobility and reshaped transportation access for generations.

- **Transit policing and fare enforcement (1970s–present):** Beginning in the 1970s, transit agencies across the United States formalized fare enforcement policies and partnered with law enforcement to police minor infractions like fare evasion, loitering, and disorderly conduct. These policies disproportionately target Black, Latine, and unhoused riders, leading to fines, arrests, and even deadly violence, while doing little to improve public safety or equitable access to transit.

LAWS AND POLICIES THAT ENDANGER OUR ENVIRONMENT AND CLIMATE

- **Infrastructure and energy policies (1940s–present):** These policies at the federal, state, and local levels allow polluting industries, highways, and hazardous waste sites to be concentrated in communities of color. This has led to long-term environmental and health harms among the people within and around these communities.
- **National Environmental Policy Act (1970–present):** This federal law requires federal agencies to assess the environmental impacts of certain significant federal actions (like infrastructure projects or land management decisions) before they begin. However, it does not grant communities real power to prevent harm. Projects like the Dakota Access Pipeline moved forward despite clear threats to Indigenous sovereignty, water safety, and public health.
- **Clean Air Act (1970–present):** This federal law set national air quality standards, but they are weakly enforced in many low-income neighborhoods and communities of color. Heavier polluters often face fewer penalties in these areas, leaving residents exposed to decades of toxic air and resulting in asthma and other health harms.
- **Disaster response and insurance inequities (1970s–present):** Federal and state disaster policies—such as Stafford Act aid programs, Federal Emergency Management Agency guidelines, and the National Flood Insurance Program—have repeatedly failed to protect low-income communities and communities of color. After catastrophic disasters like Hurricane Katrina, survivors received slower rescue efforts and less rebuilding aid, and faced discriminatory insurance practices, leaving many families displaced and financially devastated.
- **Flint water crisis (2014–present):** The predominantly Black community of Flint, Michigan was exposed to dangerous lead-contaminated water for years without residents' knowledge. Upon being revealed, it became a national example of environmental racism and government neglect. This preventable crisis resulted from Michigan's Emergency Manager Law, cost-cutting policies, and failure to enforce water safety standards.
- **Toxic waste siting and Superfund cleanup delays (1980s–present):** A legacy of redlining, industrial zoning, and environmental racism, hazardous waste sites and industrial dumps have been disproportionately located in communities of color and in low-income communities. The federal Superfund program, established in 1980 to clean up these sites, has failed to address many contaminated areas, leaving them unremediated for decades. This failure has damaged the health of surrounding

communities writ large, prolonging their exposure to dangerous toxins like lead, arsenic, and radioactive compounds.

- **Robert T. Stafford Disaster Relief and Emergency Assistance Act (1988–present):** This federal law authorizes federal disaster aid but has been criticized for discriminatory funding distribution, bureaucratic barriers, and slow responses that leave low-income communities and communities of color more vulnerable and slower to recover.
- **Energy deregulation and infrastructure disinvestment (1990s–present):** State and federal policies that deregulated energy markets and failed to require investment in resilient infrastructure have left low-income communities of color disproportionately vulnerable to power outages and climate-related crises. In 2017, Hurricane Maria devastated Puerto Rico, triggering one of the longest blackouts in US history and contributing to thousands of deaths amid grid collapse. In Texas, the 2021 winter storm caused massive outages and hundreds of deaths when the deregulated energy system failed to withstand extreme cold. In the face of climate change, these extreme weather events—and the dangers they pose to marginalized, frontline communities—will only increase.
- **Climate gentrification policies (2010s–present):** Climate adaptation and "green redevelopment" projects often increase property values and contribute to the displacement of low-income communities and communities of color instead of providing equitable protection from climate risks.

REFERENCES

1. Erakat N. *Justice for Some: Law and the Question of Palestine.* Stanford University Press; 2019.
2. Lopez RP. Public health, the APHA, and urban renewal. *Am J Public Health.* 2009;99(9): 1603–1611. doi:10.2105/AJPH.2008.150136
3. Wheeler L. Razed in the city. *Washington Post.* June 10, 2004. Accessed August 7, 2025. https://www.washingtonpost.com/archive/lifestyle/2004/06/10/razed-in-the-city/b5605a06-c32e-4748-b7b8-dbde4bff2823
4. Library of Congress. Slave code for the District of Columbia. Slavery and the Judiciary, 1740 to 1860 (digital collection). 1860. Accessed May 16, 2025. https://www.loc.gov/collections/slavery-and-the-judiciary-from-1740-to-1860/articles-and-essays/slave-code-for-the-district-of-columbia
5. National Constitution Center. Mississippi & South Carolina Black Codes, 1865. Accessed May 16, 2025. https://constitutioncenter.org/the-constitution/historic-document-library/detail/mississippi-south-carolina-black-codes-1865
6. HISTORY.com editors. Black codes. History. February 27, 2025. Accessed May 16, 2025. https://www.history.com/topics/black-history/black-codes
7. Batra Kashyap M. US settler colonialism, white supremacy, and the racially disparate impacts of COVID-19. *Calif Law Rev Online.* 2020;11:517–529. Accessed May 16, 2025. https://digitalcommons.law.seattleu.edu/cgi/viewcontent.cgi?article=1832&context=faculty

8. HISTORY.com Editors. Jim Crow laws: Definition, examples & timeline. History. April 15, 2025. Accessed May 16, 2025. https://www.history.com/topics/early-20th-century-us/jim-crow-laws

9. Clemence S. Is there racism in the deed to your home? *New York Times*. August 17, 2021. Accessed August 8, 2025. https://www.nytimes.com/2021/08/17/realestate/racism-home-deeds.html

10. Miller J. Roads to nowhere: How infrastructure built on American inequality. *The Guardian*. February 21, 2023. Accessed May 16, 2025. https://www.theguardian.com/cities/2018/feb/21/roads-nowhere-infrastructure-american-inequality

11. Kruse KM. What does a traffic jam in Atlanta have to do with segregation? Quite a lot. *New York Times Magazine*. August 14, 2019. Accessed June 3, 2025. https://www.nytimes.com/interactive/2019/08/14/magazine/traffic-atlanta-segregation.html

12. McGhee H. *The Sum of Us: What Racism Costs Everyone and How We Can Prosper Together*. One World; 2021.

13. Uggen C, Larson R, Shannon S, Stewart R, Hauf M. Locked out 2024: Four million denied voting rights due to a felony conviction. The Sentencing Project. October 10, 2024. Accessed August 7, 2025. https://www.sentencingproject.org/reports/locked-out-2024-four-million-denied-voting-rights-due-to-a-felony-conviction

14. Balmaceda J. Federal data inequities in US territories hinder inclusive and precise policymaking. Center on Budget and Policy Priorities. August 7, 2024. https://www.cbpp.org/blog/federal-data-inequities-in-us-territories-hinder-inclusive-and-precise-policymaking

15. *Shelby County v Holder*, 570 US 529 (2013).

16. Alexander M. *The New Jim Crow: Mass Incarceration in the Age of Colorblindness*. 10th Anniv ed. The New Press; 2020.

17. Little B. Does an exception clause in the 13th Amendment still permit slavery? History. March 6, 2025. Accessed May 16, 2025. https://www.history.com/news/13th-amendment-slavery-loophole-jim-crow-prisons

18. Rosales J, Walker T. The racist beginnings of standardized testing. *NEA Today*. March 20, 2021. Accessed May 16, 2025. https://www.nea.org/nea-today/all-news-articles/racist-beginnings-standardized-testing

19. Maglione F, Cachero P, Choi A, Wahid R. Black enrollment drops at top schools as affirmative action axed. *Bloomberg Law*. September 27, 2024. Accessed August 7, 2025. https://news.bloomberglaw.com/us-law-week/black-enrollment-drops-at-top-schools-as-affirmative-action-axed

20. Chao-Fong L. Elite US colleges see Black enrollment drop after affirmative action strike-down. *The Guardian*. August 30, 2024. Accessed August 7, 2025. https://www.theguardian.com/us-news/article/2024/aug/30/black-college-student-enrollment-declines-affirmative-action-strike-down

21. Lee McFarling U. Legal overreaction to Supreme Court ban on race fueling loss of diversity at medical schools. *STAT*. January 23, 2025. Accessed August 7, 2025. https://www.statnews.com/2025/01/23/legal-overreaction-to-supreme-court-ban-on-race-fueling-loss-of-diversity-at-medical-schools

22. Bennett G, Khan S, Midura K. Hundreds of migrant children remain separated from families despite push to reunite them. *PBS NewsHour*. February 6, 2023. Accessed May 16, 2025. https://www.pbs.org/newshour/show/hundreds-of-migrant-children-remain-separated-from-families-despite-push-to-reunite-them

23. Sanders T, Rabinowitz K, Conarck B. Walking while Black: Jacksonville's enforcement of pedestrian violations raises concerns that it's another example of racial profiling. *ProPublica*. November 16, 2017. Accessed August 8, 2025. https://features.propublica.org/walking-while-black/jacksonville-pedestrian-violations-racial-profiling

II. SEIZING OPPORTUNITIES FOR CHANGE

We continue our journey by examining what holds back our nation's progress toward equity and justice. We dive into the ways mindsets and narratives can uplift or undermine community health. We then explore the transformative potential of power, assurance, and evaluation to create new opportunities and drive change.

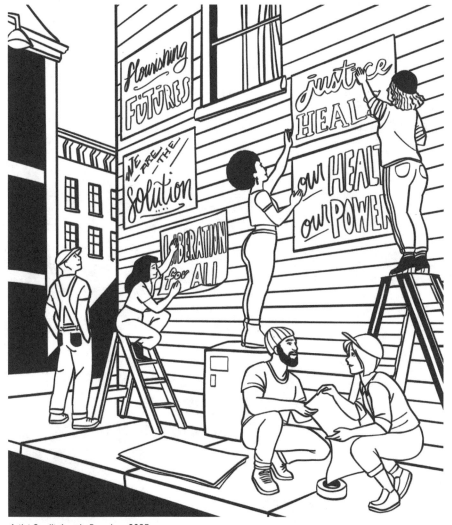

Artist Credit: Jasmin Pamukcu, 2025.
Coalitions for Change

Transforming Mindsets and Narratives to Advance Health

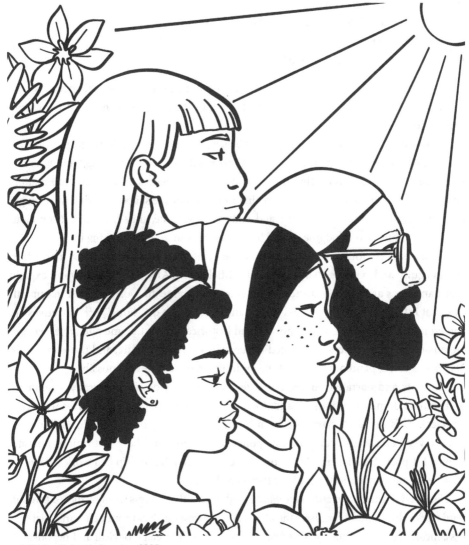

Artist Credit: Jasmin Pamukcu, 2025.

Narratives in Bloom

We have so many phobias that are so deeply seeded in our culture, and they're all reinforcing of these hierarchies of human value.... [T]hese norms, if you kind of trace them back, [are] all rooted in a story we have about whose life is more valuable.

–Ai-jen Poo, labor organizer and president of the
National Domestic Workers Alliance[1]

Some statements seem instinctively true when we hear them. You've heard phrases like these before:

- *The United States is a land of equal opportunity.*
- *Hard work determines success.*
- *People should pull themselves up by their bootstraps.*
- *I don't see color.*
- *Health is a personal responsibility.*

These phrases are repeated so often—in classrooms, media, political speeches, and everyday conversations—that they begin to sound like common sense. But familiarity should not be confused with truth.

These phrases are **mindsets**—deeply held beliefs, attitudes, assumptions, and perspectives that shape how we think about the world.[2] As assumed patterns of thinking,[3] mindsets also influence what we do—including how we interpret experiences, assess new information, and make decisions. Mindsets form early in our lives; they are shaped by what we're taught and reinforced by our environment and culture. Over time, they become subconscious filters that influence our judgments and behaviors without us even realizing it.

Mindsets don't form in isolation; they are reinforced and sustained by narratives. Racial equity and systems change advocates Michael McAfee and Vanice Dunn explain that **narratives** are "the big stories we tell ourselves about the world, rooted in our values, that influence how we process information and make decisions."[4(p10)] Narratives are rooted in shared values, cultural norms, and historical context. Some narratives we create ourselves, while others are created for us by institutions, media, and those in power. Narratives can expand our imaginations or limit what we believe is possible.

Mindsets and narratives operate in a feedback loop: Dominant narratives reinforce and amplify dominant mindsets, and dominant mindsets shape the narratives we accept or reject. This **mindset–narrative loop** influences not only how individuals think but also how systems are structured, how policies are made, and how institutions operate. Figure 4-1 provides an example of how the reinforcing relationship can work between a mindset, a narrative, and the policies they can shape.

Figure 4-1 illustrates a *meritocracy mindset*—the belief that success is only achieved through hard work. This mindset dismisses the idea that other systemic factors influence material success, including social status, generational wealth, and widespread cronyism and nepotism. It reinforces damaging narratives that frame poor people as lazy or undeserving when, in reality, they face pervasive exclusion and exploitation under systems like racial capitalism.

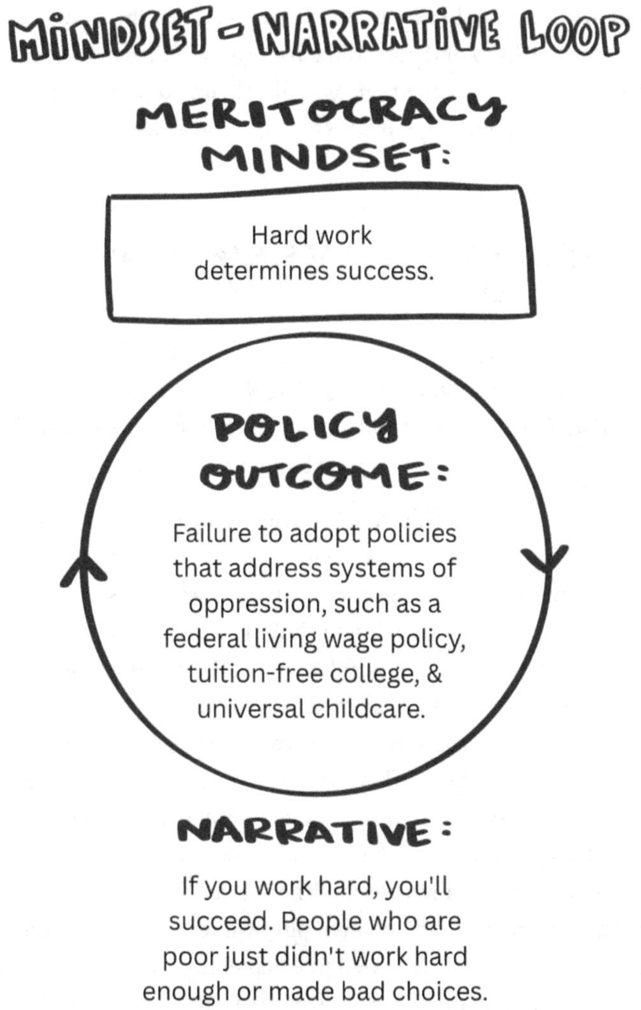

MINDSET - NARRATIVE LOOP

MERITOCRACY MINDSET:

Hard work
determines success.

POLICY OUTCOME:

Failure to adopt policies
that address systems of
oppression, such as a
federal living wage policy,
tuition-free college, &
universal childcare.

NARRATIVE:

If you work hard, you'll
succeed. People who are
poor just didn't work hard
enough or made bad choices.

Artist Credit: Jasmin Pamukcu, 2025.

Figure 4-1. The Mindset–Narrative Loop

Mindsets don't exist in isolation. We all hold multiple, often conflicting, mindsets that influence how we interpret the world—consciously or not. For instance, a *zero-sum mindset* is the belief that power and resources are finite; gains for one group must come at the expense of another. This mindset makes efforts to invest in equity seem unrealistic or unfair because if one group gains, another must lose. By contrast, an *abundance mindset* holds that there are enough resources and opportunities for everyone. This perspective makes it easier to craft solutions based on the just creation and collective stewardship of shared wealth and power.

A *punitive mindset*, reinforced by narratives and beliefs about personal responsibility, drives narratives that blame and justify punishing people for poor health outcomes—rather than addressing the structural barriers that harm health in the first place. A *restorative mindset,* by contrast, seeks to understand the root causes of harm in society and respond with accountability and care, rather than assigning blame or punishment.

To change health outcomes, we must change mindsets—and that means changing systems.

MINDSETS BENEATH THE SURFACE: EXPLORING THE ICEBERG MODEL

[W]e are going to have to learn to think in radical terms. I use the term radical *in its original meaning—getting down to and understanding the root cause. It means facing a system that does not lend itself to your needs and devising means by which you change that system.*
                                        —Ella Baker, organizer and civil rights leader[5]

Systems change is the process of shifting the underlying conditions that hold a complex problem in place.[6] It requires us to look beneath the surface—beyond individual events or outcomes—to understand the deeper forces shaping what we see. One way to do this is by examining the patterns, structures, and mindsets that drive and sustain inequity. The *Iceberg Model*[7] (Figure 4-2) offers a useful framework for this deeper analysis, helping visualize and understand the hidden layers that result in visible outcomes.

Like an iceberg, where 90% lies hidden beneath the water, most of what drives health outcomes exists below the surface. When we experience a policy failure or witness unjust health disparities, those are occurring above the waterline. Below these events are deeper layers: harmful patterns, institutional structures, and dominant mindsets rooted in systems like structural racism, sexism, and ableism. These forces are often invisible, but they are powerful—shaping laws, narratives, and even our own sense of what is normal or possible.

Take racism, for example. As discussed in Chapter 2, "race" is a social fiction with no biological or scientific foundation—yet racism is real and deadly. The false narrative that people can be ranked and valued by skin color has justified centuries of violence, exclusion, and exploitation. Racism continues to shape our systems, institutions, policies, and public narratives to this day. If we want to improve community health, we cannot implement interventions that merely scratch the surface. We must dive deeper to dismantle the mindsets that allow these systems of oppression to persist.

The Iceberg Model helps us do just that. It reveals the interconnected layers—events, patterns, structures, and mindsets and narratives—that shape the conditions for health. And as the model illustrates, the deeper we intervene, the greater our potential to create transformative, lasting change. According to the Iceberg Model,

1. **Events are surface-level symptoms.** These are visible crises that grab headlines—like a pregnancy-related death, a disease outbreak, or a surge in overdoses. They can generally be described and measured. At this level, we ask: *What is happening?*

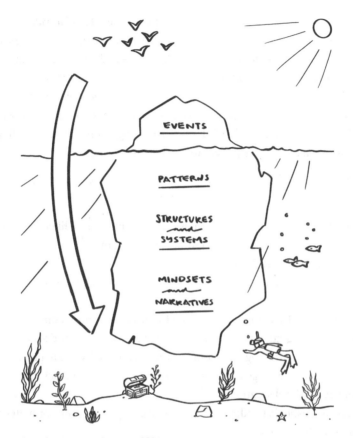

Artist Credit: Jasmin Pamukcu, 2025.

Figure 4-2. The Iceberg Model

Event-level solutions tend to be reactive: They may be important responses in the moment, but they do not transform the root causes of the problem.

2. **Patterns are symptoms that repeat.** These trends reveal that the problem is not new or isolated. At this layer, we ask: *What is repeating and recurring over time?* Solutions here are more forward-looking but may still focus on treating symptoms instead of causes.

3. **Structures and systems drive the patterns.** These include the laws, policies, practices, institutions, and power relationships that shape our daily lives and sustain health inequities. At this layer, we ask: *What's built into the system that's creating these patterns? How are these systems and structures connected? How are they interacting to keep inequity in place?* Solutions here can be proactively designed with greater ambition and vision.

4. **Mindsets and narratives shape structures and systems.** These are the deeply held beliefs, assumptions, and stories that give rise to what we believe and define what we

consider normal or acceptable. At this deepest layer, we ask: *What values, assumptions, and worldviews shape systems and structures? What are the stories that sustain them?* Solutions here have the potential to be transformative and long-lasting—but only if they tangibly transform systems and structures themselves. Just as systems of oppression and structural inequities persist independently of individual acts of prejudice, a change in hearts and minds alone won't produce equitable outcomes unless paired with concrete action. This is why it's essential to link narrative change with changes in policy, funding, and decision-making to reshape real-world outcomes.

To illustrate how the Iceberg Model can be applied, this section analyzes an important public health issue: unjust racial disparities in maternal health.*

- **Event:** Black women in the United States are three times more likely to die from pregnancy-related complications compared with white women.[8]
  Potential event-level solutions:
  ○ Require hospitals to track and publicly report racial inequities in maternal mortality rates.
  ○ Implement antidiscrimination training for health care providers.
- **Patterns:** Racial inequities in maternal mortality have persisted for decades in the United States, even when controlling for income and education level. Gaps in prenatal care, postpartum support, and emergency response continue to persist in Black communities.
  Potential pattern-level solutions:
  ○ Require all hospitals to adopt racially aware clinical protocols for maternal health.
  ○ Expand Medicaid postpartum coverage.
  ○ Invest in community-based models of care like midwifery and doulas.
- **Structures and systems:** Medicaid restrictions cut off postpartum care too early, leaving new mothers without medical support. Many women whose incomes are too high to qualify for Medicaid go underinsured or uninsured. Medical training largely ignores Black maternal health and racism in health care more broadly. Lack of paid maternity leave forces many Black women to return to work too soon, increasing health risks.
  Potential solutions at the structures and systems level:
  ○ Adopt a federal universal health care policy.
  ○ Adopt a federal paid family leave policy.
  ○ Change medical school curricula and the US Medical Licensing Examination to include efforts to dismantle scientific racism and medical racism.
  ○ Invest federal and state resources into equity-focused maternity services.
- **Mindsets and narratives:** The misleading mindset of personal responsibility frames racially unjust maternal outcomes as individual failures instead of systemic ones.

---

*The term *maternal health* is widely used in public health and health care, and we reference women here given limitations in how the data and research are framed. We acknowledge this omission and intend the example to be inclusive of all birthing people, including transgender and nonbinary individuals who give birth.

The US health care system operates on the assumption that health care is a privilege and a commodity rather than a right, leading to wealthier, insured people receiving better care. The devaluation of Black women's lives leads to a widespread neglect of Black women's care, autonomy, and health outcomes. As a result, Black women's health concerns are ignored and disrespected, their experiences are dismissed, and their health care needs are unaddressed.

Potential solutions at the mindset and narrative level:

o Use storytelling, data, and journalism to demonstrate that racial inequities in maternal health are a systemic issue—not an individual problem—that requires systemic solutions.

o Partner with leaders of social justice movements, funders, and experts on framing and narrative change to uplift the value of Black lives and to shift the mindset that health care is a right, not a commodity or a privilege.

If we want to advance equity and justice, we must focus on the base of the iceberg: mindsets and narratives. Creating new policies and structural approaches is critically necessary but not sufficient if we don't also challenge the mindsets and narratives that generate injustice in the first place.

Unfortunately, in public health, we operate from many dominant and misleading mindsets. These mindsets present as common sense, use seemingly plausible data, or even appear to be equity-friendly ideas at first glance. But beneath the surface, these misleading mindsets obstruct progress, waste resources, and pull us away from solutions that could actually move us closer to justice. These pernicious mindsets often serve those who benefit from the status quo. They offer simplistic, familiar, or comfortable explanations for complex problems—blaming individuals instead of systems and normalizing inequities as inevitable.

The next section highlights some of the most persistent misleading mindsets in public health. Recognizing them will help you maintain focus, counter distractions, and structure your work around what really matters: addressing the root causes of health inequities with clarity, purpose, and courage.

MISLEADING MINDSET: HEALTH IS A PERSONAL RESPONSIBILITY

[T]here is a very narrow focus on the individual. It's the notion that if you just pull yourself up by your bootstraps, you can make it. Systems and structures are invisible, and there is a limited sense of inter-dependence.

–Camara Jones, epidemiologist and antiracism scholar[9]

Although public health is uniquely defined by its population-level focus, our field has long been preoccupied with influencing individual behavior. We are too often focused on trying to get individuals to *do* something—to quit smoking, to eat healthier foods, or to exercise more. As a result, we've created numerous educational campaigns and interventions in hopes of changing individual people's behaviors. Behavior change theories are a central focus of public health academic curricula and research, and they are applied and reinforced in public health practice.

But **lifestyle drift**—our tendency in public health to narrowly focus on individual behavior—results in overlooking the drivers of these behaviors: "the causes of the causes."[10] Instead of confronting the root causes, systems, and structures that shape and constrain people's choices (see Box 4-1), we wrongly and repeatedly overfocus on the individual people who are doing their best to navigate complex and unjust systems. Even well-intentioned behavior-focused efforts have fallen short because they fail to acknowledge how structural racism, racial capitalism, and other systems of oppression shape people's options in the first place.[11-13]

By centering lifestyle drift in public health efforts, we perpetuate a flawed and misleading mindset: "Health is a personal responsibility"—that being healthy comes down to individual behaviors and personal choices. This mindset causes real harm. By overemphasizing personal responsibility, we reinforce stigmatizing narratives that blame the very communities we claim to serve. This damaging mindset also plays right into the hands of powerful, profit-driven industries that purposely deflect accountability and resist structural change, as illustrated by these examples:

- **Soda companies and other for-profit industries** cofounded the nonprofit Keep America Beautiful, which condemned consumers for littering and effectively shifted blame and attention from their pollution-generating activities, like the mass manufacturing of single-use plastics that pose dangers to people and the planet.[14]

Box 4-1. Root Causes Avoidance

Lifestyle drift is part of a larger phenomenon that we refer to as **root causes avoidance**—the tendency of many public health organizations and interventions to focus on surface-level factors like health behaviors or individual risk, while failing—or outright refusing—to name and confront the underlying systems that shape people's behaviors in the first place.

Root causes avoidance is exacerbated by restrictive funding structures that are routinely imposed by government agencies and philanthropic organizations. These short cycles often require rapid, overly ambitious, and quantifiable results in complex issue areas like chronic disease prevention and community violence. These unrealistic time horizons for change instead push public health institutions to measure and manage only what is immediately visible and quantifiable—like the number of home injury prevention trainings conducted, fire alarms distributed, or levels of particulate matter in the air—rather than tackling the deeper housing, employment, and environmental injustices that actually drive these outcomes.

If we hope to genuinely advance equity and justice in public health, then we must commit to continually asking, *Are we naming the root causes of health inequities? Are we directly confronting the systems of oppression and structural inequities that determine who lives and who dies?* Without a focus on directly addressing root causes, we will only continue to treat the symptoms of the public health problems, rather than being a force for real structural and systemic change.

- **Industrial food companies** insist that consumers are personally responsible for choosing low-calorie and sugar-free options while they simultaneously resist policies to regulate nutrition standards, provide resources to food-scarce neighborhoods, and prevent predatory advertising.[15]
- **Alcohol companies** place the burden of alcohol use on the shoulders of consumers by advising them to "drink responsibly," while simultaneously lobbying for policies that allow them to avoid paying taxes on billions of dollars of profits—tax dollars that could be used to support alcohol-related public health efforts.[16]
- **Influential and wealthy tech companies** promote features intended for individual users, like user privacy settings and settings to manage screen time, all the while misdirecting attention from the mental health harms of their algorithms, particularly among youth.[17]

In addition to furthering the narratives and bottom lines of profit-driven industries, this insidious mindset has undermined our own efforts to address public health problems at the policy and systems levels.[12] The *Let's Move!* initiative provides a useful example of how a well-intentioned public health campaign perpetuated misleading mindsets and harmful narratives of individual behavior—ultimately missing critical opportunities to make meaningful, systems-level changes (Box 4-2).[18-31]

As public health practitioners, we must be honest about the limits of individual behavior change as a population-level strategy. If we want to make the greatest impact, we must change policies that determine the choices people can make in the first place and transform the systems that shape the conditions of their lives. That is the only way we can create meaningful, lasting change for the people and populations we serve.

Let's replace this misleading mindset with a more just one:

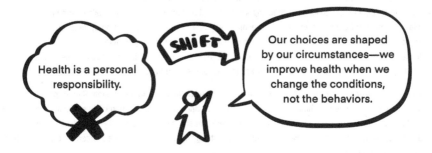

By adopting this new and more accurate mindset, we can stop blaming individuals for poor health and start holding systems accountable for creating the conditions that drive poor health outcomes. By shifting our focus from individual responsibility to systems-level accountability, we can develop more powerful solutions that address the root causes of injustice.

Box 4-2. *Let's Move!*—A Well-Meaning Public Health Intervention That Reinforced Misleading Mindsets

Launched by the Obama administration in 2010 to address childhood obesity, *Let's Move!* encouraged healthier nutrition for students, access to healthier food for families, and more physical activity for children.[18]

Encouraging healthy eating and more active lifestyles can be important, but as discussed in Chapter 1, public health interventions that focus primarily on changing individual behavior—rather than advancing equity- and justice-oriented systems change—are inevitably limited in their effectiveness. Worse, they divert attention and resources from addressing the deeper systemic forces that shape behavior, limit choices, and drive health outcomes. With this in mind, *Let's Move!* made several major missteps:

- **Overfocusing on individual behavior:** While the campaign attempted to promote healthier lifestyles, its focus on individual behavior—encouraging parents to make healthy choices and children to be more active— overlooked the systemic issues behind "obesity" rates. This put the responsibility for making "healthy decisions" primarily on parents and children.[19] *Let's Move!* also failed to address structural issues like food scarcity, underfunded public programs like SNAP, financial pressures on school free-lunch programs,[20] and corporate practices that make unhealthy food cheap and widely accessible.
- **Placing the burden of change on marginalized communities:** The campaign also included an initiative called *Let's Move! in Indian Country*, which asked Tribal Nations to "help families make healthy choices" and "create capacity for physical education, sports and outdoor recreation programs"[21]—but *Let's Move!* provided no resources in support. As discussed in Chapters 2 and 3, the federal government has a long history of genocidal policies that enabled the widespread loss of Indigenous territory, resources, and sovereignty. These policies have directly contributed to ongoing food insecurity, economic injustice, and health inequities that exist in Indigenous communities today. Given the need for redress, the federal government should have provided the necessary resources without question, while also seeking the full consent, guidance, and leadership of the Tribal Nations that chose to participate in *Let's Move!*
- **Ignoring anti-fat discrimination:** The campaign's focus on reducing "obesity" contributed to stigmatizing attitudes about body size. It perpetuated the harmful and inaccurate notion that thinness equals health and fatness equals disease. This approach ignores the fact that health is a complex, multifaceted concept that cannot be determined by body size alone (especially when assessed through the unreliable measure of BMI, as we discuss in Chapter 2). It also reinforced anti-fat discrimination and failed to acknowledge the harmful effects of this stigmatization on children's mental and emotional well-being.

Let's Move! engaged in *root causes avoidance*: It focused on surface-level factors like health behaviors while failing to name and confront the underlying systems that shape people's behaviors in the first place. It is impossible to make individual people responsible for changing systems-level problems. By creating public health interventions that place blame and burdens on marginalized people and communities—rather than on systems and structures— we are not only ineffectual but can harm the very communities we are intending to help.

To create meaningful change, *Let's Move!* should have instead confronted the unjust structures and systems that contribute to food insecurity and unhealthy environments. It should have taken on the following:

- **Economic injustice.** Decades-long cycles of layoffs,[22] wage stagnation, and the erosion of labor protections have diminished household incomes across working-class and marginalized communities. Rising costs of living, unstable employment, and a lack of access to affordable health care compound these hardships. The result is a growing divide in food access, where those who are struggling financially are often forced to rely on low-cost, low-nutrition options.[23]
- **Food apartheid.** Fresh food is generally abundant in wealthy neighborhoods and scarce in poor ones. This is a direct result of policy, planning, and private-sector decisions—both past and present—that have perpetuated racial segregation, concentrated disadvantage, and systematic community disinvestment.[24] Ultimately, this inequity means that more affluent neighborhoods have a high concentration of grocery stores while others have few or none at all.[25]

(Continued)

Box 4-2. (Continued)

- **Unjust policies.** Zoning, land use, and tax policies all contribute to poor health. Certain zoning laws have restricted commercial development—such as grocery stores—in residential neighborhoods, limiting walkable access to fresh food. Tax laws have suppressed public and private investment. In addition, governments have failed to incentivize the creation of grocery stores in urban and rural areas, instead allowing convenience stores and fast food outlets to more heavily populate these areas.[26]
- **Efforts that prioritize profits over people.** Grocery chains have refused to open stores in areas they deem unprofitable.[27] In the mid- to late 20th century, supermarket chains abandoned urban neighborhoods in favor of what they perceived would be more lucrative suburbs. In the process, they left behind vacant retail spaces. According to attorney and antitrust scholar Christopher R. Leslie, these businesses embedded anti-competitive "scorched-earth covenants" in their property deeds, barring any future owners from putting grocery stores on those sites again. This also meant that whole communities were abandoned[28] to food apartheid following the mass movement of white people from urban areas to the suburbs—a phenomenon known as *white flight*.
- **Underfunded social safety nets.** The federal TANF and SNAP programs have made healthy food more accessible and affordable for low-income families, but these programs have been consistently underfunded and remain politically vulnerable to budget cuts.[29,30]
- **Flawed policy governing food production.** Federal incentives overwhelmingly favor large-scale commodity production (corn, soy, wheat, livestock), while offering limited support for local and regional food systems. This makes it economically difficult for farmers to grow and sell healthy, locally produced foods.[31] Meanwhile, fruit and vegetable production—which is key to food justice and nutrition—receives comparatively little public investment.

Public health efforts that ignore root causes—and instead place the burden of change on individuals and marginalized communities—reinforce injustice, deepen inequities, and fail to achieve meaningful and long-lasting impact. *Let's Move!* is a cautionary tale that provides us with a valuable lesson: Our public health interventions must transform policies and systems if they are to achieve lasting, positive change. To advance equity and justice, we must commit to systems-change strategies that confront injustice at its roots, center community leadership, fully resource communities, and move us toward health and collective flourishing.

Note: BMI = body mass index; SNAP = Supplemental Nutrition Assistance Program; TANF = Temporary Assistance for Needy Families.

MISLEADING MINDSET: POOR HEALTH ISN'T ABOUT "RACE"—JUST MONEY

This fight for decent pay has, like many labor struggles before it, exposed the fact that workers of color suffer the most acute economic injustices, but most of the people harmed in a wage structure built on racism are white. And like every truly successful labor movement, it has found its reach and its strength because of cross-racial solidarity.

–Heather McGhee, author and attorney[32(p156)]

The belief that poverty alone—and not racism—is the primary cause of poor health outcomes in the United States is widespread. While classism, poverty, and unjust disparities in wealth are indeed root causes of inequity (as discussed in Chapter 3), this mindset is incomplete and misleading. In a racialized and capitalistic society, poverty is not experienced the same way by all people. Racism amplifies the pernicious and pervasive consequences of poverty in ways that make health and well-being nearly impossible.

For instance, compared with a poor white family, a poor Black family is more likely to live in a community where many other poor families have lived for decades. These are places that are described as having **concentrated, intergenerational poverty**: a pervasive form of poverty that is entrenched, neighborhood- and community-wide, and difficult— oftentimes impossible—to escape. This is because systems of oppression and structural inequities drive racial segregation, community disinvestment, and other forms of subjugation to keep it intact.

As journalist and urban policy scholar Emily Badger writes, the kind of concentrated poverty that Black families experience "extends out the door of a family's home and occupies the entire neighborhood around it, touching the streets, the schools, the grocery stores."[33] As a result, upward mobility in communities of color is not only harder to achieve, it is also more fragile and fleeting, especially for Black families.[34]

By contrast, poverty among poor white families is much less likely to be entrenched or concentrated in communities, making intergenerational advancement much more likely. In fact, poor white families tend to live in better-resourced neighborhoods than middle-class Black and Latine families.[35] These racialized differences make poverty more enduring and devastating for communities of color.

Wealth and privilege do not shield people from racism. Indeed, violence and backlash have historically followed the advancement of people of color. When communities of color have made economic gains throughout US history, they have inevitably faced violent and systemic retaliation. Examples abound. In the 1920s, white residents of Osage County orchestrated the murders of wealthy Osage Nation members to rob them of their land and oil rights.[36] During the same decade, white mobs decimated Tulsa's prosperous Black Wall Street, destroying homes, businesses, and lives.[37] During World War II, the US government incarcerated Japanese Americans en masse, stripping many families of wealth and property.[38] These events expose a pattern: Economic success has not guaranteed safety for people of color; instead, it has often triggered state-sanctioned violence, terror, and persecution.

Today, even those with high incomes, advanced education, or public visibility continue to face structural racism and the health consequences that come with it. Both research and lived experience make several lessons clear:

- **Unjust racial gaps in economic mobility remain wide.** A landmark study of 20 million children and their parents across multiple generations found that Black children whose parents were in the top 1% of earners—incomes at an average of $1.1 million— grew up to have incomes 12.4% *lower* than white children who grew up in households with similar incomes.[39] Researchers concluded that this finding "undermines the widely held belief that class, not ['race,'] is the most fundamental predictor of economic outcomes for children in the United States."[40]
- **Wealth and education don't level the playing field.** Inequities persist even when comparing wealth and education. White people who did not complete high school, for

example, have a higher median net worth than Black and Latine college graduates[41]— revealing how wealth accumulation is shaped by racial inequities, not simply personal or educational achievements.

- **High incomes don't erase unjust racial health disparities.** Even among people with high incomes, racial inequities in health persist. Despite having access to above-average social and economic resources, Black and Latine people who have a high socio-economic status report significantly worse health compared with similarly situated white people. For white people, moderate income gains over time resulted in significantly less exposure to acute and chronic discrimination and unfair treatment. But, by contrast, upwardly mobile Black and Latine people were significantly *more likely* to experience acute and chronic discrimination.[42] While economic success often shields white people from harm, for people of color, it perversely and all too often increases visibility and vulnerability.

- **Wealth and fame don't insulate against discrimination or criminalization.** High-income and highly visible people of color still face discrimination. For example, tennis champion and entrepreneur Serena Williams nearly died after childbirth due to medical providers dismissing her symptoms—an experience that mirrors research showing Black women are three times more likely to die from pregnancy-related causes than white women, regardless of income or education.[8] Other prominent people of color have shared harrowing experiences, from actor and filmmaker Forest Whitaker, who was falsely accused of shoplifting,[43] to comedian and actor Jay Pharoah, who was held at gunpoint by police while simply walking outside.[44] These stories are not anomalies; they reflect patterns of profiling, surveillance, and violence experienced by Black people across the socioeconomic spectrum.

These examples reveal that racism is not just additive to poverty; racism is foundational to how poverty is structured, reproduced, and maintained across class lines. The mindset, "Poor health isn't about 'race'—just money," is dangerous precisely because it attempts to erase this knowledge. It ignores a fundamental truth: Poor white families and poor families of color have different health outcomes, and people of color with high incomes are still subject to racism that harms their health.

But perhaps most importantly, this mindset serves a deeper political function: It undermines the very possibility of cross-racial solidarity. By treating "race" as unrelated to class, this mindset negates the way racial capitalism uses racism to divide people with shared economic interests. When racism is ignored or treated as separate from economic injustice, it drives a wedge between communities that would otherwise benefit by uniting against systems that perpetuate economic exploitation. As discussed in Chapter 2, this "divide and conquer" strategy has long been used by those in power to prevent the formation of multiracial, working-class social justice movements.[32]

In the final years of his life, Baptist minister and civil rights leader Martin Luther King Jr. helped launch the *Poor People's Campaign*—a movement built on the moral conviction that liberation requires linking the struggle against racism with the struggle against poverty. A renewed version of the Poor People's Campaign, led by ministers and organizers William Barber II and Liz Theoharis, kicked off nearly five decades later to continue the work King and his colleagues started: to build multiracial solidarity across poor communities and disrupt the economic structures that devalue human life.[45]

Ignoring "race" in conversations about poverty doesn't just distort the truth; it fractures solidarity among poor, working-class, and wage-dependent communities, making it harder for them to work together to advance common interests. To build the coalitions necessary to create positive and lasting change, we must reject this false dichotomy and embrace a mindset that recognizes how racism and economic injustice are deeply intertwined.

Let's replace this misleading mindset with a more just one:

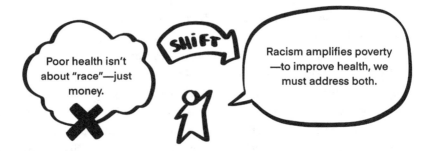

Focusing only on poverty ignores how racism shapes who is poor, which paths brought them there, and the harms they face because of it. A more accurate lens can help public health practitioners target root causes and implement interventions that simultaneously address structural racism and economic injustice.

MISLEADING MINDSET: SOME PEOPLE DESERVE POOR HEALTH

We need a world that insists upon safety and dignity for all of us—not because we are beautiful, healthy, blameless, exceptional, or beyond reproach, but because we are human beings.
—Aubrey Gordon, writer and cultural critic[46(p221)]

Another common but misleading mindset is that some individuals or groups "deserve" poor health outcomes because of their personal choices, behaviors, or life circumstances. This myth wrongly shifts blame from systems to individuals, reinforcing stigma and ignoring the many structural factors that shape health and well-being.

Rooted in broader and often racialized notions that some people deserve help and others do not, this mindset dates back to colonial and Victorian-era policies that categorized people based on perceptions of morality, work ethic, and "worthiness" of support.[47]

These policies targeted and blamed marginalized people, particularly people of color, immigrants, and disabled people. These ideas crossed the Atlantic Ocean and became embedded in US policies and attitudes, resurfacing time and again in ways that criminalize poverty and uphold structural racism. Here are some examples of this misleading mindset in action:

- **The "welfare queen" myth:** Politicians have long invoked stereotypes of laziness and fraud to weaponize racial prejudice and to justify cutting essential social service programs. The term "welfare queen"—popularized in the 1980s by then-presidential candidate Ronald Reagan—perpetuated a fictional and racist stereotype that portrayed Black women as opportunists who exploited welfare systems to fund luxurious lifestyles.[48] This false narrative discredited the reality of poverty in communities of color that was largely driven by systemic factors like redlining, community disinvestment, and wage stagnation. Moreover, "welfare queen" narratives and their offshoots undermined the value of social service programs by characterizing them as unnecessary and prone to fraud. This myth helped drive welfare "reforms" in the 1980s and 1990s, which simultaneously reduced benefits and made them more difficult to access, imposed stringent work requirements, and increased surveillance of recipients—adding additional hardship for those who were already struggling.
- **SNAP restrictions that punish poverty:** Policies that force people to meet punitive work requirements to access basic benefits through the Supplemental Nutrition Assistance Program (SNAP) harm people facing economic precarity—especially workers with unstable employment, low-wage earners, women, and people with disabilities. These restrictions reduce access to essential food assistance without actually increasing long-term employment prospects and economic mobility.[49] Other restrictions, such as prohibiting SNAP recipients from purchasing hot or prepared foods, hurt people who cannot cook for themselves, such as people experiencing homelessness or who have a disability that hinders them from preparing food.[50] These policies reinforce unfounded stereotypes about the "lazy" poor and narrow definitions of "responsible" food consumption, all the while ignoring the real-life constraints faced by SNAP recipients, further stigmatizing low-income people and their families.
- **Punishing people experiencing homelessness:** Public attitudes toward homelessness often divide people who are unhoused into the "deserving" and "undeserving"—with veterans or families deemed more worthy of help, for example, than people struggling with addiction or who have had interactions with the criminal legal system.[51] This harmful and divisive framing distorts funding priorities and policy responses, ultimately undermining access to supportive housing for all who need it. As a result, many so-called solutions to homelessness prioritize short-term shelters with limited services and no continuity of care. They rarely involve investing in long-term

solutions like *Housing First** strategies that provide people with permanent housing without preconditions and requirements, as well as comprehensive, wraparound support services as a foundation for long-term stability.

- **The persecution of immigrants:** Immigration debates are often framed in terms of "deserving" versus "undeserving" immigrants, favoring those perceived as economically beneficial—such as those with specialized expertise or advanced training—while stigmatizing undocumented individuals and people fleeing violence and poverty. These narratives are rooted in racism and legitimize the systematic devaluation and subjugation of immigrants—human beings who have inherent dignity and worth. Public figures have openly expressed preferences for immigrants from majority-white nations, while portraying Black and brown immigrants as undesirable and threatening.[52,53] Policies like the "public charge" rule reflect and reinforce systems of oppression by restricting entry into the United States based on perceived economic worth.[54] One of the most visible and violent expressions of racist nativism has been the raids carried out by Immigration and Customs Enforcement—often in cooperation with other government agencies.[55] These inhumane, military-style operations routinely bypass due process[56] and target immigrants as well as US citizens, legal permanent residents, visitors, students, and tourists.[57] The result is widespread terror and destabilization, tearing apart families and disrupting entire communities.[58,59]

The "some people deserve poor health" mindset unjustly punishes people for the impacts of systems of oppression on their lives. As public health practitioners, we must reject cruel mindsets and narratives that convey that only certain groups "deserve" to be part of our shared social fabric. Instead, we must embrace our collective responsibility to create conditions that allow everyone to flourish:

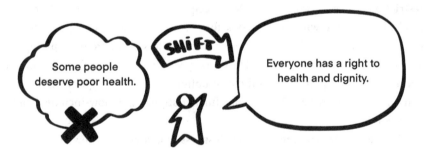

This shift moves us away from blame and toward solidarity. It reframes health, not as a reward for "good behavior" or a reflection of personal worth, but as a right to which we are all entitled and a collective responsibility rather than an individual outcome.

Housing First was developed by clinical psychologist and Pathways to Housing founder Sam Tsemberis. See Tsemberis S. Housing First: Implementation, dissemination, and program fidelity. *Am J Psychiatr Rehabil.* 2013;16(4):235–239. doi:10.1080/15487768.2013.847732

Everyone—regardless of income, identity, or life circumstances—deserves the conditions necessary to be healthy and safe, and to be treated with dignity and respect.

MISLEADING MINDSET: PROGRESS IS INEVITABLE

[H]uman progress never rolls in on wheels of inevitability. It comes through the tireless efforts and the persistent work of dedicated individuals. Without this hard work, time becomes an ally of the primitive forces of social stagnation.

–Martin Luther King Jr., Baptist minister and civil rights leader[60]

A common belief in the United States is that society is always moving forward—that social progress naturally advances with time. But history tells a different story. According to the Aspen Institute, history shows that "progress is made through the passage of legislation, court rulings and other formal mechanisms" but is inevitably "challenged, neutralized or undermined."[61] This means that progress is never linear, guaranteed, or self-sustaining. Gains in civil rights, health, and justice have been achieved through ongoing struggles that have been repeatedly met with backlash and retrenchment.

The pattern is persistent: Victories of equity and justice are almost always followed by deliberate efforts to undermine them. Examples exist across history and throughout the present day:

- **Reconstruction and Jim Crow.** The progressive victories of Reconstruction included the abolition of chattel slavery, citizenship for formerly enslaved people, and voting rights for Black men. Several Black men briefly held seats in the US Congress, and civil rights laws were adopted to address racial discrimination. However, the Compromise of 1877 effectively ended Reconstruction. It gave Rutherford B. Hayes the presidency in exchange for withdrawing federal troops from the South and leaving Black communities to be tormented by white supremacist violence. This compromise by Congress provided fertile ground for *Jim Crow*—a system of state and local laws that legalized racial segregation, oppression, and violence—to control all aspects of daily life for nearly a century.
- **The Civil Rights Movement and the rollbacks that followed.** The progressive victories of the 1960s and 1970s, achieved through the advocacy of Black activists and their allies, included the Civil Rights Act of 1964, the Voting Rights Act of 1965, and the Fair Housing Act of 1968. But these wins were quickly followed by a generations-long backlash that eroded gains in desegregation, antidiscrimination, and voting rights protection. In the decades that followed, "law and order" policies, mass incarceration, and attacks on voting rights proliferated— culminating in the Supreme Court's 2013 decision in *Shelby County v Holder*, which paved the way for a wave of new voter suppression laws that were adopted across the country.[62]

- **Reproductive rights and the repeal of *Roe v Wade*.** The reproductive rights movement of the 1960s and early 1970s achieved the legalization of abortion through the landmark *Roe v Wade* Supreme Court case. However, these advances were eroded and dismantled over successive decades—and have been eviscerated in recent years. The 2022 Supreme Court case *Dobbs v Jackson Women's Health Organization* overturned *Roe v Wade* and stripped away a constitutional right to abortion that stood for nearly 50 years. Without federal protections for abortion, women must rely on states to safeguard abortion rights amid ongoing efforts to restrict and criminalize abortion—disproportionately harming low-income women and women of color.
- **Marriage equality and anti-queer legislation.** The 2015 Supreme Court decision *Obergefell v Hodges* was a landmark victory that legalized same-sex marriage across the country. But recently, a wave of anti-queer legislation has emerged—notable for its specific targeting of transgender and nonbinary people. Laws banning gender-affirming care, prohibiting any mention of queer identities in schools, restricting participation in sports, and criminalizing bathroom access based on gender identity all reflect ongoing efforts to roll back queer rights.[63,64]
- **The 2020 racial reckoning and ongoing backlash.** In the wake of George Floyd's murder by a Minneapolis, Minnesota police officer and the COVID-19 pandemic's disproportionate toll on communities of color, 2020 saw unprecedented protests and public dialogue about structural racism. Racial justice became an openly discussed hot topic. Corporations pledged billions to support racial justice initiatives, and some institutions implemented modest reforms. But this moment was short-lived. In the years since, we've seen bans prohibiting schools from teaching students about racism and Critical Race Theory (CRT)*[65]; attacks on diversity, equity, and inclusion initiatives[66]; the Supreme Court dismantling affirmative action in higher education[67]; and widespread corporate backpedaling on financial pledges to address racism.[68] Together, these reversals reflect a systematic effort to suppress racial justice in public and private sectors throughout the United States.

Progress is not permanent, and it is not inevitable. It must be made, defended, and remade through sustained struggle. The idea that "things will improve with time" is not only inaccurate but also leads to complacency and inaction. It absolves individuals and institutions of our collective responsibility for making progress. It also undermines the

---

*Anti-CRT laws directed toward K–12 educational institutions are not only racist but also unnecessary. CRT is an advanced area of legal scholarship that is generally taught to law students. CRT is not commonly taught in undergraduate education, let alone K–12 schools.

ongoing collective mobilization required for social advancement by erasing the hard but necessary work of organizing, advocacy, and coalition-building.

Change doesn't equal progress. As discussed in Chapter 2, systems of oppression like structural racism constantly adapt over time and take on new and insidious forms. Systems and policies will always evolve, but without an ongoing and intentional focus on equity and justice, they will not change for the better.

Systems change is a dynamic process, shaped by power struggles, setbacks, and rebounds. The stronger the progress, the stronger the backlash often becomes. And without deliberate effort, even the most significant gains can be negated. But this should not cause us to lose hope; it should keep us alert and prepared to leverage lessons from history to inform new strategies that we can implement today. We can prepare by building diverse coalitions, by designing policies that are thoughtful and inclusive, and by taking a long view of our work.

We can draw inspiration from the **Seven Generations value** of the Haudenosaunee Confederacy (that includes the Mohawk, Oneida, Onondaga, Cayuga, and Seneca peoples), which calls on us to consider how today's decisions will impact those who come after us—because we are merely borrowing the world from future generations.[69]

With this in mind, let's replace this misleading mindset with a more just one:

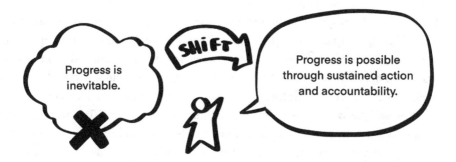

Justice is not a "natural" outcome of time; it is a product of collective, strategic, and long-term efforts in which we all must be engaged. It requires both urgency and endurance. That means recognizing the value of incremental gains and short-term solutions— not as ends in themselves, but as steps in a much longer journey. A policy change, budget win, or organizational reform may provide meaningful relief and build momentum—but only if we follow up to ask: *What's next? How do we leverage this moment to go further and deeper?*

By adopting this new mindset, we can be ready for the ongoing work required to create change. We can celebrate successes while simultaneously preparing for the resistance we will inevitably face. When we are prepared, organized, and focused on the long term, we can lay a foundation for progress that lasts.

TRANSFORMING MINDSETS TO EMBRACE EQUITY AND JUSTICE

The world changes according to the way people see it, and if you alter, even by a millimeter, the way a person looks at reality, then you can change it.
                                                   –James Baldwin, author and cultural critic[70]

To create meaningful change, we must challenge harmful mindsets and replace them with justice-centered ones. While underlying mindsets don't change overnight, they *can* shift—and with enough effort, they can be transformed. We have already seen powerful mindset and narrative shifts that demonstrate progress is possible. Consider these examples:

- **Mental health as a shared human experience.** Once stigmatized as a private burden or a moral failing, mental health is increasingly seen as a collective concern that affects everyone. As public narratives have evolved, so too has the mindset—from one of individual shame and silence to one of collective experience and responsibility. We have begun to use terms like *mental health* and *mental well-being*, rather than simply referring to *mental illness*. These terms have helped us move away from a deficit-based lens, toward a broader understanding of what it takes to have a healthy mental state. This shift has also helped expand mental health resources, reduce stigma, and integrate mental health supports into schools, workplaces, and primary care.
- **The criminal legal system as unjust by design.** For decades, mainstream narratives blamed "crime" on individuals and painted police as impartial enforcers of justice. However, advocates' sustained focus on police violence and structural discrimination has shifted mindsets and brought to light that injustice is embedded within the system itself. This shift has even influenced our language: Many of us more accurately refer to the *criminal legal system* rather than the "criminal justice system." This mindset shift has sparked conversations about decarceration, abolition, and restorative justice (see Chapter 6 for more). It's a mindset shift that moves us from individual blame to structural accountability.
- **Climate change as a justice and public health issue.** Once viewed as purely an environmental concern or esoteric scientific topic, climate change is now recognized as a crisis of justice and public health. The mindset has shifted from climate change as distant and technical to understanding it as an urgent moral issue that disproportionately harms communities of color, low-income communities, youth, and future generations. This has brought climate change to the forefront and has highlighted the leadership of youth and frontline communities—those who bear the greatest burdens of climate change—who are calling for transformative change and a sustainable, livable future.

Changing how we think can change what we do. When mindsets and narratives evolve, they create space for new policies, partnerships, and possibilities to emerge. That's why shaping mindsets must be a core competency of public health—not only as a communications strategy but also as a foundation for lasting change.

Today, our challenge is to change mindsets and narratives by telling stories that uplift intersectionality, solidarity, collective action, and transformative change. The *Narratives for Health* initiative highlights a set of powerful core messages that we can use to create new mindsets and narratives.[71] Examples of these core messages include the following:

- **Diversity is our greatest strength.** This message highlights that our differences— across "race," gender, ability, age, and more—are powerful assets. It counters the idea that equity creates division or provides unfair advantages and instead frames it as a pathway to a healthier, more inclusive society that benefits everyone.
- **Our public sphere prioritizes collective well-being.** This message reclaims the responsibility of the public sector and government to care for everyone, emphasizing that we all benefit when we invest in community health, well-being, and flourishing. It challenges privatization and "austerity logic" by asserting that public systems are essential for justice and care. It invites us to reimagine what public goods are and how we collectively govern them.
- **We have the power to transform the future.** This message centers agency and possibility, particularly in communities most harmed by injustice. It affirms that we already have the power to make the changes we want to see—that transformation is not only possible but is already underway. This frame invites collective imagination and sustained action to co-create a just future.

When we use these kinds of messages intentionally, we can open people's minds, challenge harmful assumptions, and spark change that goes beyond individual behavior. At a time of growing backlash, polarization, and disinformation, we must do more than counter misleading mindsets and harmful narratives—we must displace them entirely by offering better ones. That means telling stories rooted in solidarity, accountability, collective action, and care. And it means doing it together, across sectors, communities, and movements.

CONCLUSION

Mindsets and narratives shape public perception, inform policy decisions, and define whose experiences and needs are prioritized. As public health practitioners, we must take ownership of the stories we tell about health—what drives inequities, where responsibility lies, and what solutions are possible. Too often, those of us in public health have been reactive rather than proactive in defining the values, beliefs, and stories that characterize our work.

If we don't lead the public health narrative, others will—often in ways that distort our work, invalidate the structural and systemic causes of health inequities, and weaponize disinformation to justify harmful policies. Writer and cultural critic Aubrey Gordon warns that "if we are passive, we absorb the bias in the world around us."[46(p28)] This applies to us in public health. We must openly refute the destructive mindsets and narratives that dominate the public discourse. If we don't speak up, we allow dangerous stories to drive the creation of policies and other tools for systems change in ways that only deepen inequities.

By challenging harmful mindsets and reshaping narratives about public health problems, we can build the political and social will necessary for systemic solutions. The power of public health lies not only in data and policy but also in its ability to shape how people think about health, well-being, and the systems that govern our lives.

That starts with the stories we tell—and the mindsets we inspire. As narrative strategist and anthropologist Ella Saltmarshe reminds us, "story helps illuminate the past, present, and future, thus lighting up the paths of change."[72] We have the power to transform beliefs and create new, compelling stories that people will be eager to make real.

KEY TAKEAWAYS

 Mindsets and narratives shape how we understand the world and what we believe is possible. *Mindsets* are the deeply held beliefs, attitudes, assumptions, and perspectives that shape how we think about the world. *Narratives* are the stories we tell ourselves and each other about how the world works and what we believe to be true and possible. Mindsets and narratives operate in a feedback loop, reinforcing and amplifying one another. Together, they shape how problems are defined, which solutions are considered acceptable and feasible, and whose voices are valued.

 The *Iceberg Model* helps us see and shift the systems, narratives, and mindsets that lie beneath the surface. Many public health efforts focus only on visible symptoms, like behaviors and events. But lasting and large-scale change requires us to look deeper—at the patterns, structures, systems, and beliefs that lie beneath. The Iceberg Model helps us do just that. It reminds us that what's visible above the surface is only a small part of the story. To transform systems, we need to work below the waterline: changing institutional practices, challenging harmful narratives, and transforming the mindsets that uphold them.

 We must reject misleading mindsets that distract—and detract—from equity and justice. Misleading mindsets have long governed our approach to public health. These include erroneous beliefs and stories that ignore how our circumstances shape our health, deny the impact of racism on poverty, treat some people as deserving of poor health, and blame people for systemic failures. These misleading mindsets divert attention and critical resources away from where they *should* be invested: addressing systems of oppression and structural inequities that ultimately drive poor health outcomes.

 Progress is not inevitable—it takes preparation, endurance, and vigilance. Throughout history, whenever we've made significant gains in civil rights, health, and justice, they have been quickly met with backlash and retrenchment. It's a recurring pattern for which we can and should be prepared. Progress is not "natural" or guaranteed. It requires constant attention and deliberate effort. To advance equity and justice, we must continually build and strengthen our coalitions, push for policies that are inclusive and community-centered, and ground our work in the *Seven Generations value*—meaning that we must consider how our decisions today will impact future generations for decades to come.

 Changing mindsets is our responsibility as public health practitioners. While mindsets shape what we believe, narratives influence how those beliefs are communicated, understood, and spread. Everything tells a story— even seemingly "objective" information like data, research findings, and evaluation metrics. As public health practitioners, we can challenge dominant narratives that uphold inequity and tell new stories that reflect shared values, collective care, and the importance of systemic change. In doing so, we can transform mindsets and change what people believe is necessary and possible.

REFERENCES

1. Jones S. *America: Who Hurt You?* Who cares about the 'care economy'? with Ai-jen Poo (season 1, episode 6). August 28, 2024. Accessed August 8, 2025. https://podcasts.apple.com/us/podcast/who-cares-about-the-care-economy-w-ai-jen-poo/id1756434781?i=1000666886489
2. Buchanan A. The nature of mindsets. *Medium.* March 16, 2017. Accessed May 11, 2025. https://medium.com/benefit-mindset/the-nature-of-mindsets-18afba2ac890
3. FrameWorks Institute. Mindset shifts: What are they? Why do they matter? How do they happen? June 2020. Accessed May 11, 2025. https://www.frameworksinstitute.org/resources/mindset-shifts-what-are-they-why-do-they-matter-how-do-they-happen
4. McAfee M, Dunn V. *Governing for All: An Equity Narrative Playbook for Policymakers.* PolicyLink. 2022. Accessed June 3, 2025. https://www.policylink.org/sites/default/files/Governing%20for%20All%20Playbook.pdf
5. Baker E. The Black woman in the civil rights struggle—1969. Archives of Women's Political Communication. Iowa State University. August 9, 2019. Accessed June 7, 2025. https://awpc.cattcenter.iastate.edu/2019/08/09/the-black-woman-in-the-civil-rights-struggle-1969
6. Kania J, Kramer M, Senge P. The water of systems change. FSG. 2018. Accessed August 1, 2025. https://www.fsg.org/resource/water_of_systems_change

7. The Donella Meadows Project, Academy for Systems Change. Systems thinking resources: The iceberg model. Accessed May 11, 2025. https://donellameadows.org/systems-thinking-resources

8. Howell EA. Reducing disparities in severe maternal morbidity and mortality. *Clin Obstet Gynecol.* 2018;61(2):387–399. doi:10.1097/GRF.0000000000000349.

9. Kaiser Permanente Institute for Health Policy. How racism makes people sick: A conversation with Camara Phyllis Jones, MD, MPH, PhD. Kaiser Permanente Institute for Health Policy. August 2, 2016. https://www.kpihp.org/blog/how-racism-makes-people-sick-a-conversation-with-camara-phyllis-jones-md-mph-phd

10. Marmot M, Allen JJ. Social determinants of health equity. *Am J Public Health.* 2014;104(suppl 4):S517–S519. doi:10.2105/AJPH.2014.302200

11. Baum F, Fisher M. Why behavioural health promotion endures despite its failure to reduce health inequities. *Sociol Health Illn.* 2014;36(2):213–225. doi:10.1111/1467-9566.12112

12. Chater N, Loewenstein G. The i-frame and the s-frame: How focusing on individual-level solutions has led behavioral public policy astray. *Behav Brain Sci.* 2023;46:e147. doi:10.1017/S0140525X22002023

13. Iton A, Ross RK, Tamber P. Building community power to dismantle policy-based structural inequity in population health. *Health Aff (Millwood).* 2022;41(12):1763–1771. doi:10.1377/hlthaff.2022.00540

14. Plumer B. The origins of anti-litter campaigns. *Mother Jones.* May 22, 2006. Accessed May 12, 2025. https://www.motherjones.com/politics/2006/05/origins-anti-litter-campaigns

15. Stuckler D, Nestle M. Big Food, food systems, and global health. *PLoS Med.* 2012;9(6):e1001242. doi:10.1371/journal.pmed.1001242

16. The Lancet Gastroenterology & Hepatology. Shining a light on international alcohol industry lobbying. *Lancet Gastroenterol Hepatol.* 2022;7(4):275. doi:10.1016/S2468-1253(22)00060-7

17. De D, El Jamal M, Aydemir E, Khera A. Social media algorithms and teen addiction: Neurophysiological impact and ethical considerations. *Cureus.* 2025;17(1):e77145. doi:10.7759/cureus.77145

18. Let's Move! White House. Achievements. Accessed May 12, 2025. https://letsmove.obamawhitehouse.archives.gov/achievements

19. Etzioni A. Michelle Obama's "Let's Move" is losing its footing. *Health Affairs Forefront.* June 28, 2011. Accessed May 12, 2025. https://www.healthaffairs.org/do/10.1377/forefront.20110628.012025

20. Dillon S. Lines grow long for free school meals, thanks to economy. *New York Times.* November 30, 2011. Accessed May 12, 2025. https://www.nytimes.com/2011/11/30/education/surge-in-free-school-lunches-reflects-economic-crisis.html

21. Let's Move! Let's Move! in Indian Country: A call to action for Indian Country. 2011. Accessed May 12, 2025. https://letsmove.obamawhitehouse.archives.gov/sites/letsmove.gov/files/LMIC_CalltoActionFinal.pdf

22. Thousands of US public employees laid off in 2010. Reuters. August 30, 2011. Accessed May 12, 2025. https://www.reuters.com/article/business/thousands-of-public-laid-off-in-2010-idUSTRE77T4A9

23. US Dept of Agriculture. USDA releases study on hurdles to healthy eating on SNAP. June 23, 2021. Accessed August 4, 2025. https://www.usda.gov/about-usda/news/press-releases/2021/06/23/usda-releases-study-hurdles-healthy-eating-snap

24. Walker J. 'Food desert' vs. 'food apartheid': Which term best describes disparities in food access? University of Michigan School for Environment and Sustainability. November 29, 2023. Accessed May 12, 2025. https://seas.umich.edu/news/food-desert-vs-food-apartheid-which-term-best-describes-disparities-food-access

25. Sharkey JR. Measuring potential access to food stores and food-service places in rural areas in the US. *Am J Prev Med.* 2009;36(suppl 4):S151–S152. doi:10.1016/j.amepre.2009.01.004

26. LaFree A, Soloway M. Incentivizing fresh food retail in food deserts: Lessons learned from Pennsylvania and Maryland. Network for Public Health Law. 2021. Accessed May 12, 2025. https://www.networkforphl.org/wp-content/uploads/2021/05/Incentivizing-Fresh-Food-Retail-in-Food-Deserts-Lessons-Learned-from-Pennsylvania-and-Maryland-FINAL.pdf

27. Rowlands DW, Donoghoe M, Perry AM. What the lack of premium grocery stores says about disinvestment in Black neighborhoods. Brookings. April 11, 2023. Accessed May 6, 2025. https://www.brookings.edu/articles/what-the-lack-of-premium-grocery-stores-says-about-disinvestment-in-black-neighborhoods

28. Leslie CR. Food deserts, racism, and antitrust law. *Calif Law Rev.* 2022;110(6):1717–1776. doi:10.15779/Z38GM81P9R

29. Oliver J. TANF: Last Week Tonight with John Oliver (HBO). YouTube. June 13, 2022. Accessed May 13, 2025. https://www.youtube.com/watch?v=wJDk-czsivk

30. Bergh K. Millions of low-income households would lose food aid under proposed House Republican SNAP cuts. Center on Budget and Policy Priorities. February 24, 2025. Accessed June 3, 2025. https://www.cbpp.org/research/food-assistance/millions-of-low-income-households-would-lose-food-aid-under-proposed-house

31. Johnston KD. Agriculture on the move: Proposed actions to bolster local food systems. *Campbell Law Rev.* 2023;46:137. Accessed June 1, 2025. https://scholarship.law.campbell.edu/clr/vol46/iss1/5

32. McGhee H. *The Sum of Us: What Racism Costs Everyone and How We Can Prosper Together.* One World; 2021.

33. Badger E. Black poverty differs from white poverty. *Washington Post.* August 12, 2015. Accessed May 12, 2025. https://www.washingtonpost.com/news/wonk/wp/2015/08/12/black-poverty-differs-from-white-poverty

34. Elliott D. Two American experiences: the racial divide of poverty. Urban Institute. July 21, 2016. Accessed May 12, 2025. https://www.urban.org/urban-wire/two-american-experiences-racial-divide-poverty

35. Reardon SF, Fox L, Townsend J. Neighborhood income composition by household race and income, 1990–2009. *Ann Am Acad Polit Soc Sci.* 2015;660(1):78–97. doi:10.1177/0002716215576104

36. Grann D. *Killers of the Flower Moon: The Osage Murders and the Birth of the FBI.* Doubleday; 2017.

37. Krehbiel R. *TULSA, 1921: Reporting a Massacre.* University of Oklahoma Press; 2021.

38. US Commission on Wartime Relocation and Internment of Civilians. *Personal Justice Denied: Report of the Commission on Wartime Relocation and Internment of Civilians.* University of Washington Press; 1997.

39. Chetty R, Hendren N, Jones MR, Porter SR. Race and economic opportunity in the United States: An intergenerational perspective. *Q J Econ.* 2020;135(2):711–783. doi:10.1093/qje/qjz042

40. Keller J. Forget wealth and neighborhood: The racial income gap persists. *CPR News*. March 19, 2018. Accessed May 16, 2025. https://www.cpr.org/2018/03/19/forget-wealth-and-neighborhood-the-racial-income-gap-persists

41. Fletcher MA. White high school dropouts are wealthier than Black and Hispanic college graduates—can a new policy tool fix that? *Washington Post*. March 10, 2015. Accessed June 3, 2025. https://www.washingtonpost.com/news/wonk/wp/2015/03/10/white-high-school-dropouts-are-wealthier-than-black-and-hispanic-college-graduates-can-a-new-policy-tool-fix-that

42. Colen CG, Ramey DM, Cooksey EC, Williams DR. Racial disparities in health among nonpoor African Americans and Hispanics: The role of acute and chronic discrimination. *Soc Sci Med*. 2018;199:167-180. doi:10.1016/j.socscimed.2017.04.051

43. Thomas E. Forest Whitaker falsely accused of shoplifting: How do I explain racism to my son? *Washington Post*. February 21, 2013. Accessed June 3, 2025. https://www.washingtonpost.com/blogs/therootdc/post/forest-whitaker-falsely-accused-of-shoplifting-how-do-i-explain-racism-to-my-son/2013/02/21/164886d2-7c65-11e2-a044-676856536b40_blog.html

44. Jay Pharoah says "sorry" from LAPD cops who forcibly detained him with guns drawn is "not enough." *CBS News*. June 17, 2020. Accessed August 1, 2025. https://www.cbsnews.com/news/jay-pharoah-lapd-detained-sorry

45. Kaufmann G. The Poor People's Campaign calls out "policy violence." *The Nation*. October 16, 2018. Accessed May 16, 2025. https://www.thenation.com/article/archive/the-poor-peoples-campaign-calls-out-policy-violence

46. Gordon A. *What We Don't Talk About When We Talk About Fat*. Beacon Press; 2020.

47. Quigley WP. Five hundred years of English Poor Laws, 1349-1834: Regulating the working and nonworking poor. *Akron Law Rev*. 1996;30(1):73-128. Accessed May 16, 2025. https://www.uakron.edu/dotAsset/726694.pdf

48. Byrd A. LISTEN: Code Switch dives into the story behind the 'Welfare Queen.' *Colorlines*. June 10, 2019. Accessed May 16, 2025. https://colorlines.com/article/listen-code-switch-dives-story-behind-welfare-queen

49. Khan F. Congress is debating stricter SNAP and Medicaid work requirements, but research shows they don't work. Brookings Institution. March 3, 2025. Accessed June 26, 2025. https://www.brookings.edu/articles/congress-is-debating-stricter-snap-and-medicaid-work-requirements-but-research-shows-they-dont-work

50. Food Research & Action Center. Hot Foods Act (H.R. 3519/S. 2258) fact sheet. October 2023. Accessed June 26, 2025. https://frac.org/wp-content/uploads/Hot-Foods-Act-Fact-Sheet.pdf

51. Adams B, Welsh Carroll M, Gutierrez N. Community acceptance of, and opposition to, homeless-serving facilities. *Int J Homelessness*. 2023;3(2):156-183. doi:10.5206/ijoh.2022.2.14785

52. Pengelly M. Trump bemoans lack of immigrants from majority-white countries to the US. *The Guardian*. April 8, 2024. Accessed May 16, 2025. https://www.theguardian.com/us-news/2024/apr/08/trump-immigration-north-europe

53. Vitali A, Hunt K, Thorp F V. Trump referred to Haiti and African nations as 'shithole' countries. *NBC News*. January 11, 2018. Accessed May 16, 2025. https://www.nbcnews.com/politics/white-house/trump-referred-haiti-african-countries-shithole-nations-n836946

54. Mock B. The racism behind Trump's new 'public charge' immigration policy, explained. Bloomberg. August 14, 2019. Accessed May 16, 2025. https://www.bloomberg.com/news/articles/2019-08-14/the-racist-roots-of-trump-s-public-charge-policy

55. Ochacher J, Montoya-Galvez C, Ingram J. A majority of ICE arrests in Trump's first 5 months took place in border and Southern states, figures show. CBS News. July 31, 2025. Accessed August 4, 2025. https://www.cbsnews.com/news/ice-arrests-border-and-southern-states

56. Bustillo X. Trump wants to bypass immigration courts. Experts warn it's a 'slippery slope'. NPR. April 29, 2025. Accessed August 4, 2025. https://www.npr.org/2025/04/29/g-s1-63187/trump-courts-immigration-judges-due-process

57. Debusmann Jr B. Who has been arrested by ICE under Trump? BBC. June 11, 2025. Accessed August 4, 2025. https://www.bbc.com/news/articles/c86p821p660o

58. Barshad A. 'People are scared to go out': Fear of ICE agents forces cancellation of US summer festivals. The Guardian. August 4, 2025. Accessed August 4, 2025. https://www.theguardian.com/us-news/2025/aug/04/latino-festivals-cancelled-ice-immigration-raids

59. Dahlberg VI. ICE's military-style raid leaves immigrant communities terrorized. American Civil Liberties Union. August 29, 2019. Accessed August 4, 2025. https://www.aclu.org/news/immigrants-rights/ices-military-style-raid-leaves-immigrant

60. Oberlin College Archives. Martin Luther King, Jr. at Oberlin. June 1965. Accessed August 2, 2025. https://www2.oberlin.edu/external/EOG/BlackHistoryMonth/MLK/CommAddress.html

61. The Aspen Institute. What is structural racism? July 11, 2016. Accessed June 3, 2025. https://web.archive.org/web/20240308020323/https://www.aspeninstitute.org/blog-posts/structural-racism-definition

62. Singh J, Carter S. States have added nearly 100 restrictive laws since SCOTUS gutted the Voting Rights Act 10 years ago. Brennan Center for Justice. June 23, 2023. Accessed June 3, 2025. https://www.brennancenter.org/our-work/analysis-opinion/states-have-added-nearly-100-restrictive-laws-scotus-gutted-voting-rights

63. American Civil Liberties Union. Mapping attacks on LGBTQ rights in US state legislatures in 2024. 2024. Accessed June 3, 2025. https://www.aclu.org/legislative-attacks-on-lgbtq-rights-2024

64. Trans Legislation Tracker. Tracking the rise of anti-trans bills in the US. Accessed June 3, 2025. https://translegislation.com/learn

65. Ray R, Gibbons A. Why are states banning Critical Race Theory? Brookings Institution. July 2021. Accessed May 16, 2025. https://www.brookings.edu/articles/why-are-states-banning-critical-race-theory

66. Murray C. IBM reportedly walks back diversity policies, citing "inherent tensions": Here are all the companies rolling back DEI programs. Forbes. April 11, 2025. Accessed June 3, 2025. https://www.forbes.com/sites/conormurray/2025/04/11/ibm-reportedly-walks-back-diversity-policies-citing-inherent-tensions-here-are-all-the-companies-rolling-back-dei-programs

67. Students for Fair Admissions, Inc v President and Fellows of Harvard College, 600 US 181 (2023).

68. Harper S. Where is the $200 billion companies promised after George Floyd's murder? Forbes. October 17, 2022. Accessed May 16, 2025. https://www.forbes.com/sites/shaunharper/2022/10/17/where-is-the-200-billion-companies-promised-after-george-floyds-murder

69. Haudenosaunee Confederacy. Values. Accessed May 17, 2025. https://www.haudenosaunee confederacy.com/values

70. Romano J. James Baldwin writing and talking. *New York Times Book Review.* September 23, 1979;3:36-37. Accessed June 3, 2025. https://www.nytimes.com/1979/09/23/archives/james-baldwin-writing-and-talking-baldwin-baldwin-authors-query.html

71. County Health Rankings & Roadmaps. Narratives for Health Guide. Accessed August 1, 2025. https://www.countyhealthrankings.org/sites/default/files/media/document/NFH_Guide_0.pdf

72. Saltmarshe E. Using story to change systems. *Stanford Social Innovation Review.* February 20, 2018. Accessed June 3, 2025. https://ssir.org/articles/entry/using_story_to_change_systems

5

Equity and Justice Are a Matter of Power

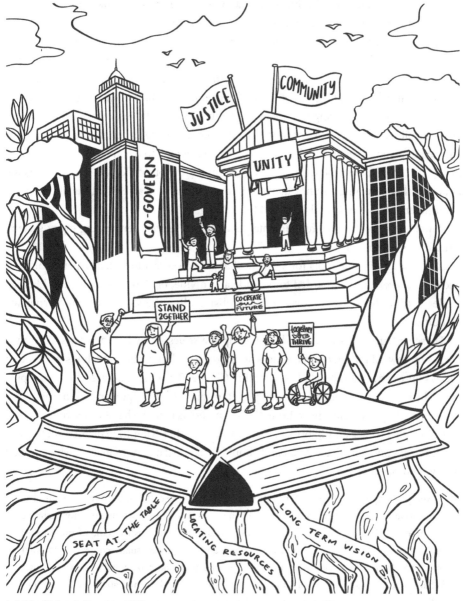

Artist Credit: Jasmin Pamukcu, 2025.

People Power

People with power don't get evicted. People with power don't get deported. People with power don't get displaced. They get to remain.
                        –Tomás Rivera, housing justice organizer and anti-displacement advocate[1]

When people think about health, they often picture personal choices—diet, exercise, or getting enough sleep. For those of us who are public health practitioners, the lens is wider. We understand that health is shaped by social determinants like housing quality, access to green space, clean air, and economic opportunity.

Yet there's a deeper, often overlooked force: power. **Power** is the ability to influence outcomes, make decisions, and control one's own destiny. It is the invisible architecture of our lives and is deeply embedded within systems of oppression and structural inequities (discussed in Chapter 3). Power is the difference between having insurance that covers preventive care and delaying treatment until you end up in the emergency room with a crushing bill. It's the difference between working a stable job with benefits and protections and being forced to get by with "under the table" wages and no recourse for harassment or injury. It's the difference between a school that nurtures your child and one that calls the police on them, turning a minor incident into a traumatizing arrest. Ultimately, power is the difference between languishing and flourishing.

Power is as present and fundamental as atoms in matter, permeating every system, structure, and experience.

And just as with the tools for systems change, power is a tool that depends on who wields it; power can be hoarded to degrade and divide, or shared to unite and liberate. Understanding how power works is key to dismantling the structures that perpetuate inequity.

These systems and structures don't just tip the scales—they *are* the scales. And they always tip toward power, determining who is positioned to thrive and who is locked into cycles of poverty, exclusion, and poor health. Chapter 3 examines how inequities are produced by systems that control access to power, resources, and opportunities. In this chapter, we turn to power itself: how it functions, who holds it, and what it can achieve.

Civil rights leader and Baptist minister Martin Luther King Jr. explained that power is not the enemy of justice—it can and should be an instrument of justice, when guided by love and purpose:

> Power, properly understood, is the ability to achieve purpose. It is the strength required to bring about social, political, or economic changes. In this sense power is not only desirable but necessary in order to implement the demands of love and justice. One of the greatest problems of history is that the concepts of love and power are usually contrasted as polar opposites. Love is identified with a resignation of power and power with a denial of love. What is needed is a realization that power without love is reckless and abusive and that love without power is sentimental and anemic. Power at its best is love implementing the demands of justice. Justice at its best is love correcting everything that stands against love.[2](p37–38)

King's vision is audacious and urgent: Justice is not possible without power, and power must be guided by love. This framing challenges us to rethink power—not as domination or control but as the capacity to enact justice. And it invites us to understand love as a moral imperative rooted in care, commitment, accountability, and a belief in the inherent worth of every person. Love is not conditional. It does not require someone to earn it, nor does it require perfection. Rather, it insists that everyone deserves to flourish simply because they are human—and justice demands intentional, collective power to make flourishing a reality.

This is public health at its best: a collective commitment and active application of love, power, and justice to create conditions in which all people can thrive.

These ideas about power may sound abstract, but as public health practitioners, we are already immersed in the dynamics of power every day. As discussed in Chapter 1, public health is rooted in social justice, and justice is always entangled with power. Whether engaging with government leaders like mayors and state health officials or connecting informally with influential colleagues and community leaders who have influence, access, and decision-shaping capacity, power is central to our work. It's part and parcel of what we do and how we get things done. But our endgame is never power for power's sake: We must build it, shift it, and share it with the communities we serve.

When we connect with partners and community members, we are shifting and sharing power to some degree. Although we commonly refer to these interactions as "community empowerment" or "community engagement," it's important that we differentiate between these terms and the deeper work of building, shifting, and sharing power.

"Community empowerment" rests on the flawed premise that power can be bestowed—especially by dominant institutions—rather than recognized as something communities already possess and have the right to exercise. This framing risks reinforcing paternalism, with outside actors deciding when and how to "empower" people.

"Community engagement" begins from a more thoughtful premise: that institutions and decision-makers must be in communication and partnership with communities. But community engagement often fails to go far enough. It stops short of actually shifting decision-making authority to communities themselves. Physicians and community health advocates Anthony Iton, Robert K. Ross, and Pritpal S. Tamber describe community engagement as "highly variable" in how it is practiced, noting that "some communities [are] merely being informed of strategies"[3(p1768)] rather than shaping them directly.

Building and sharing power involves far more than engagement; it requires intentionally shifting authority, agenda-setting, and decision-making control to marginalized communities to create lasting structural change. But to effectively create this kind of change, it is necessary to understand the basics of power.

THE BASICS OF POWER

[P]ower is real and effective in a remarkable variety of ways, some of them indirect and some hidden, and . . . indeed, it is at its most effective when least accessible to observation.
—Steven Lukes, political theorist and sociologist[4(p64)]

Fundamentally, power is about having control over one's destiny. It's at play whenever individuals or groups can influence the conditions of their lives—or are blocked from doing so. But power can oftentimes be hard to spot because it's so deeply woven into routines and relationships within our lives. Even when we don't notice it, power influences our choices, connections, and contexts. It isn't solely a matter of wealth or status, though both matter greatly. Its presence is reflected in who we know, resources we have access to, and what we can make possible.

Throughout this book, when people or communities are described as **marginalized**, it's a way of naming an abuse of power on a large scale—the result of systems of oppression that deny people access to rights, resources, and recognition. These systems—and the abuses they perpetrate—push people to the margins of civic life, public narratives, and community belonging. The margins are metaphorical edges: peripheral places far from the concentrated centers of influence, visibility, and decision-making authority. As a result, marginalized people are excluded from having access to resources and opportunities, representation in influential institutions, a voice in public discourse, visibility in mainstream narratives, and the ability to shape policies that affect their lives.

Power and marginalization have profound implications for health. Civic engagement, for example, is a commonly understood form of power that benefits not just individuals, but entire communities. Research shows that those who are civically engaged—whether through voting, volunteering, or participating in other forms of civic activism—are likely to have better physical, social, and mental well-being. And the converse is true as well: Low levels of civic engagement have been linked to poor health.[5]

The *quality of democracy*—or how well power is distributed and exercised through governance systems—is directly tied to health outcomes.[3] Inclusive civic participation—through voting, organizing, and public deliberation—is consistently tied to better health across communities. The Institute for Responsive Government's *Health & Democracy Index* finds that states with more accessible voting policies have lower uninsured rates, better mental health, and reduced infant mortality.[6] Healthier people are also more likely to engage civically, creating a virtuous cycle between health and democracy.[5]

Yet as explored in Chapter 3, this relationship between civic engagement and health has long been undermined by policies designed to strip certain communities of political power. Tactics like voter suppression, gerrymandering, voter roll purges, and other forms of voting disenfranchisement have all been intentionally deployed to negate marginalized communities' ability to influence governance and decision-making. Today, threats to democracy—such as election subversion, executive overreach, and disinformation—continue to erode public trust and restrict political power.[7] This means attacks on democracy should be understood, and responded to, as attacks on public health.

The first step toward using power in service of equity and justice is recognizing the types of power at play. The World Health Organization outlines four types of power,[8] and some community leaders have added a fifth:

- **Power over:** The ability to control or coerce others, often through hierarchy, authority, and domination. This form of power is typically unidirectional and reinforces inequitable relationships.
- **Power to:** The capacity of individuals or communities to take action, solve problems, and create change. This power grows as people gain knowledge, tools, and opportunities to influence their own lives and the systems around them.
- **Power with:** Collaborative power that emerges through solidarity, coalition-building, and partnerships. It reflects mutual support and collective strength, allowing people to accomplish more together than they could alone.
- **Power within:** The inner strength and sense of agency that comes from recognizing one's own dignity, worth, and ability to contribute. This is every person's birthright—not something bestowed by institutions—and can be strengthened through practices like *cultural affirmation* (celebrating and valuing one's cultural legacy and identities) and *consciousness raising* (building one's awareness of social and political conditions).
- **Power under:** The latent power that individuals and communities possess but do not use—whether due to internalized oppression, fear of reprisal, lack of opportunity, or lack of knowledge. In this sense, *power under* is not just about absence—it's missed or untapped potential. It can show up in situations of disengagement, learned helplessness, or failed allyship, where people who could act for change remain silent or sidelined.

Why do these distinctions matter? Understanding the types of power present in any situation helps shape effective strategies for change. If we're working within a rigid, top-down institution, for example, recognizing the dominance of *power over* might prompt us to organize *power with* others to shift decision-making dynamics.

To bring our values of equity and justice to life, we need to be aware when we are exerting *power over* in our relationships with colleagues, communities, and partners. By building and sharing *power with* the people and communities we serve, we can ensure that power is used to uplift rather than control. Power is dynamic, relational, and potentially transformative—and shifting power is essential to achieve flourishing for all.

POWER IS THE BACKBONE OF EQUITY AND JUSTICE

[M]any communities are winning fights for climate, economic, and racial justice by building grassroots political power in its many forms. Working-class communities are developing visionary demands and resources. Power structures are shifting to advance community governance and agency.

—Vivian Yi Huang, organizer and Just Transition advocate[9]

It is inevitable that shifting power to achieve collective flourishing will require confrontation and contestation, and we should be prepared for it. As abolitionist and author Frederick Douglass declared: "Power concedes nothing without a demand. It never did and it never will."[10(p22)]

Similarly, political scientist and health policy scholar Jamila Michener asserts that health justice requires political struggle. According to Michener, struggle involves both *building power*—cultivating the political capacity of those most harmed by health inequities—and *breaking power* by confronting and dismantling the institutions and systems of oppression that perpetuate injustice.[11]

The work of public health is inseparable from politics, pushback, and power because it is fundamentally about how resources, risks, and protections are distributed across society. This is why public health has never been solely about science or services. Our work raises fundamental questions about power and governance: *Who holds power? How it is used? And to what ends?* At its core, the work of public health is a reflection of how we are governed and how our society functions at large.

As public health practitioners, we have a responsibility to work in partnership with communities to build collective power, hold dominant institutions accountable, and change how we exercise power ourselves. As discussed in Chapter 1, public health goals cannot be separated from equity and justice; neither can be achieved without the other. Creating the conditions for everyone to flourish requires nurturing the power to dismantle the social, economic, and systemic barriers that produce inequities. One of the most profound of these barriers is how "race" structures access to opportunity and resources. Author and cultural critic Ta-Nehisi Coates puts it plainly: "Race is a species of power and nothing else."[12(p126)]

In public health, we can either reinforce existing hierarchies, or advance equity and justice by shifting power to communities as they shape their own futures. People in our communities already know what is shortening and sickening their lives—and what it will take to improve them. That is why we must expand what counts as evidence, learn and apply lessons from lived experience, and center the leadership of those at the margins.

Equity and justice—in both process and outcome—require community leadership. Our path forward becomes clear when communities hold real decision-making power over which public health interventions are pursued and how they are implemented.

Indigenous communities and other marginalized communities have long modeled *power with* and *power within* (see Box 5-1).[13-19] Yet despite these profound lessons,

Box 5-1. Lessons in Power From Indigenous Organizing and Resistance

Indigenous communities—with their distinct histories, cultures, and experiences—have long uplifted the importance of self-determination in promoting health and well-being. For many, self-determination includes the ability to make decisions about land use, resources, and governance—all of which directly impact health outcomes.[13] The struggle for land and resource sovereignty is especially important because it connects directly to both physical health and cultural preservation.[14]

While individual Tribal Nations may approach these issues differently, the core principle shared across many communities is that access to and control over land and resources is fundamental to health. Indigenous advocates have emphasized that health goes beyond just the physical to encompass the mental, spiritual, and emotional well-being of individuals, families, and communities.[15]

For example, food sovereignty movements have empowered communities to revitalize traditional food systems, reduce reliance on corporate food chains, and increase access to locally grown, culturally significant foods.[16] Initiatives like community land trusts, such as the Sogorea Te' Land Trust and its Shuumi Land Tax, allow Indigenous communities to secure and govern their land in ways that resist displacement and support long-term sustainability.[17] These varied approaches reflect the diversity of Indigenous cultures and the way that specific traditions and practices vary between nations.

The enduring health inequities faced by Indigenous communities are intertwined with the legacies of colonialism, genocide, and white supremacy (as discussed in Chapter 2). Land dispossession, cultural erasure, state-sanctioned violence, and the subjugation of Tribal governments have all contributed to intergenerational trauma and systemic barriers to well-being. Yet in the face of these harms, Indigenous communities continue to assert their sovereignty, revitalize traditional practices, and build systems rooted in self-determination.

Research shows that when Indigenous communities have the power to govern their lands and resources, health outcomes improve.[18] Self-determination enhances community resilience and bolsters health care, education, and other systems that align with Indigenous values and cultures.[19]

systems of oppression continue to strip marginalized people of *power to* through policies rooted in racism, colonialism, and economic exploitation. These interlocking forces disadvantage and isolate individuals—and on a broader scale, they entrench structural inequities across time and geography.

The result is a grim inheritance of layered disadvantages that accumulate, endure, and evolve—suffocating opportunity for generations. These inequities are felt in every domain of life, from housing to economic security, transportation to civic participation. The consequences are as stark as they are preventable: lives lost, health eroded, and futures dimmed by human-made inequities that undermine the full potential of society.

While community engagement is now widely acknowledged as a core competency of public health, we must move beyond tokenism, one-way requests for communities to provide "input," and surface-level consultation. The deeper and more transformative work is **shifting power**—changing who has authority, decision-making control, and access to resources.

Power shifting can occur in two key ways: power sharing and power building. **Power sharing** occurs when dominant institutions deliberately cede control, step back from the center, and uplift communities as leaders. **Power building** is what communities do to organize, mobilize, and strengthen their own collective capacity to govern, advocate, and act.

Community power cannot be manufactured by dominant institutions—it is built by communities themselves. As public health practitioners, we must support power sharing and power building. However, we must recognize that power building belongs to communities themselves. It cannot be externally engineered or bestowed from above. Communities must leverage, strengthen, and amplify the power they already have—their inherent *power within*.[20] Within institutions, our role is to stand behind—not in front of—that process by leveraging institutional power to open doors, directing resources to community priorities, and ensuring that those who are most marginalized lead the decisions that shape their health and well-being.

At the same time, shifting power to communities does not mean government can abdicate its responsibilities. Power sharing requires that public institutions remain fully engaged and supportive of communities. They should not offload essential functions onto communities already burdened with structural inequities. While governments may face constraints—such as preemption laws that limit the ability of local and state officials to enact policies that serve the the will and well-being of their communities (see Box 5-2)—they still carry public trust to act in service of the people.[21-25] That means guaranteeing the core functions and protections of governance while aligning policies, funding, and accountability mechanisms with community leadership and direction.

According to Lead Local, **community power** is "the ability of communities most impacted by structural inequity to develop, sustain and grow an organized base of people who act together through democratic structures to set agendas, shift public discourse, influence who makes decisions and cultivate ongoing relationships of mutual accountability with decision-makers that change systems and advance health equity."[26]

This is *power with*—the collective strength that comes from organizing together toward shared goals—and it grows as communities engage in power building. This kind of power requires self-determination. Communities don't just want to be consulted—they want to decide, and they expect dominant institutions to honor and implement those decisions.

As public health practitioners who consider ourselves not just allies, but co-conspirators who are deeply invested in the success and self-determination of the communities we serve, we must embrace co-creation, co-governance, and collective action. This means treating communities as full partners, valuing their leadership and lived experiences, and rejecting top-down approaches. When communities have real governing power over the decisions that shape their lives, we all benefit from improved health outcomes and a more vibrant democracy.

The *Spectrum of Community Engagement to Ownership*[27] (Figure 5-1) can help us assess how much power communities have in specific government or institutional decisions and processes—from none at all to full community self-determination. Developed by educator and artist Rosa González, the Spectrum illustrates not just whether communities are involved, but how power flows between institutions and communities. It challenges dominant institutions to shift from tokenized forms of participation to authentic power-sharing models that embrace collaboration and community.

The Spectrum challenges government institutions to move beyond simply informing or consulting communities—practices that allow them to maintain control—and to move

Box 5-2. Punitive Preemption and Protecting Public Health Power

Public health has everything to do with power: who has it, how it is exercised, and to what end. One of the clearest expressions of governmental power is **preemption**—the ability of a higher level of government (such as a state or the federal government) to override or limit the authority of a government at a lower level, like a city or county. While preemption can play a legitimate role in setting baseline protections—such as clean water standards or antidiscrimination protections—it is also commonly used to block local efforts aimed at advancing equity and justice.[21] State legislatures have increasingly preempted local policies that reflect the will and well-being of marginalized communities. This is known as **punitive preemption**, or **abusive preemption**: a form of governance where higher levels of government not only override local authority but also block policies that protect public health—and threaten to punish the lower-level government and its leaders in the process.[22]

Punitive preemption has blocked cities from raising the minimum wage, mandating paid sick leave, protecting tenants, regulating harmful industries, and responding to public health emergencies like COVID-19.[23] This misuse of power strips communities—especially communities of color and low-income communities—of their ability to govern effectively for their own health, safety, and future. This form of preemption has also given rise to more extreme measures—including penalties against local officials who defy them—as part of a broader shift toward using state power to suppress communities' self-determination.[24]

This both stifles innovation and strips communities of basic protections essential to health and well-being. When higher levels of government block local policies, they prevent jurisdictions from responding to urgent needs— like housing stability, workplace safety, and environmental health—with tailored, community-centered solutions. This undermines the foundational building blocks of public health. At the same time, they thwart promising innovations— community-driven strategies that go beyond minimum standards to address inequities and improve outcomes. Local governments are often first to witness—and respond to—the challenges their residents face, and they must have the latitude to safeguard essential protections and implement new approaches to advance equity and justice.

While responsiveness varies widely, local governments are uniquely positioned to hear neighborhood voices and act on them. And the potential is profound: when residents organize—from people's assemblies to mutual aid networks—even relatively small, community-rooted coalitions can spark meaningful policy change rooted in lived experience and collective leadership.

But we must be clear: Place-based, community-led solutions are not blanket calls for deregulation or unchecked localism that targets marginalized communities and undermines public health. After all, appeals to "states' rights" were historically used to resist federal civil rights mandates and to impose Jim Crow laws and other forms of racialized terror immediately following Reconstruction in the late 1800s and throughout most of the 20th century.[25] Such strategies reveal how legal frameworks can be weaponized to maintain unjust systems, especially under the guise of protecting "local authority." Higher levels of government should use their power to uphold people's rights—not suppress them. They should set strong equity-centered floors that no jurisdiction can fall below, while simultaneously supporting local efforts to protect, advance, and sustain equity and justice.

Like any tool of governance or any tool for systems change (as discussed in Chapter 3), preemption is not inherently good or bad, but it is also never neutral. As public health practitioners, we must always ask: *Is power being wielded to fuel inequity or to dismantle it?*

toward deeper, more authentic approaches like involvement and co-governance. But the ultimate goal is not partnership alone, it's community self-determination. In the final stage, *defer to*, institutions take on the role of supportive partner, and communities lead.

The Grassroots Power Project calls this **governing power**—the ability to control systems and decisions that shape lives.[28] Governing power reflects both *power to* and *power with*: the capacity to act and the collective strength to make change. Yet as practitioners, the Spectrum also challenges us to reflect on where we may exert *power over*—and where we can uplift the leadership of communities and serve in a supporting role.

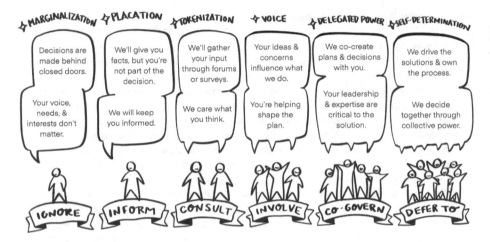

Source: Adapted with permission from González.[27]
Artist Credit: Jasmin Pamukcu, 2025.

Figure 5-1. Spectrum of Community Engagement to Ownership

The *Spectrum of Community Engagement to Ownership* can help public health practitioners assess not only how our efforts engage communities but also how power flows in these relationships:

Communities are denied access to decision-making altogether. Institutions operate behind closed doors, sometimes withholding basic information. The message is: *Your voice doesn't matter.* This results in marginalization and distrust. Activities may include internal-only meetings or disinformation campaigns. Resources are directed entirely inward—100% toward institutional administration and operations.

Institutions communicate information to the public but do not seek input or interaction. The goal is to provide updates or explanations, not to involve community members in shaping outcomes. The message is: *We will keep you informed—but it's not likely that any feedback you provide matters.* Activities include public presentations, fact sheets, town halls, and billboards. Resources remain primarily institutional: 70% to 90% for administration; 10% to 30% for promotions and publicity.

Institutions seek input from communities using various methods, but they retain full control. The message is: *We care what you think—but we'll decide.* As a result, this often feels like tokenism. Activities include surveys, focus groups, and public forums. Budgets reflect the imbalance: 60% to 80% internal; 20% to 40% for consultation activities.

Community perspectives begin to influence planning and design, signaling a shift toward valuing community voice. The message becomes: *You're helping us think and act differently.* Activities include interactive workshops, polling, and community advisory committees. Resources start to balance: 50% to 60% institutional; 40% to 50% community-focused.

 Decision-making is shared. Institutions recognize and center the community's expertise, while providing support for implementation. This is partnership, and the message is clear: *Your leadership is essential.* Activities include formal agreements with community-based organizations (such as Memoranda of Understanding or MOUs), open planning forums, and consensus-building processes. Budgets shift significantly, with 50% to 70% directed to community partners.

 Communities exercise full control over the process and outcomes. Institutions follow the lead of community-based structures and align funding, policy, and accountability accordingly. The message is: *We trust your vision and will support its realization.* Activities include participatory budgeting, community-controlled planning, and community governance—a form of collective decision-making in which community members have full authority to make decisions and guide their implementation. Most resources (80%–100%) flow to community-led efforts, ideally generating reinvestment in long-term solutions.

Many public health efforts—especially those led by government—remain stuck in the early stages of the Spectrum, where institutions share information or gather feedback without giving up control. Even when well-intentioned, these approaches leave communities without real authority and limit the potential for transformation.

Understanding Community Power: A Transportation Example

Imagine a city's department of transportation is tasked with responding to the increased traffic and road safety issues in a historic Chinatown neighborhood. By working through the *Spectrum of Community Engagement to Ownership*, we can envision possible ways that the city's department of transportation can choose to interact with the Chinatown neighborhood that they serve:

 This is the status quo. The residents of Chinatown are ignored and sidelined by the city's department of transportation. For decades, Chinatown residents have raised concerns about high-speed roads that allow people to drive through the neighborhood too quickly, poor lighting along roadways, and a lack of safety infrastructure such as wide side-walks that can accommodate wheelchairs, traffic signals, and painted crosswalks.

 The city's department of transportation simply announces that they are going to widen a road that runs through the neighborhood to address the growing traffic pressures. Residents are invited to public meetings to hear about changes that have already been decided behind closed doors. This reflects *power over*—where the government holds full decision-making authority—and also *power under*, as the department of transportation fails to use its influence to advocate for bold, community-centered solutions. As a result, residents feel excluded and distrustful, leading to disengagement and resignation; any sense of agency or belief that they can influence outcomes in government processes is stifled.

 As community pushback grows, department officials distribute surveys and hold public comment sessions. But decisions remain in government hands. Community voices are heard but not acted upon. *Power over* persists, and consultation remains largely performative. This leaves residents feeling frustrated and tokenized—especially if only the loudest or most well-connected individuals can navigate these processes and have their views heard.

 Spurred by community organizing, the city's transportation department begins cohosting listening sessions and working groups. Residents' experiences start to inform priorities, but ultimate decision-making power remains with the city agency. Here, we see early emergence of *power with*, as government begins to recognize the value of community expertise. Yet without formal power sharing, many community members still experience fatigue and skepticism about government-run processes, wondering whether their input will truly shape outcomes.

 The city's transportation department moves into collaboration with the Chinatown community, sharing decision-making authority on changes in transportation infrastructure that need to be made. The transportation department actively supports this shift by listening to, responding to, and resourcing community-driven priorities. The department and community-based advocacy organizations collaborate on a plan that will address the speeding and safety infrastructure concerns that have been shared by residents. This reflects a deeper level of *power with*, where residents and agencies are true partners, even if some institutional authority remains. Residents see tangible changes and begin to feel that their leadership, knowledge, and aspirations are genuinely valued—building trust and momentum for deeper transformation. Trust and hope emerge, making space for bolder community-led solutions.

Ultimately, residents establish a Chinatown Community Land Trust to secure permanent control over housing, retail, and cultural spaces and the roads that connect them. The residents request that the city's transportation department, health department, community development office, and city planning department play supportive roles—offering technical assistance, staffing for implementation, and grant funding—but decision-making rests entirely with the community. This represents *power to*: Residents own and govern their future, and government agencies work in service of the community with their guidance. This self-determined leadership fuels broader visions for health and equity, laying the groundwork for transformative, community-rooted change.

This example helps illustrate how community power is not static and can evolve across different stages—from full institutional control to full community governance.

This book emphasizes co-governance as a powerful and necessary shift that can help realign public health with justice and self-determination. It represents a shared responsibility to dismantle hierarchies and build new systems rooted in trust, accountability, and collective power.

At the same time, it's important to recognize that the final stage on the Spectrum—*defer to*, when communities exercise self-determination—may or may not involve co-governance with dominant institutions. Self-determination means communities exercise full agency and can decide whether or not government is at the table. Sometimes this looks like communities developing their own solutions and self-governing through structures like cooperative funds, community land trusts, and resilience hubs. In these cases, the most appropriate role for government is not to co-govern, but to step back, follow the community's lead, and direct resources in support of community-defined goals.

Defer to is not about letting communities perpetuate the exclusion and marginalization of others. As discussed in Chapter 2, self-segregated white communities chose to destroy their neighborhoods' public pools and to defund other public amenities simply to prevent Black people from benefitting from them. Deferring to communities is about allowing communities to lead in ways that uplift those who are marginalized and to work toward shared goals of health and flourishing—not to perpetuate oppression, discrimination, and subjugation.

Whether stepping into shared leadership or stepping back to follow, as public health practitioners, we must ask ourselves these questions:

- *What stage of the Spectrum of Community Engagement to Ownership do I think my team currently operates within? What about my organization?*
- *Where on the Spectrum are we—from the perspective of our community members and partners? Why?*
- *Have we been transparent with communities about where our team and organization is on the Spectrum?*

- *If we wanted to move up the Spectrum and shift more power to communities most impacted by injustice, what barriers might we encounter? How might we overcome those barriers?*
- *What concrete actions can we take to collaborate with communities in ways that move toward co-governance or self-determination?*

For public health practitioners working in government, these questions are particularly weighty. Government is meant to be of the people, for the people, and by the people. While this promise is not always realized, it creates both a responsibility and an opportunity.

It's work that begins with honesty. Accurately naming where your team or organization falls on the Spectrum can safeguard against eroded public trust and reduced government efficacy. Mislabeling a project as "co-governed"—when it truly isn't—is not only deceptive, but it also undermines credibility, damages relationships, and stalls progress. If you're only prepared to consult, for example, say so—and commit to moving forward in transparency.

TRUST IS WHERE POWER SHIFTING BEGINS

[T]he only way to build trust is through vulnerability. Trust is key in our work to end cycles of violence because when violence or harm happens, trust is one of the first things that gets broken.

–Mia Mingus, writer and disability justice organizer[29]

Building trust is the first step of shifting and sharing power. **Trust** means being seen as honest, reliable, reciprocal, and accountable—not just as an individual but also as a representative of your organization and field. For communities long harmed by policies and practices like redlining, urban renewal, and police violence, trust is rightfully and understandably difficult to earn. Deep distrust often exists between dominant institutions—especially government agencies—and communities of color because of decades of broken promises, deliberate harm and neglect, state-sanctioned violence, widespread exploitation, and the willful perpetuation of unjust policies.

Authentic collaboration requires going beyond outreach. It means listening with care, acknowledging both historical and ongoing injustices, and taking sustained action to repair harm, honor community voices, and provide redress.

Too often, we miss opportunities to build trust—especially when community members raise urgent concerns that fall outside of our jurisdiction, purview, or expertise. These moments can feel inconvenient or out of scope, but they're actually critical opportunities for us to build trust.

As a public health practitioner, this is where your role—and your obligation—comes into focus. These moments offer a defining inflection point: Dismiss the concern or embrace the opportunity to take action as a true partner. Use these opportunities to build and strengthen trust by agreeing to help, using your networks and influence to connect people with decision-makers, following through on your commitments, and demonstrating that your word can be trusted.

In fact, there are many ways to build trust with communities you serve. Here are some of the most essential:

- **Support communities on the issues that matter most to them.** Even if the concerns that are shared with you fall outside your usual scope or purview, start by listening. For example, if you're planning to ask a community to participate in a survey, initiative, or other effort, first build goodwill by addressing priorities they've already named—even if these priorities aren't within your direct control. Find a way to help communities make progress on the issues that matter to them, and they may willingly reciprocate.

- **Respond to long-standing concerns.** You'll likely find that communities have been raising urgent issues for a long time—perhaps about traffic violence, economic exploitation, unaffordable housing, or voter suppression. The specifics may vary, but the systemic patterns are familiar. Before making an ask, build trust by listening, understanding what support is needed, and offering help—especially in areas where institutions have historically been unresponsive.

- **Communicate frequently and transparently.** If plans shift or progress slows, let community members and partners know. Radio silence can feel like disregard and disrespect—and distrust grows quickly in the absence of communication. Even when there's little news to report, a brief check-in can reinforce that the relationship matters.

- **Speak plainly.** Resist the tendency to obscure your message with professional jargon, formalized institutional language, or legalese. If things go wrong, say so plainly, in the spirit of accountability. Whether you need to communicate bureaucratic delays, miscommunications, or unexpected challenges, people appreciate candor over polished excuses.

- **Show up consistently—not just when you need support.** Trust and authentic relationships are built through presence. Attend community meetings and events as a long-term partner, not just when there's a project on the table. This makes it more likely that you'll be responsive to communities' needs and that communities will be more likely to show up for you when it counts. Look for creative ways to stay connected and visible—through follow-ups, shared celebrations, or public recognition of community leadership.

- **Keep your promises.** The simplest way to build trust is to follow through. Whether it's making an introduction, sharing information, or investigating a concern—do what you said you would. Accountability starts with aligning your words and actions. Even small promises, kept consistently, can have a lasting impact.

- **Uphold commitments you're connected to.** Sometimes, a promise wasn't yours originally—perhaps it was made by your organization, your profession, or your predecessors. Honoring it now can help repair trust. It's a chance to show that things have changed and that you stand for solidarity and accountability.

Layers of distrust and hurt that have accumulated within communities over decades will not vanish overnight. Trust is built through time, humility, and sustained effort—not just by each of us as individuals, but by the teams, organizations, and institutions we represent. When we keep showing up, listening, and following through, we show communities that we are authentic, trustworthy partners in the struggle for equity and justice.

PUTTING POWER INTO PRACTICE

If you want to understand the deepest malfunctions of systems, pay attention to the rules and to who has power over them.
                                              –Donella H. Meadows, environmental scientist and educator[30]

Shifting power is both a philosophy and a practice. It means transferring access, control, and decision-making authority to the communities we serve. For public health practitioners, it begins with recognizing the power we already hold—through networks, funding, and institutional influence—and using it to support, not steer, community-led efforts.

Power shifting looks different in every context, but its core principles mean that communities should be able to advance their priorities in these important ways:

- **Setting the agenda** by naming the priorities that matter most to them.
- **Shaping decision-making** by determining who is at the table and how decisions are made.
- **Telling their own stories** to challenge misleading mindsets and destructive narratives.
- **Driving policies and controlling resources**, ensuring that outcomes reflect their needs, priorities, goals, and aspirations.

The last point acknowledges that resources are a form of power. The control of resources directly shapes which priorities and solutions are pursued, and which voices lead the way. Of all the resources we need to live well and actualize flourishing for all, funding is one of the most tangible and influential. It's often the clearest reflection of who and what we value as a society.

Communities must have access to sufficient resources to support community health and well-being—not just to survive, but to thrive. Shifting power requires both mobilizing new resources and ensuring communities have real authority over existing ones.

Resource mobilization is the practice of organizing, advocating for, and attracting new funding, partnerships, and political support to build lasting abundance—not simply manage scarcity. *Resource control* gives communities decision-making authority over how budgets and assets are used, to align with their priorities and vision. Together, these strategies move funding from transactional to transformational. When communities control the flow and generation of resources, they are better positioned to shape their own futures. That is one of the clearest ways to put power shifting into action.

Whether in resource decisions or any other arena, those most affected by health inequity must take the lead in defining priorities and shaping solutions. When communities drive the agenda, the work becomes more grounded, relevant, and credible. These are some signs you are shifting power in the right direction:

 Community leadership is central, not optional. You ensure decision-making processes and structures prioritize community voices and make space for ongoing participation. No major decisions are made without their input and agreement.

 Timelines reflect community readiness. Instead of rushing toward institutional deadlines or short-term deliverables, you respect the pace at which communities build trust, set priorities, and move collectively.

 Organizational priorities align with community-defined goals. You adapt your work to fit what communities say they need—rather than expecting them to conform to your department's or your organization's agenda.

 Funding flows directly to grassroots organizations. You provide long-term, flexible funding that allows communities—and the community-based, grassroots organizations that represent their interests—to set priorities, experiment with solutions, and make change over time.

 Power-building is resourced beyond one-off campaigns. You recognize that transformative change requires sustained investment over years, not just in brief, one-off efforts. You mobilize resources regularly to ensure funding is available for ongoing progress.

 Narratives center community dignity and leadership. You ensure communications—including reports, media, and policy briefs—are shaped by those who are most marginalized, reflecting their vision for the future rather than top-down interpretations.

Putting power into practice is ultimately about shifting the *center of gravity*—the place where decisions and power are concentrated—toward communities. In most of our nation's systems, that center of gravity sits firmly within institutions, pulled there by entrenched policies, funding structures, and decision-making practices. Shifting it means moving the weight of influence, authority, and resources to those most affected by inequities—until community leadership is not the exception but the norm.

It takes humility to release control, patience to move at the speed of trust, and courage to prioritize community needs over institutional demands. It means being transparent about limits while demonstrating a clear plan to address them. But when practiced consistently, this approach can build trust, grow credibility, and redistribute power in ways that make equity and justice both possible and durable.

WHY CO-GOVERNANCE CAN BE A GAME-CHANGER FOR PUBLIC HEALTH

If we are not prepared to govern, we are not prepared to win.

–Movement Generation[*31]

Public health's defining ambition is to protect and promote the health of entire populations (discussed in Chapter 1). But if we are honest about the challenges we face today, we must also be honest about this: Public health is underpowered.

Powerful and entrenched political, financial, and cultural forces shape our systems—from wealthy tech conglomerates that facilitate the spread of disinformation to profit-driven fossil fuel industries that shape climate policy. These dominant institutions wield influence not just through money or messaging but through the power to set agendas, shape narratives, and determine who benefits from systems and who does not. Public health, by contrast, often finds itself reacting rather than leading—struggling to set the agenda, hold decision-makers accountable, or protect hard-won progress toward equity and justice.

We are working to protect lives while playing by rules written by those who profit from injustice. To change this, we cannot rely on technical expertise or good intentions alone. We need real power. That means cultivating community power—not just in the communities we serve, but within ourselves as a collective. We must be more than experts with advanced degrees, technical training, and professionalized roles. We are experts in communities, organizing alongside others to build the collective strength needed to shift systems.

Only together—and by joining with others across backgrounds, geographies, sectors, and experiences—can we set agendas, influence decisions, and truly change systems for good. By standing in solidarity, we cultivate *power with* that can effectively confront and resist unjust interests and systems of oppression.

Power is not just about influencing decisions and policies; it's about determining whose priorities shape the future. Chapter 3 discussed how tools for systems change visualized in the Root Causes Roadmap can either be used to advance a health-affirming agenda or undermine and stymie progress. When we look at other sectors, we see stark examples of how power can be abused to drive harmful agendas, perpetuate inequity, and jeopardize health and well-being:

- **Military spending:** Despite recurring budget deficits, military budgets have been protected and expanded. Defense contractors, military leaders, and politicians form a coalition that wields enormous influence through lobbying, campaign financing, and cultural narratives about "national security." At the federal level, many public health efforts are

---

*A collective of educators and strategists, Movement Generation catalyzes transformative action for ecological and social justice.

funded through "non-defense discretionary spending" and are often cut or underfunded, while military spending is treated as untouchable and even worthy of further growth.

• **Gun control:** After tragedies like Sandy Hook and Newtown, public demand for gun control was high. Yet powerful organizations like the National Rifle Association promoted narratives related to freedom and personal safety to block meaningful reforms. Despite the overwhelming public health evidence linking gun access to violence and death, many lawmakers still refuse to act.

• **The opioid crisis:** Pharmaceutical companies manipulated research and concealed evidence about the addictive nature of opioids, prioritizing profits over public health.[32] Policymakers failed to intervene swiftly, demonstrating how power can be abused to suppress science and generate false narratives that distort public understanding and delay lifesaving action.

Each of these examples reveals how political, economic, and narrative power can override public health priorities.

Now imagine this: *What if that same amount of power and influence was held by communities, grassroots advocates, and public health practitioners committed to health justice? What if health justice—and not corporate profit or political capitulation—set the agenda for our cities, states, and nation?*

That future is not only possible. It is necessary.

Building this future requires a shift in who holds decision-making authority. It calls for governments to be accountable to communities by letting them lead and following up with support—what we refer to as *collaborative governance*.

As discussed in Chapter 3, **collaborative governance** or **co-governance** is a shared governing model in which government agencies and community members—especially those historically excluded from power—work together to shape and implement public policies, programs, and the allocation of resources. Co-governance is collaborative, formal, and deliberative.[33] This means community members are not simply consulted; they have formal governance roles, real authority, and explicit leadership in decision-making. In co-governance models, community members are central and essential to the process of shaping, implementing, and sustaining policies and systems.

Co-governance represents a realistic, transformative goal for public health—a rebalancing of power where those most impacted by inequity lead the work. Community members set priorities, shape strategies, and direct implementation. According to political scientists and policy reform strategists Hollie Russon Gilman and Mark Schmitt, co-governance "shifts power and builds trust by enabling government officials and advocates to see each other as collaborators with unique capacities and perspectives that support the other's interests and positions."[34]

In co-governance models, government agencies and institutions don't disappear; they remain essential partners. But their role shifts: from directing to supporting, from controlling to implementing. Communities set the direction, and government helps get it done.

Unlike other community-informed approaches, such as community engagement and consultation, co-governance goes further to directly confront and wrestle with issues of power, self-determination, and structural inequities. But co-governance is not the final destination. It's an essential step toward *defer to*—the stage where communities exercise full self-determination and agency. In practice, *defer to* is a long horizon, shaped by ongoing struggles to shift resources, transform institutions, and provide redress for historical injustices. Co-governance is a critical path toward that horizon. It's a way we can practice power sharing today, even as we push for deeper community self-determination in the future.

Co-governance can also help counter people's widespread mistrust of institutions.[34] By actively engaging communities in decisions and fostering transparency, co-governance can transform public perceptions of government. Rather than seeing government agencies as harmful, extractive, and adversarial entities, communities can instead see them as collaborative partners. This can result in better public and organizational policies, as well as stronger communities where government staff and community members are both well-equipped to navigate complex challenges together.

Changes that result from co-governance approaches are more sustainable because solutions rooted in community members' lived experiences—and that are coupled with backbone support and buy-in from dominant institutions like government—are more likely to endure, adapt, and receive support and investment over time. When we build structures this way, we move beyond short-term fixes and toward lasting health justice—creating communities where public health is not just something done *to* people but built *by* and *for* them.

Co-governance is a tangible way to transform systems and build trust within communities. It requires dominant institutions to be accountable to communities for outcomes and successes. It offers a path to rebuild public trust by fundamentally transforming how governments engage with the people they serve. When communities are respected, treated as full partners in decision-making, and provided with full transparency and visibility into the mechanics of processes and decisions, they are more likely to trust and support government institutions, creating a foundation for sustained civic and social progress. Co-governance provides us with opportunities to build broad and powerful coalitions composed of public health practitioners, government officials, grassroots organizers, and community members, who stand shoulder to shoulder in solidarity and work collaboratively to achieve flourishing for all.

CONCLUSION

Power is the key to improving public health at scale, and as discussed in Chapter 1, scale is one of the defining commitments of public health. It's how we shift toward long-term change that benefits large numbers of people. According to organizers and strategists

Dan McGrath and Harmony Goldberg, building power allows us to get out of "a cycle of short-term campaigns and reactive fights . . . disconnected from a broader vision or strategy for structural change."[35(p5)] and holistically transform the unjust structures driving poor health outcomes.

No matter our job titles or roles, each of us holds some degree of influence—whether through our positions, networks, institutions, funding, or access to decision-makers. Public health practitioners hold significant institutional power—far more than we may realize. But we have to ask ourselves: *How are we using our power? And how are we shifting it and sharing it with the communities that we serve?*

Shifting and sharing power means handing as much access and control to communities as possible. It means valuing community voices, insights, and experiences so deeply that our work cannot move forward without it. It means intentionally building in time—even when deadlines feel rushed—to ensure that the path we're on is really one that communities want. It requires us to challenge traditional hierarchies, invest in community governance, and ensure that public health serves as a tool for collective liberation.

But without deliberate and sustained efforts to build, shift, and share power, health interventions will continue to be temporary fixes rather than transformative solutions. Our commitment to equity and justice requires us to shift resources and decision-making capacities to communities most harmed by structural inequities.

If we want to reach our public health goals, we must upend power imbalances and stand in solidarity with the people and places most impacted by injustice. Only then can public health truly be partners in co-creation and co-governance with the communities we serve—and only then can health become a collective, unshakable priority.

KEY TAKEAWAYS

Power shapes health outcomes. Power influences every aspect of our lives. It exists within relationships and can take the form of *power over, power to, power with, power within,* and *power under.* Understanding various forms of power helps us recognize who holds it and how it operates in both our communities and organizations. Power mapping can uncover opportunities to shift dynamics— particularly from *power over* toward *power to* and *power with*—fostering collective action and nurturing equity and justice.

Power shifting is necessary to achieve our goal of all communities flourishing. Power shifting requires that dominant institutions *share power* by ceding authority, decision-making, and resource control to communities and allowing them to lead. It also involves communities' efforts to *build power* by organizing, mobilizing, and realizing their collective capacity to govern and act. Efforts to build and share power create the conditions for change by revealing effective solutions for public health problems that are born from community members' lived experiences.

We must honestly assess—and then change—how much power communities have in decision-making. The *Spectrum of Community Engagement to Ownership* helps us identify how much communities are allowed to engage in and control decisions related to issues that are relevant to their lives. It challenges dominant institutions to wrestle with the authenticity of their own processes and shift from status quo–preserving and tokenized forms of community engagement to more authentic, collaborative, and self-determined forms of governance.

Addressing distrust is a first step toward genuine relationships. Marginalized communities are understandably distrustful of government agencies and many other dominant institutions because of their role in perpetuating destructive and exploitive systems of oppression, state-sanctioned violence, and unjust policies. Before we can begin to repair relationships, we must first understand why they are in disrepair. Honest, consistent, and accountable actions can help us address layers of distrust and slowly build authentic and trusting relationships over time.

Co-governance is a tool for justice. Collaborative governance—or co-governance—involves a fundamental rebalancing of power and has far-reaching consequences. Through shared decision-making, co-governance fosters systems that are more equitable, inclusive, and responsive to the needs of marginalized communities. Co-governance models—such as participatory budgeting and advisory councils composed of community members with decision-making authority—can help ensure that marginalized communities actively shape the policies and systems that affect their lives.

REFERENCES

1. Rivera T. Convening at Chainbreaker Collective. Santa Fe, NM; June 26, 2025.
2. King ML Jr. *Where Do We Go From Here: Chaos or Community?* Beacon Press; 1967.
3. Iton A, Ross RK, Tamber PS. Building community power to dismantle policy-based structural inequity in population health. *Health Aff (Millwood)*. 2022;41(12):1763–1771. doi:10.1377/hlthaff.2022.00540
4. Lukes S. *Power: A Radical View*. 2nd ed. Palgrave Macmillan; 2005.
5. Nelson C, Sloan J, Chandra A. Examining civic engagement links to health: Findings from the literature and implications for a culture of health. RAND Corporation. 2019. Accessed August 8, 2025. https://www.rand.org/pubs/research_reports/RR3163.html

6. Hunter D, Ayers J, Mahs GRG, et al. Health & Democracy Index. Healthy Democracy Healthy People. 2022. Accessed August 8, 2025. https://democracyindex.responsivegov.org

7. Levitsky S, Ziblatt D. *How Democracies Die.* Crown Publishing; 2018.

8. Solar O, Irwin A. *A Conceptual Framework for Action on the Social Determinants of Health.* World Health Organization; 2010.

9. Huang VY. Building grassroots political power. *Stanford Social Innovation Review.* 2024. Accessed June 28, 2025. https://ssir.org/articles/entry/building_grassroots_political_power

10. Douglass F. *Two Speeches by Frederick Douglass: 1857.* C. P. Dewey; 1857. Central Library of Rochester and Monroe County, Historic Monographs Collection. Accessed August 18, 2025. https://www.libraryweb.org/~digitized/books/Two_Speeches_by_Frederick_Douglass.pdf

11. Michener J. Health justice through the lens of power. *J Law Med Ethics.* 2022;50(4):656–662. doi:10.1017/jme.2023.5

12. Coates T. *The Message.* One World; 2024.

13. Halseth R, Murdock L. *Supporting Indigenous Self-Determination in Health: Lessons Learned From a Review of Best Practices in Health Governance in Canada and Internationally.* National Collaborating Centre for Indigenous Health; December 2020. Accessed August 18, 2025. https://www.nccih.ca/495/Supporting_Indigenous_self-determination_in_health___Lessons_learned_from_a_review_of_best_practices_in_health_governance_in_Canada_and_Internationally.nccih?id=317

14. The Lancet. Indigenous health: Self-determination is key. *Lancet.* 2023;402(10400):425. doi:10.1016/S0140-6736(23)01238-2

15. World Health Organization. Global plan of action for health of Indigenous peoples. Accessed August 9, 2025. https://www.who.int/initiatives/global-plan-of-action-for-health-of-indigenous-peoples

16. Jernigan VBB, Demientieff LX, Maunakea AK. Food sovereignty as a path to health equity for Indigenous communities: Introduction to the focus issue. *Health Promot Pract.* 2023;24(6): 1066–1069. doi:10.1177/15248399231190355

17. The Sogorea Te' Land Trust. Shuumi Land Tax FAQs. Accessed June 28, 2025. https://sogoreate-landtrust.org/shuumi-land-tax-faqs

18. Joseph G. The role of sovereignty in Indigenous community-based health interventions: A qualitative metasynthesis. *Am J Community Psychol.* 2024;73(1-2):216–233. doi:10.1002/ajcp.12670

19. Roach P, McMillan F. Reconciliation and Indigenous self-determination in health research: A call to action. *PLOS Glob Public Health.* 2022;2(9):e0000999. doi:10.1371/journal.pgph.0000999

20. Health Equity Guide. Support community power building. Health in Partnership. Accessed June 3, 2025. https://healthequityguide.org/strategic-practices/support-community-power-building

21. ChangeLab Solutions. Consequences of preemption for public health & equity. July 2020. Accessed August 9, 2025. https://www.changelabsolutions.org/sites/default/files/2020-08/Consequences_of_Preemption_FINAL_Accessible_20200710.pdf

22. National League of Cities. Preemption 101: What you need to know about preemption. 2020. Accessed August 9, 2025. https://www.nlc.org/wp-content/uploads/2020/11/Preemption_101.pdf

23. National League of Cities. City rights in an era of preemption. February 22, 2017. Accessed August 9, 2025. https://www.nlc.org/resource/city-rights-in-an-era-of-preemption

24. Briffault R. The challenge of the new preemption. *Stanford Law Rev.* 2018;70:1995–2026. Accessed June 29, 2025. https://scholarship.law.columbia.edu/faculty_scholarship/2090

25. Foner E. *The Second Founding: How the Civil War and Reconstruction Remade the Constitution.* W. W. Norton & Company; 2019.

26. Lead Local Collaborative. Glossary. Accessed August 2, 2025. https://www.lead-local.org/glossary

27. González R. *The Spectrum of Community Engagement to Ownership.* Facilitating Power; 2021. Accessed June 3, 2025. https://www.facilitatingpower.com/spectrum_of_community_engagement_to_ownership

28. Grassroots Power Project. Strategic orientation for movements pursuing transformative change. Accessed June 3, 2025. https://grassrootspowerproject.org

29. Mingus M. The four parts of accountability & how to give a genuine apology. *Leaving Evidence.* December 18, 2019. Accessed June 30, 2024. https://leavingevidence.wordpress.com/#:~:text=Remember%2C%20the%20only%20way%20to,first%20things%20that%20gets%20broken

30. Meadows D. Leverage points: Places to intervene in a system. The Donella Meadows Project. 1999. Accessed August 9, 2025. https://donellameadows.org/archives/leverage-points-places-to-intervene-in-a-system

31. Movement Generation. Just Transition. Accessed May 16, 2025. https://movementgeneration.org/justtransition

32. Meier B. Origins of an epidemic: Purdue Pharma knew its opioids were widely abused. *New York Times.* May 29, 2018. Accessed August 10, 2025. https://www.nytimes.com/2018/05/29/health/purdue-opioids-oxycontin.html

33. Ansell C, Gash A. Collaborative governance in theory and practice. *J Public Adm Res Theory.* 2008;18(4):543–571. doi:10.1093/jopart/mum032

34. Gilman HR, Schmitt M. Building public trust through collaborative governance. *Stanford Social Innovation Review.* March 17, 2022. Accessed May 12, 2025. https://ssir.org/articles/entry/building_public_trust_through_collaborative_governance

35. McGrath D, Goldberg H, Grassroots Power Program. *Governing Power.* Grassroots Power Project. 2022. Accessed May 12, 2025. https://grassrootspowerproject.org/wp-content/uploads/2023/09/GPP_Book_09.22-SinglePage_Digital.pdf

Making and Measuring Change

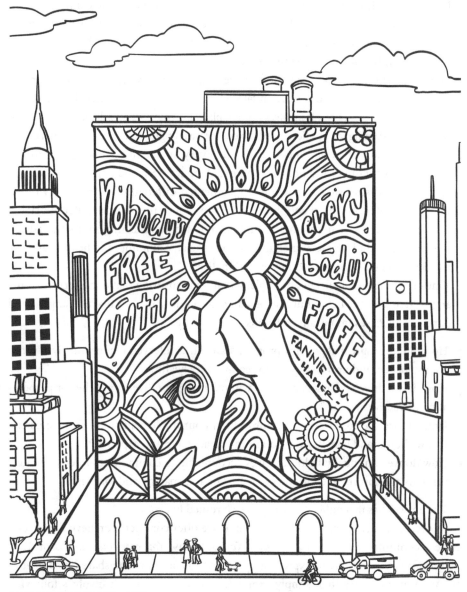

Artist Credit: Jasmin Pamukcu, 2025.

Note: Text by organizer and civil rights leader Fannie Lou Hamer.[1(p136)]

From Promise to Practice

The public health of our communities, of our states, and of our nation cannot be judged by how well the powerful, privileged, and protected are doing. We have to evaluate public health by looking at how the poor, the marginalized, the excluded, and the incarcerated are doing.
                                                                    −Bryan Stevenson, public interest attorney and author[2]

Public health is fundamentally about creating conditions that allow communities to flourish—that is, to live a good life with purpose, agency, and connection. But in the context of public health, getting closer to a world where we can all flourish requires much more than simply launching programs or adopting policies.

Implementation is where vision and strategy meet reality—where theoretical commitments to equity and justice are tested, translated into action, and operationalized through programs, policies, and practices. It involves putting plans into motion, coordinating people and resources, and adapting to specific contexts to ensure meaningful and measurable impact.

Implementation is never one-size-fits-all. Every intervention operates within a unique social, economic, and political context. A policy designed to increase access to fresh food in a disinvested area will be implemented differently in a rural town than in an urban center. An intervention developed to reduce pregnancy-related mortality must be implemented using an intersectional approach that accounts for many systems of oppression, including racial inequities in our social, economic, and health care systems. (See Chapter 2 for more on intersectionality.)

One of the biggest challenges of implementation is ensuring that our efforts not only change systems for the better but also benefit communities in ways that are tangible and enduring. This raises important questions:

- How can we ensure that policies, programs, and other interventions genuinely advance equity, justice, and universal goals for community health?
- How do we drive and assess progress without using punitive approaches or perpetuating extractive systems?
- How can we use co-governance approaches in our implementation efforts to ensure that we honor and benefit from community leadership and expertise?
- How do we continually hold ourselves accountable to communities to ensure interventions are implemented in ways that are fair, transparent, and forthright?

The answer lies in a public health approach rooted in *assurance*.

In everyday life, when we assure someone, we offer confidence, relieve doubt, and make a commitment they can rely on. We might say, *You can count on us* or *We'll see this through*—not just to express support, but to communicate shared responsibility. Assurance is more than simply expressing good intentions. It involves following through on what we say and being accountable for outcomes. It builds trust by pairing clear promises with deliberate action.

In public health, *assurance* means committing to advance the health and well-being of communities by implementing interventions that are not only effective and equitable but also grounded in trust. It challenges us to move beyond good intentions and to ask hard, necessary questions: *Are we making real, measurable improvements in people's daily lives? Are we investing our efforts and resources where injustice has created the greatest need? Are we delivering on our promises—and turning our words into concrete actions?*

Assurance is one of the core functions of public health—along with assessment and policy development—outlined by the Institute of Medicine in the 1988 landmark report, *The Future of Public Health*.[3] Originally, assurance was defined as governmental public health's authority and responsibility to ensure that conditions and services necessary for health were in place. This included implementing legal mandates, developing appropriate responses to crises, guaranteeing the availability of essential services, regulating public- and private-sector activities, and maintaining accountability by setting objectives and reporting on progress.[3]

But in the decades since the Institute of Medicine report was published, the core function of assurance has grown. Today, assurance also includes strengthening the infrastructure of public health organizations, fostering innovation through evaluation and research, ensuring a diverse and skilled public health workforce, and guaranteeing equitable access to public health services.[4-6]

Building on this evolution, this chapter defines **assurance** as the holistic responsibility to guarantee that all public health interventions—including policies, programs, services, and communication campaigns—are implemented in these ways:

- **Equitably:** Interventions actively address universal goals, rectify injustices, and provide resources according to need.
- **Effectively:** Interventions achieve their intended goals.
- **Structurally:** Interventions address the social determinants of health, structural inequities, and systems of oppression.
- **Responsibly:** Interventions use approaches that foster trust and accountability rather than causing harm or instilling fear.

Centering assurance in this way allows us to design universal interventions that benefit everyone while specifically targeting them to address the needs and priorities of marginalized communities. It requires us to work in partnership, especially with community-based organizations, to select and implement strategies that are place-based, culturally relevant, and values-aligned. Assurance also means treating feedback as essential to the ongoing evaluation and improvement of our work. Rather than using approaches that surveil or penalize people, we must gauge success by whether we are building trust, enacting community priorities, and shifting power.

To implement interventions that advance equity and justice, assurance must be our guiding approach. This chapter explores how two key aspects of implementation—enforcement and evaluation—can be reimagined for the benefit of all through an assurance-centered lens.

EVOLVING BEYOND ENFORCEMENT TO EMBRACE ASSURANCE

[T]he master's tools will never dismantle the master's house. They may allow us temporarily to beat him at his own game, but they will never enable us to bring about genuine change.
–Audre Lorde, poet and feminist scholar[7(p112)]

To ensure laws and policies are implemented, governmental public health—like other public institutions—has historically relied on enforcement. **Enforcement** refers to the mechanisms institutions use to ensure compliance with laws, rules, or policies. Governments primarily carry out the enforcement that shapes people's lives and structures the systems we live in. Although enforcement can involve monitoring, education, and accountability-centered action, it has historically and functionally relied on punitive and coercive strategies such as fines, arrests, and surveillance. These practices have disproportionately targeted marginalized communities—focusing on punishing individuals while failing to address systemic wrongdoing. Rather than operating as a tool of public accountability, enforcement more often serves as a mechanism of control that reinforces harmful power imbalances.

While oversight remains a necessary part of protecting community health, too often, public health enforcement mirrors the broader legal and criminal systems' reliance on penalties and punishment rather than support, care, or systemic change. It's a self-defeating approach—like tending a garden to help it flourish while poisoning the very soil it depends on. Some plants may wither entirely, and all will fail to thrive.

Enforcement is never neutral or impartial. It is too often carried out in ways that are discriminatory, extractive, and even violent. Similarly, public health laws and regulations have long been enforced in ways that oppress and discriminate against communities of color, poor people, and other marginalized groups.[8]

Consider Ferguson, Missouri, where the killing of Michael Brown—an unarmed Black teenager—at the hands of police in 2014 began with the enforcement of a public health ordinance. The officer claimed to have stopped Brown for his "manner of walking along roadway"[9]—a policy supposedly intended to protect pedestrian safety. As a federal investigation later showed, the law had been weaponized against Black residents, used routinely to harass and fine them, and to fuel a revenue system built on exploitation[10]—so much so that it earned the nickname *walking while Black*.[11]

Michael Brown's death became a national flashpoint[12]: A nationwide racial reckoning began, the emergent Black Lives Matter movement gained influence and momentum, and communities across the United States organized to take collective action against structural racism and state-sanctioned violence against Black people.

As public health practitioners, we must reckon with our field's own complicity in repressive policing and carceral approaches. Societally, we all operate within systems where, in the name of "health" and "safety," we have reinforced the punitive and inhumane enforcement that is fundamental to the criminal legal system. Consider these examples:

▶ **Criminalizing people in crisis.** In many cities, law enforcement remains the default response to mental health emergencies and homelessness. Police involvement often escalates situations into violent interactions that result in arrests and incarceration.[13] These punitive approaches divert attention and funding away from health-promoting strategies like expanded mental health care, trained crisis response teams, and permanent housing. They also drain resources from the very supports that can help prevent poor mental health in the first place, like ensuring people have safe and dignified homes, jobs that pay living wages, and affordable health care. Laws that criminalize public sleeping, loitering, and "panhandling" punish people who are unhoused, worsening their health and stability by subjecting them to cycles of incarceration and violence.[14]

▶ **Instituting discriminatory school discipline policies.** School discipline policies are often framed as tools to ensure safety and order. However, their enforcement frequently produces the opposite effect—particularly for students of color and students with disabilities. When discipline is administered through "zero tolerance" policies (organizational rules that mandate predetermined, often severe consequences like suspension or expulsion regardless of context) or subjective judgments about students' behavior, it reinforces exclusion and worsens health and academic inequities. These policies also ignore the underlying social conditions in students' lives, including unstable housing, poor nutrition, and experiences of abuse and neglect. Research shows that punitive discipline does not improve school safety.[15] Instead, it harms children's mental health and significantly increases the likelihood they will enter the *school-to-prison pipeline:* a system that moves students from classrooms into juvenile detention centers and other places of incarceration. This path often leads to lasting economic hardship and poor health that leaves people trapped in cycles of poverty and punishment as adults.[16-19]

▶ **Charging fines and fees that punish the poor.** Local governments too often rely on fines and fees as both enforcement mechanisms and revenue streams—a conflict of interest that not only raises ethical concerns but also undermines health and public safety.[20] Individuals can face steep financial penalties when they interact with the criminal legal system. They can be charged fines for everything from minor traffic and municipal code violations to misdemeanors and felonies. Courts then often stack on additional fees, surcharges, and expenses. When people cannot pay, they quickly become caught in a cruel cycle of mounting debt and additional punishments, including driver's license suspension, loss of voting rights, arrest, and incarceration.[21] Although the Supreme Court ruled decades ago that imprisonment for inability to pay is unconstitutional,[22] this unjust practice—which disproportionately harms low-income people of color—continues as a modern-day debtor's prison in localities across the United States.[23]

Instead of relying on punitive and violent systems of enforcement, those of us in public health—especially within government—must evolve in both our mindsets and our methods. We need to move toward more holistic, assurance-centered approaches if we are to truly promote equity, justice, and flourishing.

This shift means embracing **abolition**—not simply the absence of police and prisons, but a vision and practice for building a society where they are no longer needed. Abolition centers two core commitments: First, it addresses the root causes of harm in society so that systems of policing and punishment become obsolete. Second, it reimagines and creates new systems grounded in care, co-governance, accountability, and community well-being.[24,25] Abolition draws its name and purpose from the 19th-century movement to end chattel slavery. It connects to that legacy by dismantling modern systems of racial and social oppression and replacing them with community-based approaches that embrace human dignity.[26]

Abolition flows from a public health commitment to assurance: the responsibility to respond to harm and most importantly, prevent it, by creating the conditions that support health in the first place. As public health practitioners, we have a role to play in transforming our approaches to center abolition and health justice. This means evolving beyond the use of punitive enforcement tactics that target individuals and instead implementing strategies grounded in support and shared accountability.[8] We can embrace assurance-centered interventions by embracing a four-part *Abolitionist Framework for Public Health Practice*:

 1. Reject the use of policing and carceral systems. If we affirm that health is synonymous with flourishing—as discussed in Chapter 1—then relying on law enforcement, incarceration, and punishment is fundamentally at odds with our goals. We cannot claim to promote well-being while criminalizing substance use, dispatching police to respond to mental health crises, or punishing people for experiencing poverty and homelessness. Such enforcement efforts address symptoms without treating the root causes of the disease: the systems of oppression that perpetuate poor health and inequity.

Punitive enforcement doesn't solve oppression—it compounds and entrenches it. To effectively prevent public health problems like road fatalities, substance abuse, or homelessness, we must transform the conditions that produce them, reject the misleading mindset that "some people deserve poor health" (discussed in Chapter 4), and invest in strategies that affirm people's full dignity and humanity.

 2. Redirect resources to address root causes of injustice. As discussed in Chapter 3, systems of oppression—such as structural racism, white supremacy, and racial capitalism—block access to the resources needed for health and flourishing. But we can upend these systems of oppression by taking an assurance approach that divests from punitive enforcement and carceral systems and instead reinvests resources in health-affirming solutions, such as dignified housing, economic mobility, climate adaptation, reliable transportation, and community services.

Research shows that every dollar invested in public health and prevention can have returns ranging from 460% to 8,700%[27-30]—figures that still cannot capture the value of human lives that can be saved, now and into the future. If, as public health practitioners, we are serious about prevention, we must invest our finite time, resources, and energy into interventions that offer the greatest returns—both in terms of lives and money. That means prioritizing strategies that address root causes and create conditions for communities to become healthier and happier places to live.

 3. Center community leadership in defining and implementing solutions. As discussed in Chapter 5, public health interventions cannot be imposed on communities. They must be co-created with them and implemented in ways that elevate community leadership. Community members and the organizations that serve them are experts who have credible knowledge and invaluable expertise regarding the issues they face. An assurance-centered approach requires not just consulting communities but deferring to their leadership. This means creating formal and meaningful opportunities for residents to shape priorities, make decisions, and steer public health work.

For example, some jurisdictions have created community-led health planning boards with the authority to review, approve, and adapt public health initiatives—ensuring alignment with local needs and lived experiences. In other communities, restorative justice has emerged as a powerful alternative to the policing approaches that have consistently failed to build trust, restore relationships, or repair harm.

Restorative justice is a community-centered practice that brings together those who have been harmed and those responsible—whether individuals or institutions—in a facilitated dialogue aimed at acknowledging harm, fostering accountability, and pursuing meaningful repair. When practiced effectively, it offers people who have experienced harm a direct role in shaping the response and identifying a path forward that promotes repair and accountability.[31]

To live up to our values as public health practitioners, we must ensure that mechanisms for transparency, accountability, shared power, and ongoing dialogue are fundamental to our interventions—allowing for community-led decision-making, context-specific adaptation, and collective self-determination.

 4. Use our power to nurture communities—not extract from them. Public health has long relied on strategies that restrict, penalize, and surveil in the name of population health—taxing sugary drinks, banning smoking in public areas, and ticketing people for not wearing seatbelts. In some cases, these actions are necessary to protect health and safety. But when public health efforts come across as punitive or extractive—especially in communities already burdened by systemic disinvestment—we risk showing up as a force of control, rather than care, in people's lives.

Assurance requires us to consider not just what public health takes away but also what it gives back: *What are we putting into communities to ensure health can actually take root and grow? What are we nourishing, sustaining, and helping to thrive?* Instead of treating people as problems to manage, we must ensure that public health serves as a force for community good—catalyzing sustained resources, infrastructure, co-governance models, and power-sharing. This also means funding and implementing interventions that are expansively related to community health, such as guaranteed income initiatives, youth organizing, community land trusts, and participatory budgeting.

As public health practitioners—particularly those of us in governmental roles—we cannot simply function as authorities; we must also be neighbors, collaborators, and co-conspirators invested in communities' success. Assurance means creating the conditions for flourishing—not by extraction or control—but by building alongside communities for the long haul.

An assurance-centered approach does not mean eliminating all forms of enforcement—it means reimagining how enforcement is used and to what end. Rather than punishing and penalizing individuals and communities who have been marginalized, enforcement should be used strategically to hold systemically powerful individuals and institutions accountable. This can include corporations that pollute communities, financial institutions that engage in predatory lending, employers that violate labor laws, and landlords who neglect tenant safety. Too often, these entities treat regulatory fines and penalties as just another cost of doing business, continuing harmful practices with little meaningful consequence.

Public health organizations have a responsibility to intervene in these situations. They must work with partner agencies to both stop these injustices and use enforcement mechanisms to hold powerful institutions accountable, address the root causes of public health problems, and provide real redress—through policy change, public oversight, and compensation for communities that have been wronged.

Transforming our use of punitive enforcement methods—from controlling and extracting from communities to dismantling systems of oppression—requires a more expansive approach to assurance that is essential for public health. It also requires fundamental changes to how we invest our resources and a shift in our mindsets—our deeply held beliefs, which expand or limit what we imagine to be possible (as discussed in Chapter 4). Enforcement asks: *How do we force people to comply and penalize those who don't?* But an equity- and justice-centered approach to assurance more appropriately asks, *How can we implement interventions in ways that are effective, people-centered, and values-aligned?*

An assurance approach pushes us to reimagine public safety to be more than the absence of crime and the use of punishment for compliance. It allows us to create conditions that promote collective care, justice, and liberation in ways that help all communities flourish.

CENTERING ASSURANCE FOR EFFECTIVE EVALUATION

Once implemented, interventions must be appropriately and consistently evaluated to understand and improve their effectiveness.[32] **Evaluation** is the systematic assessment of the merit, value, or significance of an intervention.[33-35] As one of the 10 Essential Public Health Services, evaluation is a foundational mechanism through which assurance is realized. Evaluations can help us answer questions like *What do we know? How do we know? And what value does this knowledge have?**

Both research and evaluation have long been cornerstones of public health. They each enhance **learning**—our collective efforts to build shared knowledge about what's effective, what isn't, and why, so we can make meaningful improvements. But unlike research, which can generate new knowledge that may not yet have a clear application, evaluations are intended to be applicable by their very nature. Evaluation findings are generated with the express intent of being used for a specific purpose: to improve an intervention or approach and to inform future decision-making.

But much like enforcement and research, evaluation can reinforce inequities instead of remedying them if conducted without intentionality. When evaluations fail to focus on equity and justice, they risk exacerbating power imbalances, perpetuating harmful narratives, and producing misleading or false conclusions that harm community health.

Despite its potential, public health evaluation has often fallen short of advancing equity and justice. Several systemic tendencies limit its transformative potential:

▶ **Prioritizing institutional needs over community priorities.** Many public health evaluations focus on metrics dictated by funders, policymakers, program administrators, and researchers, while sidelining the insights and priorities of those directly impacted by health inequities. This top-down approach often ignores what matters most: the lived experiences, wisdom, and visions of success held by communities. When evaluations exclude community perspectives, they fail to capture what's truly working, what isn't, and why.

▶ **Focusing on individual behaviors and outcomes instead of structural change.** Too often, evaluations emphasize individual behavior changes like smoking cessation and shifts in diet, while failing to address larger and more fundamental systems of oppression that constrain people's choices (discussed in Chapters 1 and 3). This narrow lens reinforces a false narrative that health inequities result from personal failures (discussed in Chapter 4), rather than their true root cause: systemic injustice.

---

*Each of these three questions is tied to the philosophical foundations of research, specifically ontology, epistemology, and axiology. We recommend exploring these concepts further, especially if you don't mind going down a thoughtful rabbit hole!

▶ **Emphasizing short-term outputs rather than long-term transformation.** Evaluations tend to measure what can be easily captured in short grant cycles—outputs like the number of people who attended a workshop or short-term outcomes like knowledge gained by a cohort of training participants. Without resourcing longer evaluation windows, we inevitably miss large and positive ripple effects over time, like new governance models, increases in community power, changes in policies, and sustained shifts in institutional practices. The more complex the problem that an intervention attempts to address, the more time it will take to see meaningful systemic changes.

▶ **Overlooking historical and social context.** Public health interventions are not implemented in a vacuum. Histories of harm—from decades of racial segregation and discrimination to state-sanctioned violence and forced sterilization—have shaped where people live, what resources they can access, and how they relate to institutions. These legacies intersect with ongoing injustices like police violence, mass layoffs, and evictions. Together, these dynamics influence whether people feel safe participating in public health interventions, how they interpret the intentions behind them, and what outcomes are possible. When evaluations ignore this context, they risk misinterpreting findings and reinforcing the very inequities they aim to address.

Evaluation is a vital aspect of public health, but to advance equity and justice, we have to transform how it's done and what it should achieve. Rather than simply measuring outcomes, evaluation should reflect our values. An **assurance-centered evaluation** does just that: It places community needs at the center, shifts power, focuses on systems, and mutually benefits communities, as well as the institutions supporting the evaluation. When evaluations center assurance, they produce more useful, relevant, and accurate findings that support stronger interventions and healthier communities, because they take these approaches:

• **Interrogate and address power dynamics.** Evaluations are not neutral or objective. They are influenced by who decides the evaluation questions, who provides the answers, who decides what data are considered credible and valid, and who synthesizes and interprets the findings. Assurance-centered evaluation confronts these power dynamics directly. It incorporates power-sharing practices, such as inviting community members to codevelop evaluation questions, shape data collection methods, and participate in data analysis and dissemination. When evaluation centers those most impacted by health inequities, it becomes a collaborative process grounded in shared decision-making and mutual benefit.

• **Define success based on community priorities and contexts.** Rather than imposing external metrics or relying on comparisons to white populations (see Box 6-1),[36-38] assurance-centered evaluations uplift community-defined visions of success. These evaluations prioritize local goals, lived experiences, and context-specific measures of flourishing. Assurance-centered evaluations also emphasize qualitative methods—such

Box 6-1. Challenging Whiteness as the "Gold Standard" of Health

White as the default, white as the center, white as the norm, is the central part of the master narrative. The centrality of whiteness—how it constructed white versus black, legal versus illegal—hurts not only people of color who aren't white but also white people who can't carry the burden of what they've constructed.

—Jose Antonio Vargas, journalist and filmmaker[36(p77-78)]

In public health, it's common to see data about the health outcomes of people of color compared with those of white people. Sometimes these comparisons are necessary to highlight the deep inequities created by structural racism. But relying on this framing—especially without sufficient context—can quietly reinforce a deeper problem: It treats whiteness as the invisible norm—an unspoken standard against which all other groups are measured.

This comparison is problematic for two important reasons:

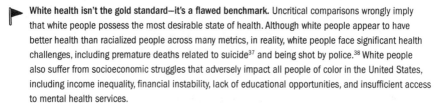 **White health isn't the gold standard—it's a flawed benchmark.** Uncritical comparisons wrongly imply that white people possess the most desirable state of health. Although white people appear to have better health than racialized people across many metrics, in reality, white people face significant health challenges, including premature deaths related to suicide[37] and being shot by police.[38] White people also suffer from socioeconomic struggles that adversely impact all people of color in the United States, including income inequality, financial instability, lack of educational opportunities, and insufficient access to mental health services.

Health inequity burdens all, even if the weight isn't evenly carried. Constantly measuring people of color against white people obscures a bigger truth: the systems of oppression that generate poor health outcomes affect us all (see Box 2-7 in Chapter 2)—they just impact people of color and other marginalized people disproportionately more than others. But while these systems may target communities of color more aggressively, they also erode the well-being of white people, especially those who are poor, disabled, queer, or otherwise marginalized.

As discussed in Chapter 1, having universal goals—fair and just outcomes that we believe everyone deserves—can help us envision a future where flourishing is possible for everyone. Universal goals can also help us identify the targeted supports that groups need to reach that future. Instead of using whiteness as the benchmark for health, we should ask, *What would it look like to set universal goals rooted in flourishing for all people? What if our goal was for everyone to live 90 or 100 years of vibrant, high-quality life? How might that change the interventions we design and how we evaluate them?*

With this reframing, the universal goal becomes the basis of comparison—not a specific racialized group. *What could be possible if we set aspirational goals, then took actions to help all people reach them?*

To move beyond using whiteness as a default standard for comparison, as public health practitioners, we must look to alternative frames—such as community-defined benchmarks, historic baseline comparisons, and international standards. These alternatives can offer more holistic, culturally relevant, and historically accurate reference points for evaluating progress toward community health goals and identifying the interventions needed for equity and justice.

When we overfocus on the disparities that exist between racial groups, we miss opportunities to demand better health and well-being for everyone. Equity and justice aren't about narrowing the gap between white people and people of color. They are about dismantling the very systems and structures that produce inequities at every level and building a society where everyone can flourish.

as stories, maps, and discussion-based insights—that offer richer, more nuanced understandings than quantitative data can offer alone (see Box 6-2).

- **Focus on improving interventions, not people.** Too often, those leading and funding evaluations frame them as judging people rather than assessing the value of

Box 6-2. The Value of Qualitative Data

In public health surveillance and evaluation, we have all too often allowed numerical data to dominate the conversation. Yet when it comes to shaping policies and approaches that genuinely reflect community needs, *qualitative data*—rooted in lived experiences, local knowledge, and personal histories—is invaluable. It helps us understand not just what is happening and to whom, but why it matters.

To illustrate how qualitative data can deepen and expand our understanding of seemingly straightforward metrics, this chapter includes real-world example from urban planning and environmental justice practitioner Taren Evans. The narrative she shares below conveys how qualitative data generates rich and unexpected information that can produce effective, community-desired solutions:

There is so much that is missed when we focus on quantitative data alone. This reality becomes apparent when taking even a cursory analysis of some of the quantitative measures that are used to inform policy.

My team and I worked on a project with local government staff to improve walkability in an area of Portland, Oregon. We began by looking at a set of environmental justice indicators in various areas, including tree canopy cover, park access, and walkability, among others. All of these indicators had a corresponding quantitative measure associated with them. Looking at these measures alone, it quickly became apparent how insufficient they were to truly understand these issues.

For example, a metric associated with measuring walkability was "intersections per square mile." However, anyone who reflects on this metric knows that it alone can never capture all the factors that go into assessing walkability. Later, at a meeting of community-based organizations, I posed the question to the group: "Does this measure alone capture everything that you think of in terms of walkability?" Of course, there was a resounding "No!" A discussion quickly ensued about all the other factors that go into determining walkability.

Community members who rely on walking as their primary means of transportation know the streets to avoid because of a lack of sidewalks, poor lighting at night, or a high volume of fast-moving traffic that makes walking feel uncomfortable. Yet looking at the singular quantitative metric of "intersections per square mile," the policy solution to increase walkability would perhaps simply be to create more intersections.

The walkability example is just one of many that highlight how quantitative metrics alone fail to capture the lived realities of impacted communities and the value of qualitative data. The dismissal of these types of data, or even the failure to recognize them as valid data, is reflective of exclusionary policymaking that devalues the experiences of low-income communities and communities of color, who experience the inequities embedded in the policies created for them each day. Too often, we have undervalued this knowledge and relegated it to the category of anecdotal or supplemental, when, in fact, we need this critical community knowledge—often presented as qualitative data—to create policy solutions that are multifaceted, value community members' unique contributions and perspectives, and meet real community needs.

Courtesy of Taren Evans, MURP. Reprinted with permission.

interventions—a perception that undermines trust and limits learning. Assurance-centered evaluation shifts the focus to improving the intervention, not the people involved. By clearly placing the focus on improving systems rather than individuals, evaluations can become tools for reflection and refinement—revealing what's working, what needs to be adjusted, and how interventions can be more equitable and effective.

• **Prioritize mutual benefit, not extraction.** Evaluations should never feel like a one-way data grab. They should have utility and benefit for the participants involved. This means engaging evaluation participants as mutually invested partners who have a say in how the evaluation is designed, how data are collected, and how evaluation results will be interpreted and used. It also means that evaluation findings should be shared with participants, given that their insights and perspectives are what make evaluations possible. When an evaluation is structured as a reciprocal process, it becomes a vehicle for shared learning and collective progress.

BUILDING EQUITY AND JUSTICE INTO EVALUATION

No matter the intervention—whether it's a vaccine distribution initiative, a diabetes education program, or a policy to expand access to affordable childcare—evaluations should be used to assess how effectively we are advancing equity and justice. We must ask, *Is the intervention changing conditions, relationships, power dynamics, and systems?*

It's not enough to document activities, track outputs, or measure short-term changes in knowledge or behavior. Our evaluations only matter if they can tell us not only what is changing and for whom but also deeper and more fundamental information: whether the intervention is meaningfully shifting the status quo, expanding what's possible, and moving us closer to justice.

To advance equity and justice, we can draw on the *Six Pillars of Assurance-Centered Evaluation* (Figure 6-1), which affirm that evaluations should have these characteristics:

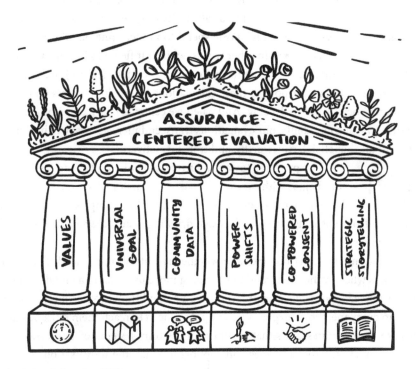

Artist Credit: Jasmin Pamukcu, 2025.

Figure 6-1. The Six Pillars of Assurance-Centered Evaluation

1. Be rooted in core values, especially reciprocity. Evaluations are inherently subjective. They are imbued with the priorities, assumptions, and worldviews of those who fund, design, and conduct them. Without intentionality, evaluations easily become extractive, taking knowledge from communities without offering anything in return. The values that govern the evaluation—and the evaluator—should be explicitly articulated and used to guide decisions. The end goal is not to simply evaluate an intervention with "rigor," but to evaluate it in ways that are values-aligned.

One essential value in evaluation is **reciprocity**—an ethical principle that emphasizes mutual respect, shared benefit, and fitting response to others' contributions. It is widely recognized across disciplines—from philosophy to social psychology—as a norm that sustains fairness, trust, and cooperation. In evaluation, reciprocity means that those who contribute their expertise and insights to an evaluation should meaningfully benefit from the knowledge, resources, and outcomes it generates. Rather than a transactional exchange, reciprocity calls for evaluators to build relationships rooted in trust, transparency, and a commitment to giving back in ways that reflect community priorities.

Epidemiologist and human rights scholar Jonathan Mann warned that the field of public health, even with all of its advanced methods of making precise measurements, was losing sight of why we measure at all: to identify and address the root causes of health inequities. As he put it: "[W]e spend too much time on 'p' values and not enough time on values."[39(p233)] In other words, while our field has become increasingly skilled at calculating statistical significance (what p values measure), we risk forgetting that the ultimate purpose of these calculations is to help us assess and improve community health and well-being. And when we center values like reciprocity, transparency, and accountability, our evaluations transcend mere accuracy to become useful, mutually beneficial, trustworthy, and transformative.

 2. Assess progress toward a universal goal. Equity- and justice-driven work begins with a *universal goal*—a vision for what everyone should be able to experience or achieve. Public health examples of universal goals can range from ensuring everyone has safe drinking water to every family attaining economic security.

Evaluations shouldn't just measure whether an intervention "works." They must also assess whether that intervention is helping move us closer to a broader, universal goal. A *targeted universalism* approach offers a helpful frame: While our goals should apply to everyone, the strategies different people need to reach them must be tailored. Because communities are situated differently within systems of oppression, some groups require specific strategies and support to reach the universal outcome. (See Chapter 1 for more on targeted universalism and Chapter 3 for more on systems of oppression.) Given this, evaluations should examine these questions:

- How effectively is the intervention advancing progress toward universal goals?
- Which groups remain furthest from those goals, and why?
- What additional strategies or resources are needed to close the gaps we see?

By building evaluations that measure progress toward universal goals—and by assessing the value of targeted approaches to reach them—evaluations become powerful tools for public health. They not only show where progress is being made but also help us chart a path forward so that every community can obtain what they need to flourish.

 3. Use *community data* to understand lived experiences. What we learn from an evaluation depends on the questions we ask—and the data we choose to value. It can be tempting to default to **quantitative data**—numeric metrics and statistics like percentages, rates, and counts—that are familiar to us and are relatively easier to acquire and analyze. But numbers alone can never be sufficient to provide complex insights into how change happens, who it impacts, and why it matters.

That's why qualitative data are essential. **Qualitative data**—rich information that includes stories, interviews, conversations, group discussions, and testimonials—illuminate changes in relationships, trust, power, and perceptions—elements that are vital to community health but are difficult to quantify. These data do what quantitative data struggle to do: "capture changes to the human experience"[40] with context and richness.

Evaluations can go further still, to embrace *community data*—a concept defined and coined by research justice advocates and scholars Mira Mohsini, Andres Lopez, Khanya Msibi, dallas haley, and Polet Campos-Melchor.

Community data are trusted and credible evidence generated by communities themselves and include all the ways communities express and document their everyday experiences and realities. Community data include stories, narratives, numbers, art, music, maps, oral histories, and firsthand accounts. These data reflect people's lived experiences, priorities, and aspirations—and must be produced on the terms of communities themselves.[41] They offer critical context about what happened in the past, what is happening in the present, who is living through these experiences, and why these experiences matter. The richness and context that community data provide cannot be found in administrative records or in government-generated statistics.

Community data cannot be extracted, collected, or controlled by dominant institutions, such as government agencies, academic entities, or funders. To obtain and use community data responsibly, evaluations must be codesigned and conducted in partnership with community power-building organizations. These partners are essential to ensure that data are gathered in ways that respect community desires, boundaries, and preferences—and that the evaluation yields tangible benefits for community members who contribute their data.

When collected and used properly, community data can inevitably improve evaluations, build trust, and ensure that findings are not only meaningful but also genuinely useful to the people whose lives and experiences they reflect.

 4. Examine changes in relationships and power. In any intervention focused on systems and structures, evolutions in relationships are among the first signals of transformative change. That means that before we can expect to see measurable improvements in health outcomes, we must first see signs that relationships and power dynamics are shifting.

An assurance-centered intervention does not solve public health challenges overnight. But it should generate trust, build stronger ties between communities and public institutions, expand community capacity, build and improve co-governance and community governance structures, and place more power in the hands of people most harmed by injustice. Without these relational shifts, public health interventions are unlikely to take root or deliver lasting impact.

Because community data are rooted in people's lived experiences, they can reveal how relationships are evolving and where power is shifting. These shifts may not always be immediately visible, but even incremental changes can open the door to more meaningful, systemic transformation. Evaluators can learn from community data to understand if power dynamics have changed, to what degree—and if the changes can be sustained. (For more on power, see Chapter 5.)

Evaluations should be designed to detect these relational shifts to understand whether power is being meaningfully shifted and shared. This means asking important questions during the design phase of an evaluation: *Are the evaluation questions and methods aligned with community priorities and ways of knowing? To what extent are community members being given real decision-making authority within the evaluation process? How are the findings being used to create new structures—such as policies, community governance bodies, and funding mechanisms—that institutionalize shifts in power?*

Stronger, more reciprocal relationships between communities and government institutions—from health departments to planning departments, city councils to mayors' offices—should be core outcomes of public health interventions. Evaluations must be intentionally designed to detect, assess, and support these relational shifts, recognizing them as necessary conditions for advancing equity and justice.

 5. Work toward co-powered consent. In public health, evaluations have many ethical considerations,[42] especially when they involve collecting information directly from people. Before they are allowed to proceed, these evaluations require approval from an institutional review board, which ensures studies meet ethical standards that protect the rights, safety, and welfare of participants. These technical requirements of ethics should be seen as the bare minimum.

Ethical evaluation begins with respect for the rights, dignity, and expertise of those whose experiences we are seeking to learn from. This means moving beyond the traditional model of *informed consent*—ensuring participants are told the risks and benefits before agreeing to participate—and aspiring toward **co-powered consent**: a participatory approach where evaluation participants influence the evaluation's design and implementation. In an evaluation that embraces co-powered consent, evaluation participants can decide *if* they will participate in an evaluation, as well as *how* their participation will be structured in the first place.

Co-powered consent draws inspiration from the *FRIES model of consent* developed by Planned Parenthood, which outlines five essential elements of genuine consent. It must be Freely given, Reversible, Informed, Enthusiastic, and Specific.*[43] Co-powered consent embraces and builds on this model to additionally prioritize agency, collaboration, and accountability.

People who agree to participate in an evaluation cannot be treated as passive subjects with *power over* imposed on them by evaluators and funders. They are active co-creators of knowledge and value, influencing everything from the evaluation's purpose to how their data are shared.

When evaluations are guided by co-powered consent, participants become partners in learning—which helps build relationships, reinforce trust, and generate knowledge that serves the communities at the heart of the work. To implement co-powered consent in assurance-centered evaluation, practitioners must take these actions†:

- **Clarify why data are being collected.** Clearly and candidly communicate the purpose of the evaluation, the value of participant contributions, and how data and findings will be used.
- **Be transparent about who will see the data.** Explain who will have access to the data, how it will be stored, and the level of confidentiality or anonymity that can be guaranteed. This includes explaining the difference between *confidential* information—where participant identities are known but safeguarded—and *anonymous* information, where data cannot reasonably be linked to specific individuals. Evaluators must be honest about what level of protection is possible.

---

*We thank cultural anthropologist and research justice scholar Mira Mohsini for uplifting the importance of the FRIES model to us.
†These recommendations for co-powered consent were adapted from data accountability agreements co-created by communities that are part of the Modernized Anti-racist Data Ecosystems (MADE) for Health Justice initiative—a partnership between the Robert Wood Johnson Foundation and the de Beaumont Foundation. The work of MADE for Health Justice is driven by community power-building organizations that are facilitating the creation of local data ecosystems that are expanding our understanding and use of civic data by centering antiracism, equity, justice, and community power. These organizations include Baltimore's Promise (Baltimore, MD), the Black Equity Coalition (Pittsburgh, PA), Coalition of Communities of Color (Portland, OR), and the Tucson Indian Center (Tucson, AZ).

- **Build consensus on how evaluation data will be collected and used.** Collaborate with evaluation participants to develop *data accountability agreements* that respect participants' boundaries, honor their autonomy, and document and define agreed-upon ways in which evaluation data will be collected and used. The process of creating data accountability agreements should include open and ongoing dialogue, negotiation, and shared decision-making to ensure that participants' rights and wishes are upheld throughout the evaluation process. Data accountability agreements are living commitments that can always be revisited, amended, and renegotiated throughout the evaluation process.[44]

- **Return findings to participants.** Share evaluation results in a timely manner and using accessible formats—such as community presentations, plain-language summaries, or visual materials. This allows participants to see how their insights shaped the work and contributed to future action. There's no need to wait until the evaluation is "over." If evaluation data are being synthesized across multiple periods over time, prioritize sharing this information with participants on an ongoing basis.

- **Credit participants based on their preferences.** Evaluations wholly depend on the knowledge, perspectives, and experiences that participants are willing to share. To honor their contributions, we must credit them in ways that reflect their wishes—whether that means providing public acknowledgment, sharing private appreciations, or maintaining their anonymity. Asking for these preferences and respecting them demonstrates that we value evaluation participants and their insights. It also affirms their agency in how their involvement is recognized.

Co-powered consent takes more time, conversation, and flexibility than traditional evaluation practices. But engaging in this process is necessary to live up to our values, to conduct evaluations equitably, and to ensure evaluation efforts result in shared benefits for all involved. When we center participant agency and treat evaluation as a collective endeavor, we strengthen the integrity of our findings and lay the groundwork for stronger relationships, deeper learning, and lasting change.

 6. Use strategic storytelling to communicate findings. The realities of human life are complex, and public health interventions must be implemented within these dynamic environments—unfolding amid shifts in political and organizational leadership, evolving funder expectations, changes in policies, and turnover within partner agencies. These conditions—combined with the longer time horizons often required for even the strongest interventions to yield measurable health outcomes—make it essential to tell a clear, consistent, and compelling story about public health work. We must be able to communicate what it aims to do and how it's making a difference.

An assurance-centered evaluation is a powerful tool for telling that story. It can provide evidence of how an intervention is contributing to systems change, shifting power, and addressing the root causes of health inequities.

As discussed in Chapter 4, narratives shape how people understand health, community, and justice. Strategic storytelling draws on these insights by using relatable, emotionally resonant narratives to influence audiences and achieve specific objectives.[45] In evaluation, strategic storytelling means communicating findings in ways that center community voices, reflect lived experiences, and speak to the purpose and progress of the intervention. Strategic storytelling can help strengthen support and keep communities and partners invested in an intervention for the long haul.

Evaluation findings are not neutral, and they don't "speak for themselves." How results are framed and contextualized shapes how they're understood, accepted, and acted upon. It's important to go beyond written reports and academic publications to utilize engaging, accessible formats such as narrative videos, digital stories, community briefings, and visually rich infographics. These tools not only make evaluation findings easier to understand but also humanize the work by showing the people behind the intervention being evaluated. They build buy-in and trust by showcasing the ways in which valuable insights are being uncovered and used in real time, ultimately supporting the intervention's longevity. When storytelling is an intentional aspect of the evaluation process, it deepens public understanding and builds the case for sustained investment and scale.

Together, these six pillars reimagine evaluation as a living practice for accountability, learning, and transformation. When we center assurance in evaluation, we create opportunities to measure impact while also building trust, shifting power, and moving closer to equity and justice. In a time when public health resources are stretched thin and political pressures are high, evaluations grounded in shared values and community partnership can help our interventions achieve their truest purpose: ensuring collective flourishing for all.

CONCLUSION

As public health practitioners, we are responsible for how we pursue change and how we assess the impact of our interventions. That means we must critically examine how we implement our interventions and how we evaluate their progress. We must ground our work and how we evaluate it within assurance: a public health approach grounded in transparency, collaboration, accountability, and mutual benefit.

Assurance asks us to make authentic promises to communities and to follow through: to act, to stay present, to build trust, and to ensure that interventions are effective, values-based, and systems-focused. Assurance-centered strategies support power shifting, co-governance, community priorities, and long-term infrastructure that enables collective decision-making. This includes creating space for communities to shape implementation, guide evaluation, and hold dominant institutions accountable for health outcomes.

Assurance isn't about public health "delivering" solutions to communities—it's about shifting who holds the power to define problems, design solutions, and make decisions. It also reminds us that we cannot do this work alone, whether as individuals, organizations, or even as a field. Advancing equity and justice through public health interventions requires collective capacity—teams of people working in alignment, bringing together diverse skills, expertise, and lived experiences, but all with a shared purpose: to improve community health and well-being. Whether it involves designing policies, implementing programs, or conducting evaluations, assurance means showing up alongside community members as partners and fellow collaborators, not as authorities.

Assurance is ultimately about trust, which is built over time based on the strength of our relationships with and within communities. When we replace punishment with partnership and extraction with reciprocity, we create the conditions for better public health, which requires deeper trust, lasting power, and a foundation for communities to flourish.

KEY TAKEAWAYS

Implementation is where our values meet reality. Any intervention is only as good as its implementation. Without equitable, effective, and community-led follow-through, even the most promising initiative will fall short. *Assurance* demands that we implement interventions in ways that are effective, systems focused, and responsible. This means planning for and monitoring not just outcomes but also the processes that shape them: *Are frontline staff equipped and supported? Are communities receiving the resources they were promised? Is the policy being implemented as intended?* Assurance-centered implementation requires us to ensure that every intervention serves and benefits those harmed by health inequities.

Assurance offers a path beyond punishment. Public health has too often relied on enforcement models that punish rather than protect—especially in marginalized communities. Embracing assurance means moving toward an *Abolitionist Framework for Public Health Practice* and away from carceral approaches: reducing reliance on punishment and control and instead building systems rooted in reciprocity, care, and collective accountability. This shift invites us to proactively design interventions that prevent harms before they occur, rather than responding with financial exploitation, criminalization, and coercion. When we center care and prevention, we create conditions where people are supported—not penalized—and where public health advances and reimagines safety and well-being.

Public health must be a source of abundance, not a force of extraction. We must reject the role of moralizing, controlling, or taking from communities in the name of health—whether through policing and punishment, blaming people's behaviors for systemic problems, or using ahistorical and context-insensitive approaches to evaluate interventions. Instead, our work must be additive and strengths-based, enriching everyday life with opportunities for health and shared prosperity. That means asking more than, *Did it work?* We must go deeper to assess and ask, *Who did it work for? Why? And how can it be improved?* When we lead with this mindset, public health becomes a true partner in creating lasting conditions for care, connection, and collective flourishing.

 Public health is strengthened by using the *Six Pillars of Assurance-Centered Evaluation.* These pillars help us stay rooted in shared values, work toward universal goals, cultivate community data, examine shifts in power, center co-powered consent, and use strategic storytelling to communicate meaningfully and move people to action. These pillars move evaluation beyond a narrow focus on efficiency or outputs. They reflect a commitment to transforming evaluation practice: ensuring that those harmed by health inequities are co-creating evaluation processes, assessing the value of interventions on their terms, and defining success based on their priorities and experiences.

 Community data are powerful, trusted, and credible evidence. Generated on the terms of communities themselves and reflecting information about their everyday lives, community data elevate and enhance both implementation and evaluation. Community data provide a richness of information, context, and evidence for decision-making that cannot be found in administrative records or government-generated statistics. These data—which can include stories, maps, oral histories, numbers, and art—are not only trusted and credible but also make the work we do more thoughtful, applicable, and solutions-oriented.

REFERENCES

1. Fannie Lou Hamer. *The Speeches of Fannie Lou Hamer: To Tell It Like It Is.* University Press of Mississippi; 2011.
2. Stevenson B. Keynote address. Presented at: American Public Health Association Annual Meeting; October 25, 2020; virtual meeting.
3. Institute of Medicine Committee for the Study of the Future of Public Health. *The Future of Public Health.* National Academies Press; 1988.
4. Perry IA. Assessment, policy development, and assurance: Evolving the core functions of public health to address health threats. *AJPM Focus.* 2023;3(1):100172. doi:10.1016/j.focus.2023.100172

5. Alang S, Hardeman R, Karbeah J, et al. White supremacy and the core functions of public health. *Am J Public Health*. 2021;111(5):815–819. doi:10.2105/AJPH.2020.306137

6. Centers for Disease Control and Prevention. 10 Essential Public Health Services. May 16, 2024. Accessed May 12, 2025. https://www.cdc.gov/public-health-gateway/php/about/index.html

7. Lorde A. *Sister Outsider: Essays and Speeches*. Crossing Press; 2007.

8. Pamukcu A, Harris AP. Health justice and the criminal legal system: From reform to transformation. *Bill of Health*. September 10, 2021. Accessed August 11, 2025. https://petrieflom.law.harvard.edu/2021/09/10/health-justice-criminal-legal-system

9. Ehrenfreund M. The risks of walking while Black in Ferguson. *Washington Post*. March 4, 2015. Accessed May 12, 2025. https://www.washingtonpost.com/news/wonk/wp/2015/03/04/95-percent-of-people-arrested-for-jaywalking-in-ferguson-were-black

10. US Dept of Justice, Civil Rights Division. *Investigation of the Ferguson Police Department*. March 4, 2015. Accessed May 12, 2025. https://www.justice.gov/sites/default/files/opa/press-releases/attachments/2015/03/04/ferguson_police_department_report.pdf

11. Hennessy-Fiske M. Walking in Ferguson: If you're Black, it's often against the law. *Los Angeles Times*. March 5, 2015. Accessed May 12, 2025. https://www.latimes.com/nation/la-na-walking-black-ferguson-police-justice-report-20150305-story.html

12. Morrison A. Michael Brown's death transformed a nation and sparked a decade of American reckoning on race. *Associated Press*. August 8, 2023. Accessed June 16, 2025. https://apnews.com/article/michael-brown-ferguson-anniversary-racial-justice-06773aab70c16bbbfd-4835be1bf6037c

13. National Homelessness Law Center; University of Miami School of Law Human Rights Clinic. *Criminalization of Homelessness and Mental Health in the United States: Shadow Report to the United Nations Human Rights Committee (ICCPR Review of the United States)*. September 12, 2023. Accessed June 3, 2025. https://homelesslaw.org/wp-content/uploads/2023/09/ICCPR-Report-2023.pdf

14. National Law Center on Homelessness & Poverty. *Housing Not Handcuffs 2019: Ending the Criminalization of Homelessness in US Cities*. December 2019. Accessed June 3, 2025. https://homelesslaw.org/wp-content/uploads/2019/12/HOUSING-NOT-HANDCUFFS-2019-FINAL.pdf

15. Hall D, Terenzi K. From failure to freedom: Dismantling Milwaukee's school-to-prison pipeline with the youth power agenda. Center for Popular Democracy; Leaders Igniting Transformation. April 2018. Accessed June 10, 2025. https://populardemocracy.org/sites/default/files/FailureToFreedom.pdf

16. Morris EW, Perry BL. The punishment gap: School suspension and racial disparities in achievement. *Soc Probl*. 2016;63(1):68–86. doi:10.1093/socpro/spv026

17. Gregory A, Skiba RJ, Noguera PA. The achievement gap and the discipline gap: Two sides of the same coin? *Educ Res*. 2010;39(1):59–68. doi:10.3102/0013189X09357621

18. Skiba RJ, Arredondo MI, Williams NT. More than a metaphor: The contribution of exclusionary discipline to a school-to-prison pipeline. *Equity Excell Educ*. 2014;47(4):546–564. doi:10.1080/10665684.2014.958965

19. Davison M, Penner AM, Penner EK, et al. School discipline and racial disparities in early adulthood. *Educ Res*. 2022;51(3):231–234. doi:10.3102/0013189X211061732

20. Sanders C, Leachman M. Step one to an antiracist state revenue policy: Eliminate criminal justice fees and reform fines. Center on Budget and Policy Priorities. September 17, 2021. Accessed June 3, 2025. https://www.cbpp.org/research/state-budget-and-tax/step-one-to-an-antiracist-state-revenue-policy-eliminate-criminal

21. Fines and Fees Justice Center. About us. Accessed June 10, 2025. https://finesandfeesjusticecenter.org/about-fines-fees-justice-center

22. *Bearden v Georgia*, 461 US 660 (1983).

23. Equal Justice Initiative. Unjust fines and fees. Accessed June 10, 2025. https://eji.org/projects/fees-and-fines

24. The Daily Show. Derecka Purnell – making the argument for abolishing the police [video]. YouTube. September 29, 2021. Accessed May 12, 2025. https://www.youtube.com/watch?v=vUtpuU4mzOM

25. Raven L, Mohapatra M, Kuo R. 8 to Abolition is advocating to abolish police to keep us all safe. TransformHarm. June 26, 2020. Accessed May 12, 2025. https://transformharm.org/ab_resource/8-to-abolition-is-advocating-to-abolish-police-to-keep-us-all-safe

26. Roberts DE. Abolition constitutionalism. *Harvard Law Rev.* 2019;133(1):1-77. Accessed August 10, 2025. https://harvardlawreview.org/print/vol-133/abolition-constitutionalism

27. Bor J. Capitalizing on natural experiments to improve our understanding of population health. *Am J Public Health.* 2016;106(8):1388-1389. doi:10.2105/AJPH.2016.303294

28. United Nations. WHO study shows $39 return for each dollar invested in fight against TB. *UN News.* March 18, 2024. Accessed May 5, 2025. https://news.un.org/en/story/2024/03/1147696

29. Miller TR, Hendrie D. *Substance Abuse Prevention Dollars and Cents: A Cost-Benefit Analysis.* Center for Substance Abuse Prevention, Substance Abuse and Mental Health Services Administration. 2009. Accessed June 3, 2025. https://www.samhsa.gov/sites/default/files/cost-benefits-prevention.pdf

30. Trust for America's Health. *Prevention for a Healthier America: Investments in Disease Prevention Yield Significant Savings, Stronger Communities.* July 2008. Accessed June 3, 2025. https://www.tfah.org/wp-content/uploads/archive/reports/prevention08/Prevention08.pdf

31. Restorative Justice Council. What is restorative justice? Accessed June 18, 2025. https://restorativejustice.org.uk/what-restorative-justice

32. Porter JM, Brennan LK, Fine M, Robinson II. The elements to enhance the successful start and completion of program and policy evaluations: The Injury & Violence Prevention Program & Policy Evaluation Institute. *J Multidiscip Eval.* 2020;16(37):58-73. doi:10.56645/jmde.v16i37.659

33. Scriven M. Minimalist theory: The least theory that practice requires. *Am J Eval.* 1998;19(1):57-70. doi:10.1016/S1098-2140(99)80180-5

34. Shadish WR, Cook TD, Leviton LC. *Foundations of Program Evaluation: Theories of Practice.* Sage Publications; 1991.

35. Milstein B, Wetterhall SF. Framework for program evaluation in public health. *MMWR Recomm Rep.* 1999;48(RR-11):1-40.

36. Vargas JA. *Dear America: Notes of an Undocumented Citizen.* Dey Street Books; 2018.

37. Suicide Prevention Resource Center. Racial and ethnic disparities: White populations. Accessed May 12, 2025. https://sprc.org/about-suicide/scope-of-the-problem/racial-and-ethnic-disparities/white-populations

38. Henderson H. Rethinking the role of race in crime and police violence. Brookings Institution. June 27, 2024. Accessed May 12, 2025. https://www.brookings.edu/articles/rethinking-the-role-of-race-in-crime-and-police-violence

39. Mann J. Human rights and the new public health. *Health Hum Rights*. 1995;1(3):229-233. doi:10.2307/4065135

40. The Praxis Project. Measuring the impact of building community power for health justice: What? Why? and How? Centering Community in Public Health—Learning Circle Brief Series, No. 2. 2020. Accessed June 3, 2025. https://static1.squarespace.com/static/5bf21032b98a7888bf3b6e21/t/5ec6c0a2e811ca37e79b284f/1590083752827/PraxisLCBrief2-Power-Praxis.pdf

41. Mohsini M, Lopez A, Msibi K, haley d, Campos-Melchor P. Introducing Community Data. Coalition of Communities of Color. 2024. Accessed August 8, 2025. https://www.coalitioncommunitiescolor.org/research-and-publications/introducing-community-data

42. Akrami F, Zali A, Abbasi M, et al. An ethical framework for evaluation of public health plans: A systematic process for legitimate and fair decision-making. *Public Health*. 2018;164:30-38. doi:10.1016/j.puhe.2018.07.018

43. Planned Parenthood. What is consent? April 1, 2024. Accessed July 9, 2025. https://www.plannedparenthooddirect.org/article/what-consent

44. Schaffer K, Porter JM. Show me the values: Centering communities and co-creation in an equity-driven evaluation. *J Public Health Manag Pract*. 2025;31(5):897–898. doi:10.1097/PHH.0000000000002187

45. Arat RF. The art of strategic storytelling: How to master it. Pip Decks. June 14, 2024. Accessed May 9, 2025. https://web.archive.org/web/20240720003131/https://pipdecks.com/blogs/storytelling/how-to-master-strategic-storytelling

III. CREATING FLOURISHING FUTURES FOR ALL

In the space between dreaming and doing, we can plan a path toward a flourishing future. In this third and final section, we explore a bold, hopeful vision for community health and offer 10 practical actions we can take in our daily work to make equity and justice a reality—now and for generations to come.

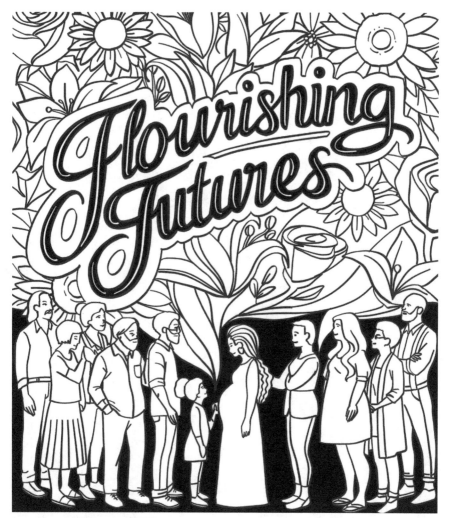

Artist Credit: Jasmin Pamukcu, 2025.
Our Inalienable Right

Envisioning and Actualizing a Better World

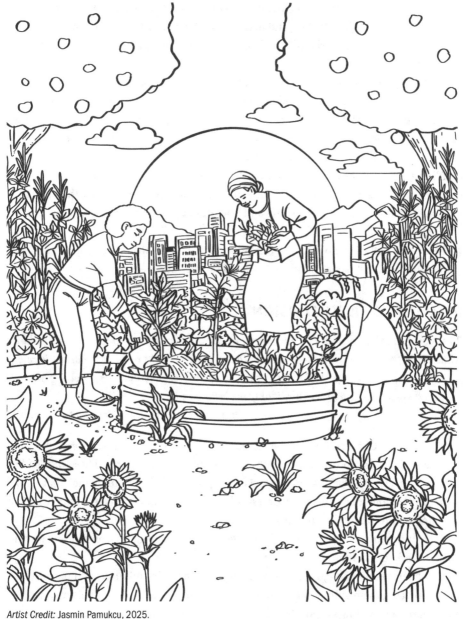

Artist Credit: Jasmin Pamukcu, 2025.

Three Sisters: Interwoven Futures

The radical imagination is not just about dreaming of different futures. It's about bringing those possibilities back from the future to work on the present, to inspire action and new forms of solidarity today.

—Alex Khasnabish, sociologist and social movement scholar, and
Max Haiven, cultural theorist and political economist[1(p3)]

Part I of this book unearthed the foundations of (in)equity and (in)justice, defining key concepts related to equity, justice, and health—and how these terms have evolved; examining the intertwined histories of "race," racism, and public health; and exposing the root causes of health inequities.

Part II explored opportunities we can seize for change: how *misleading mindsets* and damaging narratives undermine equity, justice, and well-being; how policy, power, and *co-governance* shape health on a large scale; and how *assurance*—a core function of public health—is essential for implementing and evaluating public health interventions.

This third and final part focuses on creating flourishing futures for all. It involves building a vision for health, equity, and justice—rooted not only in identifying problems but also in creating new possibilities and reimagined systems. It is a vision that invites us to imagine a future where flourishing and liberation are not distant dreams but day-to-day realities.

This book will then close with a final chapter that turns that vision into action, as a culmination of the lessons and insights shared throughout.

ELEMENTS OF A BOLD VISION

To vision futures is to conjure something that sits outside of your time and circumstance while being firmly rooted in the moment. To listen for the calls of what is not yet here but waiting just in the wings. Visioning is the uncovering of potential. It's revealing what is already there and trying to become, if only we believe in it.

—Prentis Hemphill, organizer and therapist[2(p11)]

As discussed in Chapter 4, public health approaches have too often reinforced harmful mindsets that sustain inequities rather than dismantling them. These *misleading mindsets*—such as blaming individuals for poor health or implying that some communities "deserve" worse outcomes—obscure a fundamental truth: Our lives and our fates are profoundly interconnected.

Such mindsets fuel separation and erode empathy, preventing us from finding ways to imagine and build a flourishing future.

To advance equity and justice, we must upend destructive mindsets and narratives—while replacing them with new ones that are compelling and inspiring. This involves not only improving existing systems but also daring to reimagine and build new ones that are rooted in compassion and solidarity.

To guide this work, we can turn to the *Three Threads of Vision*—essential strands woven into justice movements' collective purpose and aspirations. We position ourselves to realize transformational change when our visions are grounded in imagination, discipline, and audacity:

Imagination: the courage to dream beyond what currently exists. Feminist writer and cultural critic bell hooks reminds us, "What we cannot imagine cannot come into being"[3(p14)]—that ultimately, imagining new futures is not a luxury or distraction. Vision gives us direction, helping us resist injustice by saying no to harm while also offering a compelling *yes*—toward new systems and ways of being that affirm life. As we dream up the future, we must also open space for others to dream, especially those whose energy is consumed by survival. Imagination must be democratized: shared and nurtured, so that the futures we build reflect our collective hopes.

Discipline: the daily practice of staying the course, rejecting distractions, and maintaining focus on our goals. Organizer and abolitionist Mariame Kaba teaches that "hope is a discipline."[4] This is an active and often difficult practice. Although we face injustices that have long been entrenched, we must have the persistence to envision a better future—and to continue moving forward to make that future a reality. This manifests as a daily decision to use our courage and energy to do the work of creating the world we want.

Audacity: the bravery to question the systems we have inherited and to dream beyond them. Anthropologist and activist David Graeber reminds us that the structures we live under—our institutions, hierarchies, and rules—are not inevitable or unchangeable: "The ultimate hidden truth of the world is that it is something that we make, and could just as easily make differently."[5(p89)] Health inequities are not natural; they are human-made and can be changed. This means we can unmake them—and create something better in their place.

To move people to action—especially in the face of fear, fragmentation, and overwhelm—a bold vision names what we're up against while grounding us in what we are working toward. When we articulate a compelling vision, we inspire and sustain collective action in specific, meaningful ways. Transformative visions have the power to acknowledge oppression without being limited or defined by it; invite people into collective and connected purpose; combine emotional resonance, moral clarity, and actionability; and endure and adapt over time.

Acknowledge Oppression Without Being Defined by It

As public health practitioners, we have had to mobilize alongside our allies in response to seemingly unrelenting crises—the forced separation of children from their families at the US-Mexico border,[6] the outbreak of the COVID-19 pandemic,[7] widespread evictions of renters on a national scale,[8] and the murder of George Floyd and its aftermath.[9,10]

These moments reflect a deepening pattern of systemic injustice. We see it in efforts to erase populations—people of color, nonbinary people, and trans people—from federally funded research and datasets.[11] We see it in the rollback of abortion access and reproductive rights[12]; bans on evidence-based harm reduction programs[13]; and the rise of discriminatory deportation policies that target and terrorize immigrants regardless of documentation or legal standing.[14] We see it in the censorship of health-related education and resources.[15]

Our responses to these crises have been powerful, but not always consistent or coordinated. Mobilization has often been reactive, fragmented across disciplines and geographies, and shaped by the urgency of the moment rather than a shared long-term strategy.

These injustices are real and pressing. But as we confront them, we must also sharpen our ability to respond with both immediacy and foresight. The pace of policy change, disinformation, and political backlash demands that we act swiftly—but not at the expense of vision. We must be building toward longer-term goals, even while we are actively responding to acute crises.

Consider the example of immigration policy: Certainly, we are responding today to stop children from being torn from their parents and protect families from being deported in ways that sow fear and violate basic rights. But we must also imagine and work toward a world where all families—regardless of citizenship status—are centered in policy and practice, where migration is met with care and compassion, and where immigration is no longer entangled in carceral systems. That vision also requires reckoning with the role the United States has played in global instability—through military actions, economic exploitation, and climate disruption—that forces people to flee their homes in the first place.[16]

In addition to reactive and rapid response, we must also hone our ability to do proactive future-shaping. Just Transition advocates call this dual focus *stopping the bad* and *building the new*.[17]

Invite People Into Collective and Connected Purpose

A truly inclusive vision gives everyone a place in a future we are building together—and a responsibility to help create it. Transformative movements articulate a shared purpose that connects people across lines of "race," class, geography, and ideology. This kind of vision doesn't flatten differences but honors them while revealing how our struggles are intertwined.

Consider *The Poor People's Campaign: A National Call for a Moral Revival*—an anti-poverty justice movement.[18] Rooted in the unfinished work of Baptist minister and civil rights leader Martin Luther King Jr. and many others, the campaign frames poverty, structural racism, ecological devastation, and militarism as interlocking injustices. Its demands—"federal and state living-wage laws, equity in education, an end to mass incarceration, a single-payer health-care system, and the protection of the right to vote"[19]—are not siloed issues but part of a broader moral vision. By naming these connections, the campaign invites people to see themselves not just as victims of injustice or allies to others, but as co-creators of and co-conspirators in the creation of a more just society.

A guiding vision that unites us with a shared purpose can help us recognize connections between different forms of injustice, uncover our common interests, amplify our collective strengths, and motivate us to advocate for changes that benefit everyone.

Combine Emotional Resonance, Moral Clarity, and Actionability

Sometimes, powerful tools in our toolbox, like rigorous research and detailed policy proposals, can work against us when it's time to inspire people to act. Movements don't win on technical precision or facts alone. Sociologist and economist Manuel Pastor emphasizes that successful movements are built not just on interests and transactions, but on vision and values that resonate emotionally and morally.[20]

Movements succeed not just by presenting facts or critiques, but by connecting to shared values like dignity, safety, and belonging. This inspires the collaboration and connectedness that make movements durable and transformative. As Pastor puts it, "Just as markets reward and teach us to pursue self-interest, movements reward and teach us to act mutually."[19]

A compelling vision combines this emotional resonance with a feeling that something is doable or achievable. It offers people a way to act on their values—to translate moral clarity into tangible change. That means pairing bold ideas with concrete strategies, clear demands, and structures that invite participation.

Consider the *Marriage Equality Movement*, which catalyzed what sociologist and social demographer Michael Rosenfeld calls "the greatest transformation of public opinion in US history."[21(p8)] In the late 1990s and early 2000s, support for same-sex marriage was politically risky and publicly unpopular—most mainstream politicians opposed it.[22] While organizing and advocacy had been underway for decades, a more dramatic shift occurred from 2008 to 2015, when marriage equality moved from a marginalized demand into a widely embraced civil right.[21]

Advocates didn't just argue for legal recognition; they made a moral case for love, dignity, and family—values that resonated across ideological lines. That emotional clarity—paired with coordinated legal strategy, compelling narratives in popular culture,[23] and persistent grassroots organizing—helped shift public sentiment so rapidly that by the time the Supreme Court legalized same-sex marriage nationwide in *Obergefell v Hodges* (2015), many of the same politicians who once opposed it were celebrating the decision.

This was a testament to how movements can win when their vision connects moral clarity to actionable demands. When our vision speaks to what people care about most—and shows them how to act on it—we build movements that are not only inspiring but also irresistible and unstoppable.

Endure and Adapt Over Time

A transformative vision usually won't be static—it will be resilient enough to withstand backlash, flexible enough to integrate new insights, and deeply rooted enough to shape culture, policy, and institutions over the long haul. Movements that endure imagine a better future while simultaneously creating mechanisms to sustain themselves. This requires investing in leadership development, narrative infrastructure, and long-term organizing—mobilizing to meet the moment and also building for generations to come.

Consider how the reproductive rights movement evolved into reproductive justice. Coined in the 1990s by Black women activists,* *reproductive justice* reframed the struggle from a narrow focus on legal access to abortion toward a holistic vision of the human right to bodily autonomy, to have children or to not have children, and to raise children in safe, sustainable communities.[25(p9)]

This framework expanded the movement's reach and relevance, linking it to racial, economic, and environmental justice, and grounding it in lived experience. Its evolution has influenced policy debates, public health frameworks, and community-led initiatives, while also equipping the movement with a vision capable of adapting and persevering through shifting political landscapes.

LESSONS IN VISION

How can we bring these lessons to public health? Fortunately, we are not starting from scratch. Across social justice movements, powerful visions have emerged that challenge systems of oppression and offer bold alternatives rooted in care and community. These movements help us reimagine what collective flourishing can look like and how we might build systems that truly support it.

These next examples show the transformative potential of justice-centered visions. Each offers insights that can deepen our understanding and practice of public health.

Just Transition

Just Transition is a vision-led framework grounded by the principle that a healthy economy and a healthy environment can and must coexist.[26,27] It calls for a shift from an extractive, racialized economy—one that sacrifices people and planet in pursuit of ever-growing profits—to a generative economy rooted in dignity, sustainability, and shared prosperity. As author and activist Naomi Klein writes, "Climate change isn't an 'issue' to add to the list

---

*The term *reproductive justice* was developed by Black women who formed Women of African Descent for Reproductive Justice in 1994. The cofounders are community leaders and racial justice advocates Toni M. Bond Leonard, Rev. Alma Crawford, Evelyn S. Field, Terri James, Bisola Marignay, Cassandra McConnell, Cynthia Newbille, Loretta Ross, Elizabeth Terry, "Able" Mable Thomas, Winnette P. Willis, and Kim Youngblood.[24]

of things to worry about . . . It is a civilizational wake-up call . . . telling us that we need an entirely new economic model and a new way of sharing this planet."[28(p25)]

Originally developed by labor advocates to protect workers during industrial shifts, Just Transition has been embraced by diverse, multi-movement collaborations that include those advocating for health broadly, as well as climate and reproductive justice.[29] In recent years, it has gained prominence as a central demand of youth-led climate movements such as *Fridays for Future*[30] and has been recognized by international bodies like the United Nations and the International Labour Organization as essential to shaping equitable and sustainable transitions.[31,32]

Just Transition is now a globally relevant vision and framework that emphasizes transnational solidarity and the interconnectedness of our economic and ecological systems. It makes explicit the links that exist between our health, climate catastrophe, environmental degradation, and the global structures of profit-driven exploitation that drive them.

Multiracial Democracy

Multiracial democracy is the vision for a future in which the United States at last lives up to its founding promise of a "government of the people, by the people, and for the people."[33] It is a model of governance designed for a racially diverse society—one where everyone's rights are protected and all communities have real power to shape their futures.

Realizing this vision requires us to reckon with the reality of our nation's past and present: a country built on stolen land, stolen labor, and stolen lives. It also requires us to wrestle with—and meaningfully redress—the many ways in which white supremacy and structural racism are perpetuated within our nation's systems of government and governance. But it also offers a path forward: the *transformation of democracy*, a reimagined and revitalized form of governance in which all people—especially those who have been racialized and subjugated by multiple systems of oppression—are central to decision-making.

As racial equity and systems change advocates Michael McAfee and Ashleigh Gardere write, "We the People must become the founders of a nation yet to be realized—the opportunity of our generation."[34] This reframes democracy not as a static inheritance but as a living project we are all responsible for shaping.

Political theorist and civic educator Danielle Allen points to the Declaration of Independence as a guide for how to continually refound our democracy—through deliberate commitments that bind us together. In her words, "solidarity cannot be built without principle."[35(p98)] The solidarity of multiracial democracy demands widening the circle of belonging, sharing power across all communities, and making equity and justice the foundation of our collective future.

Gender Liberation

Gender liberation imagines a world where everyone has the freedom to express, define, and live their gender without fear or violence. It centers *bodily autonomy*—the right of all people to make decisions about their own bodies, lives, and futures—and encompasses the struggles for abortion access, gender-affirming health care, and reproductive justice. These are core public health issues, deeply tied to access, dignity, and safety.

Led by trans, nonbinary, and queer communities, gender liberation benefits everyone by freeing us all from rigid roles and expectations. Poet and performance artist Alok Vaid-Menon uplifts the lessons of trans people throughout history, whose "possible impossible lives" are in fact "templates of everyday, embodied practices of freedom."[36]

All people experience gender in unique ways, and all people thrive in societies where gender diversity is celebrated—not policed or punished. Whether someone identifies as trans, cisgender, nonbinary, genderfluid, agender, intersex, or has any other self-defined experience of gender, the freedom to express oneself in dignity and to live fully is a shared human need. Gender is lived individually, but liberation is sustained collectively.

Gender liberation calls us to create systems that affirm our autonomy, protect our identities, and embrace the wide diversity of what it means to be human. It reminds us that health is not just physical; it's also about freedom, safety, and belonging.

Disability Justice

Disability justice affirms that all bodies and minds are valuable. It reframes disability from a personal deficit to a social and political experience—the result of how we can or cannot move through the world, and the barriers that have been built into environments, policies, and systems. It envisions a future where disabled people—especially disabled people of color, queer disabled people, and others at the intersections—lead the transformation of society.

Coined and developed by disabled queer and trans members of the performance collective Sins Invalid, disability justice moves beyond a narrow focus on access or compliance to confront the ways ableism, racial capitalism, and other systems of oppression are intertwined.[37(p15)]

Dismantling ableism benefits all struggles for justice because, in the words of writer and disability justice organizer Mia Mingus, "it undergirds notions of whose bodies are considered valuable, desirable and disposable."[38] Disability justice challenges the expectation that disabled people must adapt to unjust environments and, instead, calls for society itself to change.

In the vision set forth by disability justice advocates, difference is a natural, expected part of human life rather than a flaw to be corrected. The movement calls us to build communities where access, autonomy, and dignity are not special accommodations but woven into the fabric of everyday life, to the benefit of all. A future shaped by disability justice is one where all people, of all bodies and minds, are valued and cared for.

Land Back

Land Back envisions a future where Indigenous peoples reclaim stewardship over their ancestral lands and waters. It centers sovereignty, cultural resurgence, and dismantling colonial systems that continue to harm Indigenous communities and all other communities of color. While Indigenous resistance has taken many forms across history, from protecting sacred sites to revitalizing languages, Land Back offers a focused vision: returning land to Indigenous peoples as a foundation for self-determination, health, and cultural resurgence.

Supporting Land Back means recognizing the deep connection between Indigenous health and Indigenous land, language, and governance. In the words of Swinomish Elder and Community Environmental Health Specialist Larry Campbell, "Our health comes from our culture and our culture comes from our lands, our waters. To make good decisions, these connections must be respected."[39]

Land dispossession was not just a loss of territory; it was a catastrophic disruption to food systems, spiritual practices, and lifeways that sustained health and community for generations.

Land Back is not a one-size-fits-all demand. It is a framework for repair that can take many forms: comanagement agreements, the return of public lands, restoration of sacred sites, and investments in Indigenous land trusts. It acknowledges that real repair will require shifts in ownership, governance, and resources—pushing us beyond symbolic gestures like land acknowledgments. Land Back means correcting historic injustices, restoring Indigenous sovereignty, and building a future rooted in self-determination, justice, and care for the land itself.

Each of these movements articulates powerful new futures and invites us into a collective vision of equity and justice. As public health practitioners, we are directly and inexorably linked with these struggles. We can stand in solidarity with these movements by aligning our work with their values, amplifying their demands, and learning from their leadership. By embracing visionary frameworks and committing to justice, we can reimagine what's possible for our work—and help turn bold ideas into lived reality.

BUILDING A BOLD VISION THAT REIMAGINES PUBLIC HEALTH

There's nothing new / under the sun, / but there are new suns.
                                        –Octavia Butler, writer and science fiction trailblazer[40]

As public health practitioners, we excel at identifying threats—from acute hazards like lead exposure to systemic injustices like housing segregation. These efforts have led to real and meaningful victories—more children growing up free from preventable diseases, more families living in safe homes, and more communities gaining access to clean water, nourishing food, and protective policies that safeguard fundamental rights.

On the other hand, we have also perpetuated cycles of negativity where we have defined communities solely by unjust health disparities and deficits. Public health narratives too often focus on the harms communities endure—such as gun violence, chronic illness, and premature death—without recognizing the full humanity and the strengths, wisdom, and aspirations that all people and communities hold.

Author and therapist Prentis Hemphill notes that trauma can keep us locked in short-term survival thinking, preventing us from imagining new possibilities.[2] Without vision, we risk narrowing our sense of what is achievable. We stay mired in the problems of the status quo rather than imagining and realizing a better future we can build together.

Identifying threats and improving conditions is necessary, but insufficient. Diagnosing injustice is not the same as dismantling the systems that perpetuate it. In public health, we have a unique vantage point: We witness how social determinants, historical harms, and present-day policies intersect and intensify, determining who gets to live a long, healthy life and who does not. But it is not enough to see these patterns ourselves. We must make them visible to others, illuminating the deep interconnections between health, power, justice, and liberation.

We need a bold, galvanizing vision to guide public health moving forward. This vision can serve as an aspirational and collective imagining of the healthier, more just world we are striving to build. A compelling vision helps us move beyond documenting harm to fueling hope, action, and accountability. Inspired by social justice movements, community leaders, and the insights of scholars and advocates, this chapter offers a set of core values to anchor a new vision for public health that we can craft together.

This is not a blueprint or a framework but is instead a set of basic ingredients—principles to reflect on, refine, and grow in community. At the heart of this vision are values that affirm dignity, recognize worth, and create the conditions for communities to flourish.

Universal Dignity

Every person has inherent **dignity**—intrinsic value, worth, and deservingness of respect and fair treatment simply because they are human. Acknowledging that dignity is universal and that everyone has inherent value and worth means honoring people's strengths, dreams, and contributions—while refusing to reduce anyone to their identities, appearance, or health conditions.

Dignity is both individual and collective: Communities, too, have the right to be valued, respected, and supported in their ability to thrive. Flourishing depends not only on material resources but also on recognition and belonging. Dignity scholar and cultural sociologist Michèle Lamont writes that "whether groups are recognized and afforded dignity is *just as* important [as money and power] to their flourishing as human beings, just as vital to their drive to be all they can be. This is a radical idea . . . in our materialist, individualist, and achievement-oriented societies."[41(p4)]

When public health efforts affirm the value of every individual and community, we move beyond preventing harm to promoting flourishing. A vision rooted in dignity rejects narratives of *scarcity*, *disposability*, and *blame*. It calls on us to center *abundance*, *belonging*, and *care*.

A flourishing future recognizes that health is not a privilege to be earned through attributes like wealth, productivity, citizenship, "race," gender, or ability—it is a right rooted in our shared humanity.

Solidarity

Solidarity recognizes that injustices are interconnected—and so must be our responses. It challenges us to move beyond charity or saviorism toward relationships grounded in mutual respect, shared fate, and collective liberation. Solidarity is empathy in action: It compels us to actively show up and stand alongside others, even when their struggles are not our own.

As journalist and novelist Eduardo Galeano reminds us, "solidarity is horizontal"[42]; it is not a gift bestowed from above, but a commitment to struggle side by side. Racial justice leader and author Linda Sarsour adds that solidarity is also a form of self-protection: "Do we speak when the most vulnerable are under attack? We must for two reasons: Number one, it's the right thing to do. And two—trust me when I tell you—it's also a protection for you, because they're not far from us."[43]

In public health, this means building and sustaining alliances across communities and justice movements—because our collective future depends on it.

Care and Connection

One of the most profound lessons from COVID-19 is that our collective health is deeply interdependent. Public health crises like pandemics hit hardest where our social fabric is weakest.[44] We are only as healthy as our least valued and least cared-for neighbor.

Collective care refers to a shared responsibility for each other's emotional, physical, and social well-being within communities, organizations, and movements. It is the antithesis of hyper-individualism, which insists that we remain isolated and solely responsible for our own survival. Collective care affirms that connection is the foundation of health, safety, and justice. As writer and disability justice advocate Alice Wong reminds us: "We must build a world that acknowledges our interdependence with one another so no one ever falls through the cracks."[45]

In a reimagined vision for public health, care is not rationed to people according to their perceived economic value or personal merits. It is universal, abundant, and freely given. As Martin Luther King Jr. observed, "We are caught in an inescapable network of mutuality, tied in a single garment of destiny. Whatever affects one directly, affects all indirectly."[46] Collective care honors that reality. It also reminds us that even the most ideal policies cannot substitute for the trust, reciprocity, and solidarity that emerge from strong, mutual networks of care.

None of us is truly safe until all of us are safe—and care must be at the center of how we govern, allocate resources, and protect one another. When care is woven into the very design of our systems, it protects us in moments of crisis while also creating the conditions for all communities to flourish.

Self-Determination

Flourishing requires the ability to shape the course of one's own life and community. **Self-determination** is the ability of individuals and communities to define and pursue their own vision of health, safety, and well-being on their own terms. In international law, self-determination is recognized as a collective right of peoples to determine their political status and control their economic, social, and cultural development. In public health, it functions as both a principle and a practice rooted in respect for autonomy, lived experience, community power, and the right to direct one's own future.

Self-determination is not the same as unchecked individualism—it is a relational, justice-oriented framework grounded in mutuality, accountability, care, and consent. It recognizes that autonomy is shaped by context, and that true freedom requires collective conditions that make choice and dignity possible. Anthropologist and policy scholar Diane Smith notes that settler colonial states attempted to "reduce the 'collective self' of First Nations . . . to 'selfish' (individualistic) determination."[47(p7)] By contrast, self-determination—understood as a collective and cultural right, alongside the principle of personal autonomy—offers an alternative to the individualism and isolation imposed by settler colonial frameworks.

We have many teachers: from Indigenous movements for sovereignty, to disability justice frameworks of interdependence, to reproductive justice's commitment to bodily autonomy. In public health, self-determination requires moving beyond programs designed "for" communities toward policies, institutions, and investments led and governed by communities themselves. It calls us to center lived experience, honor local knowledge, and shift power to those who have been deeply harmed by inequities. When communities define their own priorities, the solutions are more sustainable and more effective in advancing health and well-being.

Accountability

In a reimagined public health future, **accountability** is both a personal and structural obligation to honor our commitments, to take responsibility for our decisions, and to face the consequences of our actions. Accountability is not about assigning blame but is instead about pursuing transformation and repair. It requires openness, honesty, and courage, especially in the face of harm or discomfort.

Characteristic of her interest in where people come from and who they are accountable to, organizer and civil rights leader Ella Baker once asked, "Who are your people?"[48(p13-14)] As public health practitioners, our answer must always be: the communities harmed by injustice. Accountability means creating real mechanisms and relationships through which communities can hold us responsible for serving with integrity, humility, and care.

True accountability is inseparable from power. Community power is a collective resource to be shared and grown. Without shifting power, authority, and decision-making control to communities, accountability becomes performative rather than transformative.

A public health system rooted in accountability nurtures *power with:* It means we are fully backing communities in organizing, advocating, and building systems that generate flourishing. Accountability and power call us to move from paternalism to partnership—to follow community leadership with humility, transparency, and courage.

Truth and Redress

Health inequities are the living legacies of stolen land, stolen labor, and stolen lives. The only way we can improve the health of our communities today—and prevent future harm—is by confronting the past openly and honestly.

Redress, the act of rectifying past harms and injustice, begins with truth and moves to action. We cannot repair what we are unwilling to see, much less confront it directly. As writer and cultural critic James Baldwin put it, "Not everything that is faced can be changed; but nothing can be changed until it is faced."[49]

A shared future demands an unflinching understanding of history—not a selective and sanitized version, but an honest reckoning with how injustice was deliberately built into our systems and our society. Truth-telling is the first act of redress. It creates the foundation for accountability, trust, and collective action—all of which are vital to advancing public health and movements for justice.[44]

Redress then requires tangible and meaningful actions: returning land, reinvesting in communities harmed by policy violence, dismantling exclusionary systems, and shifting power to those long denied it. Redress means making amends for the past to liberate our future. A public health vision grounded in redress recognizes that collective flourishing is only possible when we face history honestly—and act boldly to repair its consequences.

Joy and Hope

A transformative vision of public health centers joy and hope as essential sources of energy, adaptability, and connection. This is what sustains us through dark and challenging times, since even the most committed advocates risk burnout, cynicism, or despair. Determination and grit can take us far—but they are finite.

Joy can be a form of resistance—from *Black joy*[50] to *queer joy*[51]—it is a deliberate, life-affirming act of connection and possibility. As poet and activist Audre Lorde writes, "The sharing of joy, whether physical, emotional, psychic, or intellectual, forms a bridge between the sharers."[52(p56)] This joy becomes a way to reclaim narrative, affirm existence, and build solidarity. It replenishes our spirits and expands our capacity to pursue long-term goals, build creative solutions, and unite across differences.

Hope is what keeps us going—not because we possess it, but because we practice it. Abolitionists and organizers Kelly Hayes and Mariame Kaba write, "To practice active hope, we do not need to believe that everything will work out in the end. We need only decide who we are choosing to be and how we are choosing to function in relation to the outcome we desire, and abide by what those decisions demand of us."[53] This hope is not passive or naïve—it is "a source of comfort to the afflicted but also a strategic imperative."[53] Active hope allows us to adapt, to imagine, and to move forward with clarity and purpose.

Together, joy and hope become the practice of vision—a way to resist fear and build the world we want. Even when joy is elusive, hope can anchor us. And when joy surfaces, it deepens our capacity to dream, connect, and sustain the work ahead.

We need a vision of health and flourishing that is expansive, inspiring, and rooted in the lived realities and aspirations of communities themselves. Justice movements show us that a different world is not just possible; it is already being imagined and built, and we can all be a part of it (Box 7-1).[54-70]

Box 7-1. Models of Bold Vision in Public Health Practice

We are living through a time of both crisis and possibility. Our communities, our rights, our planet, and the conditions we need to be healthy and thrive are under attack. At the same time, peoples' movements for justice and equity are building powerful bases and visioning liberated, health-affirming futures. To navigate this moment, we need clear strategies and a strong ecosystem capable of forging a path forward together.
        —Selma Aly, Asamia Diaby, and Julian Drix, public health advocates and organizers[54(p9)]

Across the country, communities are already using bold visions to guide the creation of audacious, community-led strategies to advance health, equity, and justice. These efforts respond to immediate needs while also setting a broader, aspirational vision for what flourishing can look like:

- **St. Louis tenants organizing for housing justice.** In a city long shaped by racial segregation and disinvestment,[55] tenants responded to unsafe conditions—like lead poisonings, asthma-inducing mold, and sewage backups—to hold landlords accountable, and they ultimately reclaimed their right to safe housing. Through forming Tenants Transforming Greater St. Louis, they developed a 10-year strategic vision for code

(Continued)

Box 7-1. (Continued)

enforcement. They collaborated with the city to adopt policies addressing habitability; ensured tenants were regularly informed of landlords' code violations; and established a tenant relocation assistance fund.[56] Their work affirms that housing is foundational to health and a universal right.

- **Swinomish Tribe visioning health through Indigenous values.** The Swinomish Indian Tribal Community in Washington, located on ancestral Coast Salish lands along the Salish Sea, has long faced threats to its cultural and environmental lifeways—from colonial displacement to climate change.[57] The Tribe developed Indigenous Health Indicators, a visionary framework that redefines health through Coast Salish values. It goes beyond biomedical metrics to include cultural practices, environmental stewardship, and spiritual well-being.[58] This work has guided climate adaptation strategies, youth education, and food sovereignty efforts like a community garden, seasonal produce, carts, and the first modern clam garden.[59-61] The Swinomish Tribe shows us that health is holistic—rooted in sustainability and self-determination.
- **Appalachia's Pansy Collective building mutual aid and cultural power.** Pansy Collective began in Asheville, North Carolina as a trans-founded art, music, and community hub.[62] During COVID-19, it became a mutual aid network, distributing food, medical supplies, and emergency funding across the region. After Hurricane Helene, Pansy Collective rapidly mobilized with Mutual Aid Disaster Relief and local venues to distribute essential aid—often reaching remote communities before government responders.[63] As one viral meme put it, "You know our systems are broke when 5 gay DJs can bring 10k of supplies back before the national guard does,"[63] expressing both the radical, everyday mutuality of marginalized people and burden of infrastructure collapse under racial capitalism. This nimble, community-rooted response reflects a vision of health grounded in cultural belonging, self-determination, and collective care.
- **Connecting climate and health in LA County.** LA is home to one of the largest populations of people of color in the United States and has long suffered from some of the nation's worst air pollution[64]—conditions that disproportionately harm Black and brown communities.[65] In response, the county's Department of Public Health launched the Office of Environmental Justice and Climate Health, tasked with partnering with frontline communities to codesign climate justice strategies—reducing heat exposure, investing in green spaces, improving air quality, and promoting health equity.[66,67] By inviting communities to lead in shaping climate resilience, this office and countywide strategy embodies an expansive vision for health that weaves together racial, economic, and environmental justice into an ambitious, regional sustainability plan.
- **Reshaping food systems through the Black Farmer Fund.** Black people built the foundation of US agriculture through centuries of enslaved labor. Despite briefly owning as much as 19 million acres by 1910, land dispossession and systemic discrimination—including by USDA—have reduced Black land ownership to less than 1% of total US farmland today.[68,69] The Black Farmer Fund in New York demonstrates a bold reimagining of food systems by building collective power for Black farmers and food business owners in the Northeast.[70] Through democratic governance and community wealth-building, it invites us to envision a food system where communities are the stewards of their own health and economic futures.

These stories show that vision doesn't have to live in the far-off future, the imagination of community leaders, or the pages of scholarly publications. Bold, bright futures are both imaginable and within reach. Governments and institutions have a role to play—but that role must be responsive, ranging from active co-creation to stepping back and supporting without centering their own priorities.

Communities across the country—and countless others—invite us to move beyond technical fixes and embrace community-led visions as the foundation for new, more just systems.

Note: LA = Los Angeles, California; USDA = US Department of Agriculture.

THE PATH AHEAD

Another world is not only possible, she is on her way. . . . [O]n a quiet day, if I listen very carefully, I can hear her breathing.

–Arundhati Roy, author and activist[71(p75)]

For us to genuinely embrace a positive new vision for health in the communities we serve, we must see ourselves not just as individuals working in a field of practice and scholarship but also as a collective force that is helping to drive a movement. This means expanding our vision beyond the silos in which we work and engaging in shifting power, changing narratives, and building coalitions. It means shifting from a reactive stance—responding to crises after they happen—to proactively shaping a future where justice, dignity, and well-being are at the center.

As public health practitioners, we are trained in pragmatic disciplines like epidemiology, biostatistics, program design, and policy analysis—areas of practice that focus on measuring and assessing what is immediately before us. While these skills are essential tools of the trade, they often leave us with little room to dream up new futures, imagine what might be possible, and invite others to work with us to make this vision a reality.

When we are focused on providing essential services that address acute problems—helping people to meet basic needs, such as obtaining healthy food, safe housing, preventive services, and safety—it can be difficult, if not impossible, to zoom out and envision something more. But transdisciplinary scholar and educator Ruha Benjamin encourages us to start "imagining and crafting the worlds you cannot live without, just as you dismantle the ones you cannot live within."[72] A bold vision for public health cannot simply encompass conditions where people can survive—it must be one where they can create, connect, and thrive. As public health practitioners, we cannot afford to only focus on preventing harm. We can—and must—become a movement of bold vision, of joy and justice, of collective care and hope, and of flourishing and possibility.

REFERENCES

1. Khasnabish A, Haiven M. *The Radical Imagination: Social Movement Research in the Age of Austerity.* Zed Books; 2014.
2. Hemphill P. *What it Takes to Heal: How Transforming Ourselves Can Change the World.* Random House; 2024.
3. hooks b. *All About Love: New Visions.* William Morrow; 2000.
4. Kaba M. *We Do This 'Til We Free Us: Abolitionist Organizing and Transforming Justice.* Haymarket Books; 2021.
5. Graeber D. *The Utopia of Rules: On Technology, Stupidity, and the Secret Joys of Bureaucracy.* Melville House; 2015.

6. Pamukcu A, Sheehy H. The epidemic of trauma at our border and in our communities was caused by policy. The solution? Better policy. ChangeLab Solutions. July 16, 2018. Accessed August 18, 2025. https://medium.com/changelab-solutions/immigration-policy-trauma-3b09e1a1a0b9

7. Honein MA, Christie A, Rose DA, et al. Summary of guidance for public health strategies to address high levels of community transmission of SARS-CoV-2 and related deaths, December 2020. *MMWR Morb Mortal Wkly Rep.* 2020;69(49):1860–1867. doi:10.15585/mmwr.mm6949e2

8. McCarty M, Perl L. Federal eviction moratoriums in response to the COVID-19 pandemic. Congressional Research Service. March 22, 2021. Accessed August 18, 2025. https://www.congress.gov/crs-product/IN11516

9. California Pan-Ethnic Health Network. Racism as a public health crisis. July 14, 2020. Accessed August 18, 2025. https://cpehn.org/what-we-do-2/our-networks/racism-as-a-public-health-crisis

10. American Public Health Association. Addressing law enforcement violence as a public health issue. November 13, 2018. Accessed August 18, 2025. https://www.apha.org/policy-and-advocacy/public-health-policy-briefs/policy-database/2019/01/29/law-enforcement-violence

11. Dall C. Removal of pages from CDC website brings confusion, dismay. CIDRAP. February 3, 2025. Accessed August 18, 2025. https://www.cidrap.umn.edu/public-health/removal-pages-cdc-website-brings-confusion-dismay

12. Benjamin GC. Supreme Court's overturning of *Roe v. Wade* jeopardizes the health of all Americans. American Public Health Association. June 23, 2022. Accessed August 18, 2025. https://www.apha.org/news-and-media/news-releases/apha-news-releases/2022/abortion_sc

13. de la Guéronnière G, Shaffer M. Recent federal and state policy developments important to syringe service programs and what may be next. Legal Action Center. March 2023. Accessed August 18, 2025. https://www.lac.org/assets/files/final-SSP-issue-brief.pdf

14. Aleaziz H. How the Supreme Court made legal immigrants vulnerable to deportation. *New York Times.* May 31, 2025. Accessed August 18, 2025. https://www.nytimes.com/2025/05/31/us/politics/supreme-court-immigrants.html

15. Brooks R. Taking a stand against book bans. *Monitor on Psychology Magazine.* July 1, 2025. Accessed August 18, 2025. https://www.apa.org/monitor/2025/07-08/fighting-book-bans-censorship

16. Kinzer S. *Overthrow: America's Century of Regime Change from Hawaii to Iraq.* Henry Holt and Company; 2006.

17. Movement Generation, Justice & Ecology Project. *From Banks and Tanks to Cooperation and Caring: A Strategic Framework for a Just Transition* [zine]. Movement Generation. 2016. Accessed June 16, 2025. https://movementgeneration.org/justtransition

18. Poor People's Campaign. Poor People's Campaign: A National Call for Moral Revival. October 2, 2019. Accessed May 7, 2025. https://www.poorpeoplescampaign.org

19. Cobb J. William Barber takes on poverty and race in the age of Trump. *The New Yorker.* May 7, 2018. Accessed May 7, 2025. https://www.newyorker.com/magazine/2018/05/14/william-barber-takes-on-poverty-and-race-in-the-age-of-trump

20. Greater Washington Community Foundation. Book group recap: Solidarity economics with Dr. Manuel Pastor. December 13, 2022. Accessed August 11, 2025. https://www.thecommunityfoundation.org/news/book-group-recap-solidarity-economics-with-dr-manuel-pastor

21. Rosenfeld MJ. *The Rainbow After the Storm: Marriage Equality and Social Change in the US.* Oxford University Press; 2021.

22. Morini M. Same-sex marriage and other moral taboos: Cultural acceptances, change in American public opinion and the evidence from the opinion polls. *Eur J Am Stud*. 2017;11(3). doi:10.4000/ejas.11824

23. Nakamura R. How 'Will & Grace' had a real-life political impact on marriage equality. *The Wrap*. September 28, 2017. Accessed August 17, 2025. https://www.thewrap.com/will-grace-real-life-political-impact-marriage-equality/

24. Women of African Descent for Reproductive Justice. Reproductive justice founders list. Community Commons. Accessed August 11, 2025. https://www.communitycommons.org/entities/715101e1-9e29-4fd7-a526-a2940c42eba7

25. Ross LJ, Solinger R. *Reproductive Justice: An Introduction*. University of California Press; 2017

26. Movement Generation, Justice & Ecology Project. Just transition. Movement Generation. Accessed May 12, 2025. https://movementgeneration.org/justtransition

27. Just Transition Alliance. What is just transition? Accessed May 12, 2025. https://jtalliance.org/what-is-just-transition

28. Klein N. *This Changes Everything: Capitalism vs. The Climate*. Simon & Schuster; 2014

29. Pamukcu A, Harris AP. Health justice and just transition. *J Law Med Ethics*. 2022;50(4):674–681. doi:10.1017/jme.2023.7

30. Corbett J. Fridays for Future plans global climate strike during COP30 in Brazil. Common Dreams. July 29, 2025. Accessed August 18, 2025. https://www.commondreams.org/news/cop30

31. United Nations Framework Convention on Climate Change. Just Transition & Sustainable Economies Day, 4th Capacity-building hub. United Nations. November 11, 2022. Accessed August 18, 2025. https://unfccc.int/pccb/4CBHub/JTDay

32. International Labour Organization. From vision to practice for a just transition for all: A cross-regional policy dialogue on energy, sustainable finance, and enterprises for inclusive policy-making and enhancing. March 10, 2025. Accessed August 18, 2025. https://www.ilo.org/resource/other/vision-practice-just-transition-all

33. Lincoln A. Gettysburg address delivered at Gettysburg Pa. Nov 19th, 1863. Library of Congress. Accessed August 12, 2025. https://www.loc.gov/item/rbpe.24404500

34. Gardere A, McAfee M. A letter: Our founding opportunity. PolicyLink. July 4, 2022. Accessed August 11, 2025. https://www.policylink.org/our-founding

35. Allen DS. *Our Declaration: A Reading of the Declaration of Independence in Defense of Equality*. Liveright Publishing; 2014.

36. ALOK. The cross-dressing laws never ended: Why we must #degender fashion. This Is an Intervention. March 9, 2021. Accessed September 6, 2025. https://thisisanintervention.org/en/intervention-04-release-an-introduction/longread-04-alok

37. Piepzna-Samarasinha LL. *Care Work: Dreaming Disability Justice*. Arsenal Pulp Press; 2018.

38. Mingus M. Changing the framework: Disability justice. *Leaving Evidence*. February 12, 2011. Accessed May 7, 2025. https://leavingevidence.wordpress.com/2011/02/12/changing-the-framework-disability-justice

39. Swinomish Climate Change Initiative. Community Environmental Health. Swinomish Indian Tribal Community. Accessed August 18, 2025. https://www.swinomish-climate.com/community-environmental-health

40. Butler OE. Parable of the Trickster (unpublished manuscript). Quoted in: Canavan G. There's nothing new / under the sun, / but there are new suns: Recovering Octavia E. Butler's lost

parables. *Los Angeles Review of Books*. June 9, 2014. Accessed August 8, 2025. https://lareviewofbooks. org/article/theres-nothing-new-sun-new-suns-recovering-octavia-e-butlers-lost-parables

41. Lamont M. *Seeing Others: How Recognition Works and How It Can Heal a Divided World*. Atria/ One Signal Publishers; 2023.

42. Manrique J. Eduardo Galeano. *BOMB Magazine*. April 1, 2001. Accessed August 25, 2025. https://bombmagazine.org/articles/2001/04/01/eduardo-galeano

43. Sarsour L. Keynote address. Presented at: MADE for Health Justice Spring Convening; April 16, 2025; San Diego, CA.

44. Harris AP, Pamukcu A. Fostering the civil rights of health. In: Burris S, de Guia S, Gable L, Levin D, Parmet WE, Terry NP, eds. *Assessing Legal Responses to COVID-19: COVID-19 Policy Playbook*. Public Health Law Watch; 2020:279–284. Accessed August 11, 2025. https://www. publichealthlawwatch.org/covid19-policy-playbook

45. Wong A. My life is in my caregivers' hands: Disability advocate Alice Wong's vision for a new approach to health care. KQED. December 9, 2022. Accessed August 11, 2025. https://www. kqed.org/news/11934545/my-life-is-in-my-caregivers-hands-disability-advocate-alice-wongs-vision-for-a-new-approach-to-health-care

46. King ML Jr. Letter from a Birmingham Jail. April 16, 1963. Accessed May 7, 2025. https://www. africa.upenn.edu/Articles_Gen/Letter_Birmingham.html

47. Smith D. Thematic introduction: Concepts, issues and trends. In: Smith D, Wighton A, Cornell S, Delaney AV, eds. *Developing Governance and Governing Development: International Case Studies of Indigenous Futures*. Rowman & Littlefield; 2021:109–118.

48. Ransby B. *Ella Baker and the Black Freedom Movement: A Radical Democratic Vision*. University of North Carolina Press; 2003.

49. Baldwin J. As much truth as one can bear; to speak out about the world as it is, says James Baldwin, is the writer's job as much of the truth as one can bear. *New York Times*. January 14, 1962. Accessed August 17, 2025. https://www.nytimes.com/1962/01/14/archives/as-much-truth-as-one-can-bear-to-speak-out-about-the-world-as-it-is.html

50. Nichols E. Black joy: Resistance, resilience, and reclamation. National Museum of African American History and Culture. Accessed August 12, 2025. https://nmaahc.si.edu/explore/ stories/black-joy-resistance-resilience-and-reclamation

51. Luong M. The art of queer joy. *YES! Magazine*. June 29, 2023. Accessed August 12, 2025. https:// www.yesmagazine.org/social-justice/2023/06/29/queer-joy

52. Lorde A. *Sister Outsider: Essays and Speeches*. Crossing Press; 2012

53. Hayes K, Kaba M. Hope is a practice and a discipline: Building a path to a counterculture of care. *Nonprofit Quarterly*. February 19, 2024. Accessed August 12, 2025. https://nonprofitquarterly. org/hope-is-a-practice-and-a-discipline-building-a-path-to-a-counterculture-of-care

54. Aly S, Diaby A, Drix J. The five dimensions of inside-outside strategy: A guide for public health and social movements to build powerful partnerships. Health in Partnership. April 29, 2025. Accessed May 7, 2025. https://humanimpact.org/wp-content/uploads/2025/04/Five-Dimensions-GUIDE.pdf

55. Cooperman J. The color line: Race in St. Louis. *St. Louis Magazine*. October 17, 2014. Accessed August 12, 2025. https://www.stlmag.com/news/the-color-line-race-in-st.-louis

56. Health in Partnership. ST. Louis case story: Don't let the bed bugs bite. July 8, 2025. Accessed July 8, 2025. https://www.healthinpartnership.org/resources/st-louis-case-story-dont-let-the-bed-bugs-bite

57. Intercontinental Cry. The Swinomish Nation: Stewards of the Salish Sea and Coast. *IC Magazine*. Accessed August 12, 2025. https://icmagazine.org/indigenous-peoples/swinomish

58. Donatuto J, Campbell L, Gregory R. Developing responsive indicators of Indigenous community health. *Int J Environ Res Public Health*. 2016;13(9):899. doi:10.3390/ijerph13090899

59. Swinomish Indian Tribal Community. Community Environmental Health Program. Accessed August 12, 2025. https://www.swinomish-nsn.gov/health-and-wellness/page/community-environmental-health

60. Swinomish Indian Tribal Community. Clam garden. Accessed August 12, 2025. https://www.swinomish-nsn.gov/fisheries/page/clam-garden

61. NOAA Fisheries. Swinomish clam garden to bolster littleneck clam populations. NOAA. November 30, 2022. Accessed August 12, 2025. https://www.fisheries.noaa.gov/feature-story/swinomish-clam-garden-bolster-littleneck-clam-populations

62. Albury W. Asheville's Pansy Fest showcases city's queer artists. *Tuner Music Magazine*. August 20, 2019. Accessed August 12, 2025. https://tunermusicmagazine.com/2019/08/20/asheville-pansy-fest-19

63. Soper BV. We are the relief: How queer Appalachian mutual aid showed up after Helene. *Them*. October 22, 2024. Accessed August 12, 2025. https://www.them.us/story/queer-appalachian-mutual-aid-helene-gay-queer-djs-faster-than-national-guard-fema-asheville-western-north-carolina

64. US Census Bureau. Los Angeles County, California - profile. Accessed August 12, 2025. https://data.census.gov/profile/Los_Angeles_County,_California?g=050XX00US06037

65. Schlossberg JA. When air pollution becomes a health equity issue. *UCLA Health*. November 1, 2021. Accessed August 12, 2025. https://www.uclahealth.org/news/article/air-pollution-health-equity-los-angeles.

66. Los Angeles County Department of Public Health. Climate change and health equity: Strategies for action report. Accessed May 16, 2025. http://publichealth.lacounty.gov/eh/docs/about/climate-change-health-equity-strategies-action-report.pdf

67. Los Angeles County Department of Public Health. Office of Environmental Justice and Climate Health. Accessed September 6, 2025. https://www.publichealth.lacounty.gov/eh/about/environmental-justice-climate-health.htm

68. Tshabalala P. A brief history of discrimination against Black farmers—including by the USDA. *The Equation*. August 27, 2024. https://blog.ucs.org/precious-tshabalala/a-brief-history-of-discrimination-against-black-farmers-including-by-the-usda

69. Black Farmer Fund. Accessed May 16, 2025. https://www.blackfarmerfund.org

70. Zinn H. *Talking About a Revolution: Interviews With Michael Albert, Noam Chomsky, Barbara Ehrenreich, bell hooks, Peter Kwong, Winona LaDuke, Manning Marable, Urvashi Vaid, and Howard Zinn*. South End Press; 1998.

71. Roy A. *War Talk*. South End Press; 2003.

72. Benjamin R. Is technology our savior—or our slayer? TEDWomen 2023. November 2023. Accessed August 18, 2025. https://www.ted.com/talks/ruha_benjamin_is_technology_our_savior_or_our_slayer

8

Ten Ways to Put Equity and Justice Into Practice

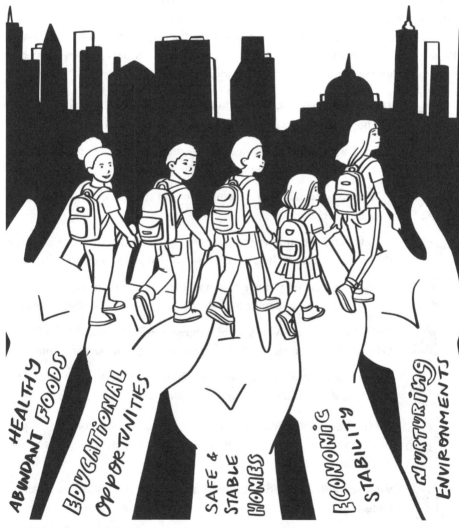

Artist Credit: Jasmin Pamukcu, 2025.

Building Blocks

We say, "Things were really bad back then. Slavery was wrong, we can admit that now. Jim Crow was a bad idea; we shouldn't have done those things. Things aren't all the way equal right now, but they're getting better, and they will be better in the future. . . The arc of the universe is long. It bends toward justice." No, it doesn't. Unless you bend it. It doesn't bend on its own.

–Nikole Hannah-Jones, journalist and author[1]

As discussed throughout this book, equity and justice are not simply aspirational ideals—they are living commitments that we must actively apply to our daily decisions, relationships, and responsibilities.

This chapter is designed to help synthesize the history, insights, data, and lessons shared throughout this book and distill them into discrete actions. It offers 10 specific ways we can advance equity and justice in our daily work:

 1. Learn our legacies, use our full latitude. Uncover the histories, harms, and hopes that got us here—and act boldly to address them.

 2. Lead with values. Let values guide every decision. When values come first, vision can become reality.

 3. Take on systems, not symptoms. Confront and challenge the root causes of health inequities.

 4. Communicate and casemake for change. Frame problems clearly, name the need for justice explicitly, and tell stories that build power and possibility.

 5. Stand in solidarity, move as a movement. Support struggles for justice beyond our own—and unite for bold, people-powered transformation.

 6. Shift and share power. Ensure communities bearing the brunt of injustice lead decision-making. Uplift community ingenuity and solutions.

 7. Organize and mobilize resources. Fund what matters. Unlock, align, and expand investment in communities long denied their fair share.

 8. Implement *inside–outside* strategies. Advance shared goals by bridging institutional and community power. Transforming systems requires coordination and trust.

 9. Make equity and justice routine. Embed equity and justice into planning, budgeting, operations, and collaboration—until bold becomes standard.

 10. Reimagine public health. Use imagination, discipline, and audacity to rewrite the rules. Redefine public health as a force for joy, justice, and liberation.

These 10 practices are not a checklist or a step-by-step formula. They are ongoing, interrelated approaches that require reflection, courage, patience, and experimentation.

What is being asked of us all as public health practitioners is often not easy, and there won't always be a single "right" answer for every situation. But these practices can help guide our thinking and actions over time. We can use them to navigate complexity and enhance our work—particularly in dynamic and evolving contexts.

1. LEARN OUR LEGACIES, USE OUR FULL LATITUDE

Uncover the histories, harms, and hopes that got us here—and act boldly to address them.

As discussed in this book, health inequities are not accidental, nor did they arise overnight—they are the result of generations of policies, decisions, agendas, and power imbalances that have all reinforced each other over time. If we want to create meaningful change, we must first understand the contexts and forces that got us here.

Learning our legacy means we must take these steps:

 Uncover the histories of the communities we serve. Every place has a backstory: events that indelibly shaped the trajectories of communities— from segregation to integration, factory closures to union victories, environmental injustices to park expansions. Yet we must proactively seek out these histories because many have been undocumented, misrepresented, or intentionally erased. Ignorance of this context can signal disinterest in people's lived realities, deepen distrust, and put us at risk of repeating harm. Whether we realize it or not, our knowledge of a community's past affects our present ability to build trust and engage authentically with those who live there (see Box 8-1).[2-23]

Box 8-1. Why Local History Matters for Public Health Today

Every community sits atop a layered history. That history—whether widely known or intentionally buried—shapes relationships, power dynamics, and people's willingness to trust institutions today. By grounding our work in place-based historical contexts, we honor people's realities and open the door to the possibility of meaningful relationships.

Consider these examples of pivotal, but often unknown histories, where local events have had long-lasting, intergenerational effects on people and places:

▶ **Wilmington, NC (1898):** White supremacists violently overthrew an elected local government that was largely composed of Black officials. This act of racial terror, which resulted in the deaths of scores of Black people—who were the only casualties—went unmentioned for well over a century, but is now considered "a landmark in North Carolina history."[2] The coup d'état sparked a mass exodus of Black people from the city,[3] decimated the number of Black registered voters in the state,[4] and helped usher in the Jim Crow era and all of its devastating effects.

▶ **Tulsa, OK (1921):** White mobs—led by the Ku Klux Klan, deputized by the Tulsa Police Department,[5] and aided by the Oklahoma National Guard—carried out a "coordinated, military-style" campaign where they

(Continued)

Box 8-1. (Continued)

bombed, burned, and destroyed the prosperous Greenwood neighborhood known as *Black Wall Street* over 2 full days. The *Tulsa "Race" Massacre*, as it is now known, describes a massive act of racial terror that resulted in hundreds of deaths and the obliteration of homes and businesses. It is one of the largest discrete acts of racial violence in US history.[6] White city officials not only spun the story to blame Black residents for the destruction but also tried to block recovery through racist zoning laws and legal obstruction. Yet residents defiantly rebuilt.[7] Decades later, Tulsa paved over Greenwood as part of "urban renewal" campaigns, compounding the trauma and damage.[8] This violence lives on today—in ongoing trauma,[9] lost generational wealth, diminished incomes,[10] and the continued struggle for recognition and justice.

Watsonville, CA (1930): White mobs attacked and killed Filipino farmworkers in a week of racially motivated assaults known as the *Watsonville Riots*. The attacks began in a dance hall—where Filipino men socialized and mingled with white women—and continued on to 5 days of large-scale violence that sparked riots in other California cities.[11] This fueled anti-Filipino sentiment and exclusionary immigration policies. Decades later, more than 1,500 predominantly Filipino farmworkers—organized by labor organizer and former farmworker Larry Itliong—launched the *Delano Grape Strike* to demand fair wages and better working conditions.[12,13] Despite the progress of that movement—including the powerful solidarity between Filipino and Latine communities—today's farmworkers still face unsafe conditions rooted in these labor exploitation systems.[14]

San Francisco, CA (1966): Trans women of color and drag queens led the *Compton's Cafeteria Riot* in the Tenderloin neighborhood—an act of resistance against police violence and the criminalization of queerness. Multiple unjust laws, such as those against "female impersonation," made everyday gender expression illegal—from makeup to shirts with buttons on the "wrong" side. The Compton's Cafeteria Riot occurred 3 years before the *Stonewall Riots* in New York City, New York, which is often cited as the start of the modern queer rights movement.[15] But that overlooks a longer history of trans leadership and queer resistance, often in places where queer culture thrived despite persistent oppression. These local histories show us who has led change—and why mistrust in institutions still runs deep in the present day. Today, Black and brown trans women in San Francisco still face violence, housing instability, and health care discrimination.[16,17] Trans-led initiatives like the Transgender District reclaim space and power in response to that legacy.[18]

Philadelphia, PA (1985): After firing more than 10,000 rounds of ammunition into a row house for more than an hour,[19] the Philadelphia Police Department dropped a bomb onto the West Philadelphia home of MOVE, a communal Black liberation organization, triggering a fire that killed 11 people—including 5 children—and destroyed more than 60 homes, leaving around 250 people without housing. Firefighters stood by while the fire burned.[20] No city representative was ever prosecuted, and it wasn't until 2020 that the city council formally apologized.[21] In 2021, Philadelphia's health commissioner was forced to resign after it was discovered that he disposed of at least 1 victim's remains without notifying their family.[22] This history continues to undermine relationships between communities and the city, while casting a long shadow of trauma over survivors and Black residents.[23]

These histories are not distant or healed wounds. They are alive in the landscapes, institutions, and relationships we navigate today. As public health practitioners, we must understand and actively address local context within our work in ways that are relevant, respectful, and rooted in repair.

Reckon with our institution's impact. These are long and complex legacies. Organizations like hospitals, nonprofits, and government agencies have both built and damaged relationships over time. Missteps, broken promises, failures to act, and overtly unjust actions—some deliberate, others neglectful—have shaped how communities perceive us and our work. While some communities recall moments of support, others remember institutional backing of segregation, labor exploitation, or the demolition of beloved neighborhoods. We carry these legacies into every room, even if they occurred before our time, and whether we are aware of them or not. Educating ourselves about this legacy is the first step toward trust, repair, and accountability.

 Learn from lived experience. Community members—elders, grassroots leaders, advocates, workers, and long-time residents—hold vital insights about what has been successful, what hasn't, and what's truly needed. Our work begins by seeking out conversations with people in the communities we serve. We build genuine relationships when we enter into dialogue about community priorities and preferences and when we ask questions long before proposing solutions. Most importantly, we must act on the guidance we receive.

 Acknowledge our positionality and act responsibly. In public health, we're often seen—or see ourselves—as "objective experts" or "neutral presenters of data." But as this book emphasizes, "neutrality" and "objectivity" are myths, and expertise is not limited to academic or technical knowledge. Our roles, identities, and lived experiences come together in a dynamic interplay of power and privilege, shaping how we move through the world and form our worldview. This is **positionality**: the ways our insights and beliefs are informed by intersecting contexts like our backgrounds, professional experiences, and lived realities. Positionality is unique and situational: how others see us depends on their own positionalities and may shift across time, place, environment, and relationships. Just as it influences how we're perceived, it also shapes the perspectives we bring to our work—affecting whose voices we amplify, whose needs we prioritize, and how we interpret information. Acknowledging our positionality is essential to engage communities effectively, authentically, and respectfully.

 Reclaim public health's social justice roots. Justice is one of the *Four Commitments of Public Health* and is fundamental to our efforts to advance community health and well-being (see Chapter 1). Breakthrough improvements in public health—from clean water to safer workplaces to dignified housing—have been achieved by social movements that were committed to community health and refused to accept injustice. Yet the field of public health abandoned this powerful legacy, choosing professionalization and clinicalization over advocacy and community accountability. Now, we have an opportunity to reclaim that legacy. We must radically evolve and restructure our processes, relationships, decision-making, and organizational goals to embrace the transformative change that justice demands. We must stand in solidarity with today's justice movements to protect hard-won gains that are in danger of being lost. Public health is about the flourishing of all people—and because our roots are in social justice, we already have the moral high ground. We must lead with courage and conviction by refusing "neutrality," naming injustice explicitly, and aligning our work with our values.

Learning our legacy is only half the challenge. The other half is exercising our full latitude. This means understanding the boundaries of our roles as well as their full potential, which should not be confused with legal limitations. Sometimes, we assume that we can't take important action—like speaking about policy or equity—when in fact, there are no rules that prohibit this. Likewise, in certain roles, we may not be allowed to lobby for or against a specific bill. But it is entirely legal—and necessary—for us to educate policymakers about public health issues and to advocate for the creation of new policies that save lives.

Far too often, we place limits on ourselves that exceed what any law or policy actually requires. We retreat preemptively—voluntarily conceding our ability to advance strategies that are fully within our purview. And in doing so, we shrink the potential of our organizations and ourselves. This is a form of *power under*, when we fail to use or surrender power that we already have. (For more on power, see Chapter 5.)

Historian and author Timothy Snyder warns against **anticipatory obedience**—preemptively conforming to imagined demands of authority before any explicit directive is given. He writes, "Do not obey in advance. Most of the power of authoritarianism is freely given."[24(p17)]

In times like these, individuals and institutions often anticipate what a more repressive authority might demand and then comply before even being asked. These actions merely teach dominant power—across individuals, institutions, and systems—what it can get away with: abuses of *power over* like coercion and intimidation. And it can place others in a continual position of *power under*, resulting in learned helplessness and defeatism.

We should never volunteer to surrender our power. Instead, we must take the time to explore what is fully within the scope of our roles—with all their limits and capabilities—rather than fearing something *might* be prohibited. We can then test our perceived limits thoughtfully, carefully, and strategically.

Within every role, there is room to act—often far more than we think. This is true both in times of calm, when the status quo feels stable and unquestioned, and in moments of volatility, when threats—whether political, organizational, or societal—press in from all sides. Although the temptation to retreat or to stay small can be strong, we must resist it.

2. LEAD WITH VALUES

Let values guide every decision. When values come first, vision can become reality.

Chapter 7 discussed discussed the importance of having a bold vision that reimagines public health. If vision is our destination, then values are our compass. In public health—where the stakes are high and the context politically charged—leading with values helps us navigate complexity without losing direction.

Whether we are leading a project, a program, a department, or an entire organization, our values provide a foundation for accountability and principled decision-making.

Values are not always universally shared, even within the same organization. Individuals may hold personal values that differ from institutional ones, and navigating that tension requires open dialogue, mutual respect, and a willingness to address underlying assumptions. Understanding where values converge—and where they diverge—can help teams move forward with greater clarity and cohesion.

At the organizational and institutional level, we can begin by identifying three to five core values. These should be clearly defined and thoughtfully translated into everyday practice. This clarity is essential to hold ourselves and our teams accountable. *Core values* cannot be mere aspirational slogans; they must be specific principles that lead to actionable commitments. These commitments guide how we show up, how we work with others, and how we make decisions. Consider these examples:

- If *equity* is a core value, we must set universal goals, allocate resources according to need, and shift power to community members so that they have decision-making authority over interventions and strategies.
- If *collaboration* is a core value, we must foster authentic relationships across sectors and spaces, co-creating interventions with community partners and communicating honestly and openly about successes and setbacks alike.
- If *reciprocity* is a core value, we must ensure that community partners feel that the energy and expertise they contribute to our work is valued and community members directly benefit from interventions and evaluations that are only possible because of their involvement.

Powerful and effective values can't be quietly tucked away in a mission statement or strategic plan—they must be developed collaboratively, consulted often, and embedded into routine operations.

Living our values means aligning them with our individual and institutional choices—routine decisions as well as those made in moments of tension and uncertainty. Upholding our values also requires ongoing self-reflection: *Are we using our power responsibly? Are we honoring the commitments we've made to our communities and each other? Are our values visible not just in what we say, but in what we do?*

Here are some practical ways to put our values into action:

 Make our values visible. We should share our values openly with staff, partners, and community members—and revisit them often. For example, we might open each of our presentations with a slide describing our values or begin meetings with a quick check-in on which values feel most relevant to items on the day's agenda. We can also feature our values prominently on organizational websites, social media channels, or publicly facing reports. When our values are clearly communicated and consistently present, others can both align with and hold us accountable to them.

Model values openly and accountably. Those of us in positions of power have a unique opportunity and responsibility to demonstrate core values—in staff meetings, in strategic planning discussions, and in community forums. If *transparency* is a core value, we might hold regular open forums where issues are discussed with staff and partners, and we could share meeting notes to provide context and rationales for decisions. If being *community-driven* is a core value, we could codesign programs with community members, invite them to serve on advisory boards, and incorporate their perspectives into final decisions. When leaders embody shared values, they invite and influence others to do the same.

Use values to guide decision-making. No matter our role, each decision point is an opportunity to pause and ask: *Does this course of action align with our values?* If it doesn't—or if there's an unclear answer—we should follow up by asking: *What would it take to get into alignment with our values?* These questions must apply across the board, from high-level strategy to daily operations like hiring, budgeting, setting priorities, and pursuing partnerships.

Revisit values to resolve conflict and navigate uncertainty. When tensions arise, internally or with partners, values offer clarity and a shared path forward. If a team is unsure how to distribute funding, valuing *equity*—seeking to rectify injustices and providing resources according to need—can point the way forward. If an organization faces political pressure to abandon an initiative that benefits marginalized communities, values of *courage* and *integrity* encourage us to stay the course and make the case for why the work must continue—and even expand. In moments of change and challenge, values ground us and guide us toward principled action.

Invite ongoing feedback, then act on it. Regular check-ins with staff, partners, and community members can help us understand how well our values are showing up in practice. We can ask: *Are we living up to the values we claim? Are they showing up in our interactions with you? Where are we falling short, and how can we improve?* When we receive constructive feedback, we should respond with meaningful changes and communicate them transparently. If a change isn't possible, we can explain why, share what we've learned, and explore other ways to address the concern. Inviting input and following through is accountability in action.

Use values to assess our organization's focus. The *Apple Tree Model* offers a visual way to understand *equality, equity, justice,* and *liberation*—not as a linear continuum, but as overlapping values and approaches that coexist and often strengthen one another. It helps us assess and honestly face where our organizations and institutions sit within the model, and how they are operating. For example, we might ask ourselves: *Are we focused on providing equal access, providing resources* *according to need, dismantling barriers, or reimagining the system entirely?* By being able to answer this, we clarify both our current stance and our potential for transformation.

 Connect vision and values. Vision is the irresistible future we strive toward—something bold and transformative beyond the limits of the status quo (See Chapter 7 for more on visioning). Values guide the daily work of bringing that future to life. They define what we refuse to normalize and help us make impactful decisions, especially when the path is unclear or contested. When we act in alignment with our values—like *justice, care,* and *accountability*—we ensure that the future we're building reflects not just our goals but our ethics.

When our values are clearly defined and actively practiced, they create a sense of shared direction. They build trust—throughout teams, across partnerships, and with the communities we serve. Leading with values keeps us rooted in purpose and helps us move forward with clarity and conviction.

By staying true to what we stand for, we can strengthen our relationships, our work, and our resolve—even under the most challenging of circumstances.

3. TAKE ON SYSTEMS, NOT SYMPTOMS

Confront and challenge the root causes of health inequities.

Poor health outcomes—from heart disease to deaths by suicide—only tell part of the story. They reveal what's happening, but not how we got here. These outcomes are symptoms of deeper systemic forces like structural racism and colonialism. To make these connections visible, Chapter 3 introduced the *Root Causes Roadmap* to visualize how public health issues are the visible manifestations of powerful forces operating below the surface.

Looking deeper prompts us to ask important questions:

- *What systems and structures are producing and reproducing these poor health outcomes?*
- *How have misleading mindsets reinforced the negative outcomes we see?*
- *How have tools for systems change—like policies and budgets—been used to unfairly advantage some communities while disadvantaging others?*

The starting point is unearthing the root causes of the health inequities we're working to address. Once we've diagnosed the root causes, we must act by challenging harmful systems, telling better and more health-affirming stories, and shifting power to support equity and justice. There are several discrete actions we can take to confront the systems that drive poor health:

 Dig deep to expose the root causes. It's tempting to respond to health inequities with comparatively quick fixes: more services, better outreach, new programs. But these are just the symptoms of underlying forces that shape what we can see. We must get to the root causes—systems of oppression and structural inequities—that are producing and reproducing these outcomes. For example, high rates of asthma in a neighborhood may prompt more clinics, but the root cause might be nearby industrial pollution, zoning laws, and chronic disinvestment. Transforming systems is only possible if we trace outcomes back to their origins and address the conditions that created them.

 Name the systems that drive inequity. Our work is incomplete at best—and harmfully complicit at worst—if we fail to name the systems of oppression, unjust policies, and power imbalances that are producing poor health outcomes. For example, when we create data reports, we must explicitly state that "race" is a social construct with no biological basis and name *racism*—not "race"—as the root cause of unjust health disparities. If we don't name these causes clearly, others will fill in the blanks—often with narratives and explanations that are scientifically baseless, detached from historical reality, and destructive to public health and society at large. (See Chapter 2 for more on the origins of "race" and *scientific racism*.)

 Recognize the interconnectedness of systems. Systems of oppression don't operate in isolation—they reinforce one another. *Intersectionality* helps us see how these overlapping systems show up in people's daily lives, compounding advantage for those with multiple forms of privilege and compounding harm for those who live at the intersections of marginalization. For example, *intersectional data analysis* can help us identify which populations face multiple barriers—such as housing insecurity, discrimination, and limited access to care. Consider the Minnesota Department of Health, which used intersectional analysis of student survey data to reveal that queer youth of color—especially those unsure of their gender identity—faced rates of sexual violence more than four times higher than their peers, informing more precise prevention strategies.[25] Understanding and naming these connections can help us codesign solutions that better respond to the complexities of lived experience.

 View health expansively. Public health is anything that advances human flourishing and well-being[26]—so anything that endangers health is fully within our purview. That could be policies driving gentrification and displacement,[27] plans to build a landfill with the potential to pollute drinking water,[28] efforts to bulldoze acres of forest to create a police training facility,[29] or efforts to purge registered voters from the rolls.[30] These moments are all opportunities to build coalitions across issue areas, support community-led resistance to unjust policies and decisions, and bring public health data and framing into spaces where health is not normally or formally part of the conversation.

 Engage across sectors. No industry, organization, or government can achieve its goals without addressing public health. A school district aiming to boost academic outcomes must confront food insecurity and mental health.³¹ A city working to enhance its transportation system needs to consider air quality and pedestrian safety.³² That means, as a public health practitioner, there is no "staying in our lane"—because our lane is human flourishing. Whether testifying at a city council meeting, joining a climate justice coalition, or supporting voting rights advocacy—we're doing public health work. This understanding can bolster us when we face pushback, skepticism, or discomfort for showing up in unexpected spaces, pushing boundaries, or doing things differently in collaboration with our partners.

 Watch for feedback loops and unintended consequences. Systems are dynamic, and changes in one place can ripple out in unexpected ways. A *feedback loop* occurs when an action sets in motion a cycle of consequences that circles back to the original action—supporting or undermining the goal, often escalating over time. For example, increasing policing to improve pedestrian safety can lead to a *negative feedback loop* of continual surveillance and criminalization of Black and brown communities. By contrast, redesigning streets to slow traffic can create a *positive feedback loop*: Safer spaces encourage walking, which builds community presence and further enhances safety. Our values must guide every phase of our work—from planning to implementation—so we can anticipate how systems will respond and adapt accordingly.

 Transform misleading mindsets. These are the deepest and most stubborn layer of systems change. Beneath policies and practices lie the beliefs, assumptions, and values that shape them. These misleading mindsets—like *individualism*, the *meritocracy myth*, or *scarcity*—are often invisible but are incredibly pervasive and powerful. Changing them is the most foundational work of systems transformation. It's also the hardest work, because it requires shifting culture, narrative, and worldview—efforts that take time and require ongoing collaboration. But when we change how people understand the world, we unlock new possibilities for what can be built within it.

 Identify leverage points within systems. All systems have places where a small shift can create a big change. As introduced in Chapter 4, the *Iceberg Model* reveals that the deeper we go—from events to patterns, structures, and underlying mindsets and narratives—the greater the potential for lasting impact. Consider a *surface*-level action of documenting local pedestrian fatalities. *Patterns* then reveal deaths are concentrated in historically redlined neighborhoods. A *systems* response could be advocating for a Complete Streets law that prioritizes infrastructure improvements in disinvested areas. At the deepest level, we could challenge the dominant *narrative* that safety is solely an individual responsibility—reframing it as a matter of public interest and the product of policy and design. Multilevel intervention makes systems change powerful and enduring.

 Anticipate pushback—and keep going. Transformative change will inevitably face opposition from those who are maintaining rigid organizational cultures, implementing entrenched and unjust policies, and working to ensure the status quo remains unchanged. But setbacks and failures are signs that we're pushing boundaries and engaging in the complexity of systems change. To stay impactful and growth-oriented, we need to cultivate *brave spaces*—structured environments that encourage us to engage in principled dissent, name discomfort, and candidly reflect on our work—not just when things go well, but especially when they don't.* Brave spaces aren't free-for-alls; they're anchored in shared commitments to equity and justice. They are necessary to help us be persistent in our efforts, learn from setbacks, and continue moving forward with conviction and purpose.

Transforming entrenched systems will not result from any one action, individual, or organization—it's the product of coordinated efforts across roles, sectors, and communities. No single policy, meeting, or decision will rewrite the rules on its own. Our ability to use different leverage points will depend on our own influence, the power and alignment of our partners, and timing—whether or not there is a window of opportunity for change.

Even seemingly small changes, when aligned with broader shifts within a system— such as evolving political climates, emerging mainstream narratives, or pivotal cultural moments—can gain momentum and change entire systems. What starts as a minor shift in one place can ripple outward, reshaping mindsets and narratives, influencing policy, and expanding what people believe is possible.

Strategic actions, aligned with values and committed partners, can spark whole movements toward justice. When we work together as a coalition of public health practitioners, community leaders, and movement builders, we can generate the collective power necessary to transform the systems that shape our lives.

4. COMMUNICATE AND CASEMAKE FOR CHANGE

Frame problems clearly, name the need for justice explicitly, and tell stories that build power and possibility.

Words shape our beliefs, and our beliefs shape action. That means the language we use has real power: It can confuse, alienate, and reinforce harm—or it can clarify, inspire, and mobilize. Advancing equity and justice requires precise and purposeful language that reflects our values and helps us move toward a flourishing future.

As discussed in Chapter 1, terms like *equity* and *justice* are not vague platitudes or interchangeable buzzwords. They have distinct meanings that require specific actions. Using them purposefully means being clear about what we're saying, understanding who

---

Safe spaces prioritize protection, validation, and respite for those who have experienced harm or marginalization, supporting healing and solidarity. *Brave spaces*—coined by educators and facilitators Brian Arao and Kristi Clemens—intentionally invite discomfort and principled risk-taking to enable growth, cross-difference dialogue, and confrontation of power and privilege, while maintaining mutual respect and care.[33,34]

we're addressing, and why it matters. Clarity helps us push back when important terms are misused or diluted, or when something important is going unsaid.

We apply this understanding through *strategic communication:* adapting our language to different audiences and contexts without compromising the integrity of what we mean. This is not the same as watering down our messages or abandoning our values. It means expanding our ability to communicate effectively, meeting people where they are, and opening paths for new ways of thinking. But to achieve this, we must know our audiences, clarify our goals, place the focus on people, and show how targeted efforts can achieve universal goals—while creating benefits for all.

For example, in a conversation with a decision-maker, we might lead with *equity* if we believe that speaks to their values. But depending on the context, we could also frame our work around shared goals: that everyone deserves an opportunity to live in a safe, thriving neighborhood. We might begin with universal aspirations—such as *Every child deserves to travel to school safely* or *Everyone should have safe drinking water in their homes*—and then build toward a deeper conversation about why targeted actions are necessary to achieve those goals.

Precision and intention in our language strengthen our work. But it's not the words that matter the most, it's the shared meaning behind them.

Promoting and protecting community health requires building a compelling case using strategic framing and rich, credible data—trusted evidence drawn from people's stories and experiences—to persuade people, mobilize support, shift understanding, and drive policy change. This approach draws on the strategic casemaking principles developed by social scientist and author Tiffany Manuel.[35]

Casemaking, in this context, is not just about presenting facts—it's about telling the right story and telling it in a way that resonates with audiences, makes structural injustices visible, and illustrates the shared benefits of equity and justice.

Through effective communication and casemaking, we can create openings for change in specific ways:

 Reframe from crisis to opportunity. Abolitionists and organizers Kelly Hayes and Mariame Kaba share the sobering reflection: "Our work is full of truths that should be unthinkable—yet the mere recitation of these facts does not move people into the streets. . . in some cases, it prompts people to turn off the television."[36(p20)] Instead of only presenting dire facts and figures, we must highlight real solutions. For example, rather than simply saying that suicide is a leading cause of death for youth and young adults in North Carolina,[37] we make a stronger case by explaining how thousands of suicides can be prevented by increasing the minimum wage by just one dollar,[38] providing supportive social spaces for youth, and investing in job training for young people.[39] Moving from problems to possibilities conveys that meaningful solutions are both urgent and achievable.

Connect through emotion and empathy. Public health is about people—not just data points. We must help audiences feel the human stakes behind health inequities. For example, instead of focusing on eviction's hardships, we might share how stable housing helped a family access preventive care, reduce chronic stress, and reconnect with community. Even when describing trauma and harm, our stories should still center dignity, adaptability, and care. Empathy-driven narratives can shift public perception, reduce stigma around health conditions, and build solidarity across groups. They remind us that, when it comes to community health, there is no "them" to be kept at arm's length. It's about all of *us* flourishing together.

 Build broad support with pragmatic persuasion. Equity and justice work succeeds when there is wide support, engagement, and investment across sectors. Not everyone will be moved by moral arguments alone, but many respond to social or economic benefits. For example, a city council may vote to expand affordable housing to reduce emergency department visits and lower costs borne by taxpayers. Business leaders might support paid sick leave because it boosts productivity and reduces turnover. Casemaking means connecting the dots: thoughtfully and intentionally linking equity and justice goals to others' values and interests. By clearly showing how justice benefits everyone—including the bottom line—we can build coalitions and momentum for meaningful change.

 Turn moments into momentum. Public health decisions often hinge on timing—whether it's a funding opportunity, legislative window, or crisis that's captured public attention. Casemaking is most effective when it strategically connects to these moments. We must be ready to respond quickly, anticipate pivotal opportunities, and actively set the agenda. For example, if a city is revising zoning laws, that presents an opening to advocate for environmental health protections. If youth mental health is dominating headlines, it's strategic to push for increased funding for schools to support youth and their families. We must be ready to respond but also bold enough to lead proactively.

 Connect the dots between health and systems. Most people don't automatically see how systems of oppression produce health inequities. Our role is to make these connections clear by pairing data with lived experience, historical context, and systems analysis. For instance, instead of simply documenting higher asthma rates in some certain neighborhoods, we can explain how multiple layered injustices—redlining, exclusionary zoning, industrial siting, and disinvestment—created the hazardous air conditions that endanger health and drive up asthma rates. When we zoom out and put outcomes in context, we help people see the full picture. As public health practitioners, we have the ability and responsibility to bridge evidence with compelling communication to help people draw thoughtful, informed conclusions.

Transform *misleading mindsets*. Effective community health work requires challenging harmful mindsets and assumptions that shape public discourse. (See Chapter 4 for more on this.) If we get drawn into insidious debates about who "deserves" health—like whether housing and basic care should be available to substance users if they aren't seeking institutionally defined "recovery"—we reinforce narratives that some people are expendable. These lose-lose conversations stem from misleading mindsets like *punishment* and *conditional worth*. We must reject them and offer more compelling alternative mindsets rooted in *care* and *universal dignity*. These health-promoting mindsets are exemplified by *Housing First* approaches, which provide immediate, unconditional housing. Not only does this demonstrate that housing is a human right—rather than a reward for specific behaviors—but it improves housing stability, health outcomes, and dignity for people experiencing homelessness.[40,41] When we affirm that everyone deserves safety and support, we reject the zero-sum thinking that endangers health.

 Demonstrate benefits for everyone. A major obstacle to advancing public health is the misleading mindset of *zero-sum*—the idea that helping one group must come at the expense of another. The *Curb-Cut Effect* challenges this by showing that interventions designed for marginalized groups ultimately benefit everyone. Curb cuts were originally championed by disability rights advocates to improve access for wheelchair users, but this improvement ultimately helped others, from parents with strollers to workers with carts. This pattern extends across public health. Environmental protections,[42] guaranteed income,[43] paid leave,[44] antidiscrimination policies,[45] free school meals,[46] affordable housing[47]—the list goes on—all lead to shared benefits across society. Showing this is how we can shift mindsets toward *collectivism* and *abundance*, counter scarcity-based narratives, all while building broader, more durable support.

 Speak so people can understand—and feel understood. Too often, as public health practitioners, we default to using abstract jargon like *relative risk, incidence,* and *transtheoretical model*. While specific to our field, these are terms that rarely, if ever, connect to what people truly care about or reflect how they actually talk about their health. If we want to be seen as caring and connected, rather than aloof and overly professionalized, we must speak to people in words that resonate broadly and connect to core desires such as *safety, dignity, stability,* and *prosperity*. Instead of "comorbidities," we could say *having more than one health problem at the same time*. Instead of saying "rate," we could talk about *how many people are affected over time*. As discussed in Chapter 1, shared meaning matters more than using the same words. By speaking plainly, we can build trust, deepen connection, and open the door to shared understanding.

Include calls to action. People are more likely to support our work when they know what to do and believe their actions matter. Casemaking should end with specific, achievable calls to action. For example, *Share your perspective with local leaders about how paid sick leave affects community health. Join the campaign for clean water in our community. Tell your story at our next town hall for fair wages.* Be honest about the scale and complexity of the challenge—but also help people see that change is possible. Clear, compelling calls to action show that people's voices, experiences, and efforts can make a real difference. When people understand how they can contribute, they're more likely to engage and help move solutions.

As public health practitioners, we must actively shape the narrative and push for structural change by intentionally and effectively connecting the dots for people. This is of paramount importance in a time of rising disinformation, backlash, and scapegoating—when the truth alone is not enough to move people, and silence is complicity.

Casemaking is an ongoing process that demands boldness, adaptability, and a commitment to long-term change. By building this capacity in public health, we can turn pushback into momentum and awareness into action.

5. STAND IN SOLIDARITY, MOVE AS A MOVEMENT

Support struggles for justice beyond our own—and unite for bold, people-powered transformation.

Public health is not neutral—nor has it ever been. It is inherently political, shaped by the narratives, policies, and power structures that surround us. From vaccines to gun violence, sex education to syringe services programs,[48] gender-affirming care to climate disaster prevention, public health strategies to address these pressing issues are routinely politicized. This is not because they lack evidence but because they challenge entrenched interests.

At its best, the work of public health is the work of saving lives and improving well-being on a large scale, grounded in rigorous evidence and shaped by lived experience. (See Chapter 1 for more on the defining characteristics of public health.) This should not be political. Yet it often is, because power and ideology shape whose health is prioritized and whose futures are protected.

Public health decisions affect entire communities. This means they inevitably intersect with—and often confront—the interests, ideologies, and priorities of those in power, from elected officials to corporate executives.

If our work is always political—and will always be politicized—what then?

The answer is that we must rediscover public health's social justice roots and embrace the transformative possibilities of practicing public health as a movement. By this we mean **social movements**: collective efforts by groups of people to challenge existing conditions, demand change, and reshape society. They can emerge in response to injustice or unmet needs and often mobilize outside formal institutions to build power and solidarity. When these movements are justice-oriented, they aim not only to reform systems but also to transform them[49]—redistributing power, resources, and recognition to those who have been historically marginalized.

But not all movements expand justice. Some movements—like the backlash against Reconstruction that followed the Civil War, the rise of mass incarceration, and ongoing attacks on democracy—have deepened systems of subordination and control. Movements are powerful vehicles for change, and the direction of that change depends on the vision and values driving them.

Social movements for justice, by contrast, have driven progress on every major public health issue—from labor protections to clean water. Our greatest public health victories, in fact, have come not from neutrality but from *solidarity*: when we've organized and mobilized with moral clarity and stood alongside communities to demand change.

We cannot simply issue guidance or publish reports from afar. We must be present in the streets, in the clinics, in the classrooms, and in the halls of power. We must use our voices and institutions to do what movements do: shift what people believe is possible and drive concrete, community-led change. To advance equity and justice, we must move with the boldness of a movement, and we must move in solidarity with others. Movements disrupt the status quo, build collective power, and imagine bold solutions that dominant institutions alone often cannot or will not pursue. To do this, we must commit to these actions:

Embrace a movement mindset. As public health practitioners, we often approach our work through a lens of policy, programs, and data. But lasting change also requires the work of *movements*—collective efforts that involve organizing, building narrative power, and uplifting grassroots leadership. Movements push forward visionary and universal ideas—like the campaign for a $15 minimum wage,[50] tuition-free public college,[51] and reparations for the intergenerational and enduring injustices stemming from chattel slavery[52]—that reframe public debates and force dominant institutions to respond. Reorienting as a movement creates opportunities to cultivate new allies, identify unexpected partners, and build broad coalitions rooted in shared values and collective care. By thinking of public health as a movement—and not merely a professional area of practice—we can reclaim public health's social justice roots, make authentic connections with advocates and movement leaders, and meaningfully improve people's lives.

Join forces across movements. Solidarity strengthens every struggle. A movement to advance health justice is inseparable from other justice movements, including those pushing for racial, economic, gender, climate, and disability justice. When these struggles align and unite, we build collective power for transformative change. As a field and as a movement, public health must demonstrate solidarity. We must help people see themselves as part of the movement for health justice—whether in government, academia, philanthropy, the nonprofit or private sectors, or directly within communities. This means embracing an expanded understanding of our scope—one that includes traditional public health, as well as partnerships and practices that may be new to us. All of us must show up with tangible support: sharing useful data, leveraging convening power, listening deeply, and using institutional resources to advance a shared agenda.

 Defend and improve democracy. When communities have real power to shape their futures, health outcomes improve. But democracy, however imperfectly structured within our nation, must be protected from erosion and actively expanded to meet the full promise of *we the people*. A health justice movement must confront voter suppression, support civic engagement, and build new democratic practices rooted in participation and *power shifting*. Improving democracy means taking a stand and ensuring that all people—especially those harmed by health inequities—can lead, decide, and transform the conditions of their lives.

 Focus on material improvements to daily life. As public health practitioners, we must deliver visible, concrete change—especially for those who have been marginalized and oppressed. Our work should lead to tangible improvements in people's lives that they can see and care about, such as safer streets, more affordable housing, and better access to health care. We must plainly show how our efforts make people freer, healthier, and more secure. This means framing public health as a shared endeavor, where each person's well-being is tied to the health of the whole. When someone asks, *Why should I care if someone else's child is vaccinated?* or *How does affordable housing make my neighborhood better?* we must be ready to answer with moral clarity and practical evidence: that public health is about mutual interdependence. Our health is connected, and better health for those most in need of care is protective for us all. By making tangible benefits of public health clear, we can inspire action and build lasting support.

 Build and be accountable to a base. Working at a large scale can be powerful. But one limitation of population-level work is that it can treat communities as statistics or demographic categories, rather than real people with names, relationships, and agency. Building a base changes that. In movement terms, a **base** is an organized, connected group of people who share common interests and goals, trust one another enough to act collectively—even under pressure—and whose leadership guides priorities and strategies. Our base can look different depending on role and context. Our base in public health is diverse and expansive across the social determinants of health. Consider community health workers embedded in neighborhoods or local tenant associations mobilizing around housing conditions, safety, and access to care. Public health department staff, too, can be a base when organizing around shared commitments, co-governing with communities, and pushing for structural change from within their institutions. A base is not necessarily the same as who we serve. It's the people we can mobilize—those who support us, hold us accountable, and whose lived experiences and collective wisdom guide us.

We can more fully realize the promise of public health by viewing it not just as a profession but also as a movement. Public health is most powerful when it stands in solidarity with other justice movements.

Not everyone can engage in direct advocacy, but all of us can think like movement-builders. This mindset invites us to reimagine our roles—what we do, how we do it, who we do it with, who we do it for, and what we believe is possible. We're not simply implementing programs or tracking metrics—we're contributing to a broader struggle for justice.

This shift expands our alliances, sharpens our purpose, and unlocks a different scale of impact. The future of public health depends on our willingness to stand with movements for justice: to listen, to learn, to act, and to build power together.

6. SHIFT AND SHARE POWER

Ensure communities bearing the brunt of injustice lead decision-making. Uplift community ingenuity and solutions.

Power is not a zero-sum game. It can be built, cultivated, expanded, and shared. In public health, this means recognizing that collective power—*power to* act together and *power with* community—is essential for transformative change.

Building collective power ensures the longevity of equity and justice efforts, preventing them from being fully dependent on—or undermined by—any one leader, intervention, or institution. Instead, they become embedded, self-sustaining realities. Shifting power is different than accumulating individual or organizational authority. It means building and sharing influence and decision-making in partnership with communities and strengthening relationships to the point where we, as a movement, can set shared agendas and achieve shared goals.

If we manage, direct, inform, or influence anything in our role, we hold some degree of power. Power is relative, influenced by our professional roles, institutional affiliations, and social identities—whether we acknowledge them or not. Understanding where power is concentrated, who holds it, and how it can be shifted and shared is a foundational skill for advancing equity and justice.

As discussed in Chapter 5, only communities themselves can do power building because institutions and other external entities cannot confer power on communities. Efforts to *build power* require communities to nurture and enhance their own innate capacity to organize, mobilize, advocate, and act. As public health practitioners, we must shift power that we hold to communities and bolster their power-building efforts by providing funding, in-kind resources, and access to decision-making spaces and platforms.

Simultaneously, in our public health roles, we must fulfill our responsibility to *break power*—to confront dominant institutions that perpetuate and profit from injustice. This means exposing systemic harms and calling out those responsible, such as pharmaceutical companies that price essential medications beyond reach and agribusinesses that flood communities with ultra-processed foods. It also means collaborating with partners who can use different tools for systems change—like regulatory policies and civil law mechanisms—to impose meaningful consequences on those who endanger public health, obtain justice and redress, and deter further harm.

The work of *shifting power* and ensuring communities have authority, decision-making control, and access to resources allows us to *share power*—to co-govern alongside communities as they lead. It is long-term and iterative work, but it always starts somewhere. Here are some helpful places we can begin:

 Identify and map power, then shift it. A first step to understanding power is to conduct a *power analysis*—a structured and collaborative process that can help us map where influence and authority are concentrated in an institution, system, geographic area, or across a policy landscape. This kind of reflection can uncover hidden dynamics and imbalances, indicate key influencers and gatekeepers, focus organizing efforts, and reveal opportunities for strategic decision-making.

 Create structures for community governing power. Authentic co-governance is the difference between performative engagement and genuine power sharing. If we want to transform systems, communities must be able to make decisions and trust that those decisions will be implemented with integrity. We can support this shift in power through governing bodies that move beyond temporary or "rubber-stamp" advisory roles and instead have real, sustained decision-making authority. The *Spectrum of Community Engagement to Ownership* helps identify how much power a community truly has in any process (as discussed in Chapter 5). Community governance structures can be transformative for advancing health, especially when dominant institutions, like government and philanthropy, take on redefined roles. We must be supportive partners in implementation, not primary decision-makers. This means backing communities that want to move beyond *co-govern*—where decisions are made collaboratively—and toward *defer to*, where community members lead and we follow their guidance.

 Leverage law and policy to make justice a reality. Law and policy have long been abused to uphold systems of oppression and concentrate dominant power (see Chapter 3), but they can also be reclaimed as tools for justice and inclusion. To transform public health systems, we must embed community priorities into the very structures that govern our lives. This means engaging in advocacy while building community capacity to lead it—training community members to navigate legislative, regulatory, and administrative processes, and collaborating with legal advocates to codevelop strategies that challenge harmful practices, assert rights, and shift power. This includes drafting legislation, influencing rulemaking, filing lawsuits or petitions, and using public comment periods to elevate community voice.

 Take the long view to build durable power. We reject short-termism and transactional approaches by anchoring our work in long-term strategy, deep relationship building, and community infrastructure. Every campaign and policy win—or even setback—should contribute to a broader, multigenerational arc toward justice. This requires operational commitments like multiyear plans, succession strategies, community-led implementation, cross-sector coalitions, leadership development pipelines, and mechanisms for shared governance and accountability. By investing in shifting and sharing power—even in areas outside our direct focus—we strengthen an adaptable ecosystem of organized, community-led groups that can show up across issues and sectors.

When we treat power as a collective asset and a force for justice, we move beyond temporary wins toward lasting change. Power that is shared, resourced, and accountable can reshape the systems that govern daily life in ways that are beneficial and transformative. This is how we can build strong and enduring foundations for community-led change—where the ability to act, decide, and build the future is not concentrated in a few hands, but belongs to the many.

7. ORGANIZE AND MOBILIZE RESOURCES

Fund what matters. Unlock, align, and expand investment in communities long denied their fair share.

If equity and justice are truly priorities, they must be backed by **resources**: tangible commitments of money, materials, labor, relationships, and infrastructure that can be mobilized to advance a goal. But like any other tool—from language to policy to data—resources are not neutral. They are built or extracted, shared or hoarded, weaponized or wielded to shift power. Indeed, it's difficult to imagine how resources could ever be neutral in a country whose wealth and influence were built on stolen land, stolen labor, and stolen lives.

The resources that move through our communities carry weighty histories and the potential to either perpetuate harm or redress it. How we direct, organize, and redistribute resources is not simply a technical or administrative matter—it is a political act. This means we must advance two interconnected efforts:

- **Allocating the resources we already control** in ways that are values-aligned, strategic, and coordinated.
- **Organizing and mobilizing new resources**—public, private, and philanthropic—to build lasting infrastructure for equity, justice, and transformative change.

When we talk about resources, the one that most readily comes to mind is money. As author and activist Edgar Villanueva writes, "Money should be a tool of love, to facilitate relationships, to help us thrive, rather than to hurt and divide us. If it's used for sacred, life-giving, restorative purposes, it can be medicine."[53(p9)] In this sense, money can be used to tend to the wounds of colonization, racism, and extraction.

But we must resist the temptation to romanticize money. Like any medicine, it must be administered with intention and care. Resources—whether financial, political, or relational—are tools for power-building when they are placed under community control. When we align resource allocation with community priorities and mobilize new investments toward their visions, we not only meet immediate needs, we redistribute power, address past harms, and strengthen the capacity for justice in the long term.

Budgets are a clear place where words and values meet reality, functioning as financial documents as well as moral statements—revealing what we care about, what we prioritize, and who we are willing to invest in. We often approach budgeting with zero-sum thinking: that a bigger slice of the pie for one program, issue area, or organization means that others must suffer and accept a smaller one. But what if we refused to limit ourselves to the slices we have and instead put our energy toward increasing the size of the entire pie?

We know that conversations about public health funding are fraught. Our field has been underfunded for decades and is at the mercy of volatile politics and shifting priorities. Local governments and nonprofits compete for limited, restricted funding.

Instead of accepting extractive approaches to funding, we can embrace a *regenerative* mindset—one that grows resources and relationships rather than depleting them. If we choose to work collaboratively, strategically, and proactively, we can expand the resources and possibilities available for all of us to make health and flourishing a reality.

Resource mobilization is critical: It means we must not only budget differently but also demand and expand what is possible. We can take these steps to change our approaches while resourcing equity and justice, both now and into the future:

Invest resources with intention. No matter the size of our budget, we can choose to resource communities harmed by injustice. Within our spheres of influence, we hold the power to operationalize equity through how we allocate and spend. This means making values-driven decisions: funding grassroots and power-building organizations, sustaining funding commitments over the long term, supporting community-led initiatives, and providing capacity-building supports like technical assistance and leadership development.

Reimagine, redesign, and diversify funding opportunities. There are many opportunities in our work to use funding processes to shift power and share resources. Our organizations should avoid being overly prescriptive; we may define the goal, but applicants propose the strategies and solutions. We must ensure that funding pools, contracts, and requests for proposals intentionally include businesses and organizations led by people of color, women, queer and trans people, and other historically excluded groups. Applications and selection criteria for grants and contracts should be written in plain language, with clear and transparent review processes that engage people with diverse lived experiences and perspectives.

 Build shared values into operational budgets. If equity and justice are truly core values, then our budgets must reflect these values across departments and projects. This could look like allocating funds for language interpretation, providing paid roles for community members, and supporting frontline staff through funding technical assistance and capacity-building. Financial processes should incorporate participatory budgeting, shared decision-making, and other co-governance practices—giving community members real authority to set priorities and decide where resources go. Equity and justice cannot just be programmatic goals; they must be embedded in how we plan, spend, and share.

 Compensate community expertise. Community members are experts in their own right, and their time, labor, connections, and knowledge must be fairly compensated. Budgets should include dedicated line items for stipends, honoraria, and contracts—recognizing that if we truly value community contributions, we must be willing to pay for them. Failing to do so perpetuates inequity and extraction and reinforces power imbalances.

 Organize for long-term, structural investments. To help the seeds of equity and justice take root and grow, we must direct government funding and philanthropic dollars toward intergenerational change. The most transformative public health solutions are those that address the systems that fuel health inequities, and they require sustained commitments over time—not fragmented short-term grants. Those of us who have positional power within government agencies and philanthropic institutions must push for long-term investments that confront systemic problems. That means resourcing solutions that go beyond treating symptoms to dismantling the structures that produce inequity in the first place.

 Coordinate for sustained impact. Long-term investments only succeed when paired with cross-sector coordination and alignment across levels of government. Public health depends on the strength of interconnected systems—from health departments to schools, from transit agencies to grassroots organizations. To mobilize sustained funding and support, we need proactive strategies like building coalitions, aligning priorities, and ensuring that our partners have the resources they need to implement long-term, health-promoting solutions. We must make a consistent, compelling case to elected officials, agency leaders, and the public: Investing in public health is a long-term investment that always pays off.

Support community ownership and wealth-building. Truly resourcing equity and justice requires investing in models that shift assets, decision-making power, and economic opportunity directly to communities. That means sustainably resourcing cooperatives, community land trusts, mutual aid networks, and other forms of collective ownership within communities. Organizer and advocate Nia Evans says this of the Boston Ujima Project, which channels capital into resident-approved businesses through a community-led investment fund: "We're not just trying to redistribute wealth—we're trying to redistribute power."[54] By funding long-term autonomy and self-determination, we can help resources stay rooted and grow within communities.

 Invest in communities rather than extracting from them. Although public health is a generative field that is focused on population-level benefit, we can also be perceived as a force for control and restriction. We must be thoughtful about how our field can be harmfully portrayed as concerned more with taking than giving: imposing restrictive dietary guidelines, shaming substance use, and enforcing home occupancy limits. We must ask: *How are our efforts additive, rather than extractive? What investments are we making that bring connection, hope, and tangible benefit to communities?* We should not allow ourselves to be defined by what we remove, but instead by what we build and sustain. By zooming out, we can reorient ourselves around adding value and joy to communities—like green spaces, well-resourced schools, affordable housing, reliable public transit, and dignified jobs. Our contributions must affirm health, foster fulfillment, and improve the material conditions of daily life.

Public health has long been expected to do more with less. But equity and justice invite us to push against zero-sum thinking, extraction, and deficit mindsets to create more—more opportunities to grow our resources, more possibilities for investment, more shared power, and more infrastructure to sustain systemic change. Intentional, place-based work—grounded in local history, leadership, and accountability—can be a powerful starting point. (See Box 8-2 for a local example of how allocating and redistributing resources can provide redress for historical harms and promote health.[55-60])

In a society shaped from its founding by racial capitalism, how we spend money—and how we organize to expand and democratize resources—is one of the clearest reflections of our true priorities. If an institution or organization claims to advance equity and justice, its financial decisions, and its efforts to mobilize new resources, should be among the strongest evidence of that commitment.

8. IMPLEMENT *INSIDE-OUTSIDE* STRATEGIES

Advance shared goals by bridging institutional and community power. Transforming systems requires coordination and trust.

Transformative change in public health—especially change that addresses the root causes of health inequities—requires coordinated and collaborative efforts within institutions and across communities.

Box 8-2. Funding Health Through Reparations

In 2019, Evanston, IL became the first city in the United States to provide publicly funded reparations to Black people as a way of addressing generations of racist policies.[55] This local program was innovatively funded by a municipal cannabis sales tax (and later supplemented by a real estate transfer tax). The initiative directed millions in housing grants—$25,000 per household—to Black residents harmed by historical redlining and housing discrimination.

This funding strategy was designed to address injustices driven by the "War on Drugs,"[56] which disproportionately criminalized Black communities, drove mass incarceration nationwide, and manufactured criminal records that have been used to limit Black people's voting rights,[57] curtail Black economic mobility by burdening people with immense debt,[58] and decrease Black people's life expectancy.[59] By rechanneling cannabis tax revenue toward reparations, Evanston made a clear statement: Resources once used to harm can be intentionally invested in restoration and redress.[60]

Because stable housing is an essential social determinant of health, the reparations initiative also represents a public health intervention. By increasing Black homeownership and reducing housing insecurity, it lowers risk for chronic stress and illness and builds community wealth. In early 2023, the city expanded eligibility to include unrestricted cash payments—a form of guaranteed income—in direct response to resident feedback.

Evanston's approach is a compelling example of participatory governance and resource mobilization in action—leveraging local funding, legal authority, and community codesign to create a sustained, reparative, and health-promoting investment that addresses past harms and moves toward shared prosperity.

An **inside-outside strategy** is a long-term strategic approach that involves trust-building and collaboration between those working on the *inside* (within dominant institutions like government agencies, universities, and philanthropies) and those working on the *outside* (in community power-building organizations, grassroots agencies, advocacy networks, and justice movements). Together, these strategies leverage a dynamic set of tactics to reshape systems, structures, policies, and practices in ways that directly improve people's lives.[61]

Inside-outside strategies leverage institutional access and community insight to drive change that neither positionality—inside or outside—could achieve alone. At their best, these collaborations are greater than the sum of their parts. The goal of an inside-outside strategy is not merely cooperation, but *synergy*—wins for equity and justice that emerge from collaborations of people and organizations that achieve much more together than they could on their own. This approach challenges traditional power dynamics and embraces fluidity. When planned with intention and foresight, inside-outside strategies evolve and continue as roles shift, relationships change, and individuals go to new jobs and carry their knowledge across sectors. The strength of these strategies relies on intentional relationships, the recognition that no single organization holds all the answers, and the ability to navigate the constant motion of an ecosystem of changemakers.

Public health practitioners can use inside-outside strategies to shift power, advance community health, and protect hard-won gains—regardless of the political climate or social circumstance. Public health advocates and organizers Selma Aly, Asamia Diaby, and Julian Drix note that, when conditions are favorable, an inside-outside strategy can catalyze "policy victories that push the boundaries of what is considered possible," and conversely, during cycles of retrenchment and backlash, "it serves as a critical tool for defending communities, protecting rights, and safeguarding past wins."[61(p12)]

Inside-outside strategies can look different based on the organizations and people involved, as well as the context. To bring this into our work, we must commit to these collective practices:

Build relationships across organizations, sectors, and levels. Relationships—not just formal partnerships—are the foundation for the ongoing collaboration required of inside-outside strategies. Regardless of our positionality, we must intentionally cultivate relationships with people across sectors and at every level, from interns to executives. Trust is built over time through reliable, reciprocal, and accountable action—not during a campaign or crisis, but over time. Strong, authentic connections expand our insight, access, and influence. There's a world of difference between showing up to a city council vote without context and having a trusted relationship with a staffer who can walk you through the agenda, perspectives, and processes. Our success depends on investing in relationships as a core strategy.

Embrace complementary roles. Every person has unique powers and constraints resulting from their role and positionality—and we must communicate those clearly. We can both push, and allow ourselves to be pushed, on assumptions about what our roles can and cannot do. Insiders bring institutional access, connections, positional power, technical expertise, insight into processes, and resources. Outsiders mobilize people power, apply strategic pressure, shape public narratives, hold institutions accountable, and say what insiders cannot. For example, community advocates can build public support for a policy and recommend policy language, while staff inside institutions open policy windows and broker key meetings. When both sides understand, respect, and strategically leverage each other's roles, they can be bolder and more effective than either could be alone.

Align early and stay connected. Shared strategy is essential, even when tactics differ. To collaborate effectively, we must have a shared understanding of what we will collectively accomplish and how we will move our work forward. We can set ourselves up for success by naming root causes and defining success—whether that's shifting power, changing policy, or improving daily life for community members in a specific way. Disagreements are inevitable—and can be generative, and even beneficial, if handled with care and respect. When all parties are grounded in shared purpose and strategy, it becomes easier to navigate tensions and move forward together. Together, the right pressure applied at the right moment can transform systems.

Plan for tension and conflict. In an inside-outside strategy, we don't have to agree on everything—or present a united front in every space—to work together toward a shared goal. Sometimes we may align privately but take different public stances, depending on our roles, audiences, or strategic needs. What matters is transparency, mutual respect, and trust. Relationships with people across institutions can open space for informal, mutually beneficial sharing and conversation. For example, a community organizer may share early insights with a health department staffer about an upcoming campaign, or a program officer might flag a timely opening—like a board discussion or funding cycle—so partners can shape the conversation with new data and insights. These informal exchanges deepen trust and increase the potential for transformative, community-rooted impact.

 Build capacity for rapid response and strategic pivots. Setbacks and sudden shifts—like leadership changes, policy reversals, and public health emergencies—demand agility. Inside–outside partners must be ready to pivot quickly and strategically. This means cultivating nimble decision-making structures, maintaining open lines of communication, and regularly assessing the landscape together. We won't always agree on the best course of action, but when we understand each other's constraints and priorities, we can act with greater intentionality and alignment. Strategic pivots may involve changing tactics, reframing narratives, or reconfiguring roles. When we are adaptable, strategic, and grounded in shared goals, we can weather disruptions and seize unexpected openings with confidence and cohesion.

 Build collective muscle for co-governance. A successful inside-outside strategy doesn't just win campaigns—it builds lasting capacity for communities, coalitions, and institutions to share power and make decisions together. This includes expanding co-governance structures, co-creating internal policies that formalize shared decision-making with community partners, and dedicated space and resources for communities to lead the long-term stewardship of our collective work.

 Protect public health gains. In moments of backlash and retrenchment, defending what we've already won is essential. Those working within institutions (on the inside) must uphold and implement existing policies, defend budgets, and resist rollbacks. Meanwhile, community organizers and advocacy groups (on the outside) must mobilize public support, apply pressure, and create political and economic consequences for those who attempt to undermine progress. But by working together, insiders and outsiders can strategically safeguard public health gains, including reproductive health programs, climate change initiatives, harm reduction services, and public investments in equity and justice. By organizing within and across institutions—and ensuring our efforts are aligned, complementary, and persistent—we can collectively resist rollbacks and protect policy wins that bolster community health.

Celebrate wins and plan for setbacks. Inside–outside strategies take time, effort, and collective energy—so any win, however small, deserves recognition. Progress may come in unexpected forms, such as a coalition formed around a failed bill that built lasting infrastructure for future organizing. At the same time, change is not linear. Political winds shift, policy windows open and close, and people cycle in and out of roles—requiring strategic adaptation, and sometimes a complete reset. We must continuously nurture our relationships, invest in coalition strength, and plan for leadership transitions. This is how inside–outside strategies stay adaptable, withstand backlash, and continue to move forward over time.

 Invest in capacity and infrastructure for the long haul. Inside–outside strategies need durable, behind-the-scenes infrastructure that rarely makes headlines or gets highlighted in press releases. But it's what makes progress possible: flexible, long-term funding for community power-building organizations and service providers, dedicated staff time within institutions, and shared tools for coordination. Funders and institutional partners must help sustain the work by prioritizing and resourcing the capacity of the entire ecosystem, not just individual projects or campaigns. When we invest in and bolster the scaffolding of collaboration—like coalition infrastructure, data systems, and community-led planning processes—we strengthen our collective ability to act boldly, consistently, and with staying power.

Inside-outside strategies don't require perfect conditions; they are strategic approaches we can use to generate and sustain progress toward shared goals across difference, institutions, roles, and time. They offer concrete and collaborative ways to build solidarity, advance justice, and improve community health.

As public health practitioners, we are uniquely positioned to lead with this approach. Our purpose is rooted in social justice, and our field spans sectors, disciplines, and political contexts. Many of us already build coalitions, work across institutional boundaries, and navigate between systems and communities. But when we do this work with intentionality—and recognize ourselves as part of a larger movement and an interconnected ecosystem of changemakers—we deepen our impact and cultivate lasting, collective power for change.

9. MAKE EQUITY AND JUSTICE ROUTINE

Embed equity and justice into planning, budgeting, operations, and collaboration—until bold becomes standard.

One of the greatest threats to equity work is that it often depends on individual champions rather than being built into institutions and systems. If the work disappears when a staff member leaves or a project ends, it was never truly institutionalized.

The goal is to integrate equity and justice into everyday operations—how we plan, fund, implement, allocate, evaluate, and collaborate—so thoroughly that it becomes standard practice. This ensures that successors don't just maintain the work—they view it as fundamental to what public health is and how it should function. The more we build equity and justice into routines, operations, and accountability structures, the more likely it is to take root and endure. Over time, practicing equity and justice can become so normalized that we can't imagine working any other way.

While policies and regulations are necessary for the process of institutionalization, our values don't become real through the written word alone. Equity and justice are actualized through daily practice: in the questions we ask, the relationships we cultivate, the processes we establish, the data we prioritize, the ways we engage communities, and the decisions we make. Equity and justice are not just about *what* we do—but *how* we do it.

While this chapter broadly explores practical ways to advance both equity and justice, the following recommendations specifically focus on how to make equity routine, recognizing that—while equity and justice are linked—justice has other distinct and overlapping ways of being actualized.

We focus here on equity because it's an essential starting point, especially for those of us working within dominant institutions like government agencies, foundations, and universities. Embedding equity into our everyday practices is both tangible and achievable. When we make equity routine, we create a critical foundation for advancing justice and, ultimately, achieving liberation.

To make equity a regular, enduring part of our work, we must take these actions:

 Institutionalize and document equity in writing. For equity efforts to survive beyond the tenure of individual staff, shifts in organizational priorities, or changes in political administrations, we must commit them to writing. Equity should be codified across all dimensions of organizational life, including policies, strategic plans, program protocols, job descriptions, standard operating procedures, hiring processes, procurement guidelines, and evaluation plans. Each role carries a responsibility for equity. It must be everywhere, not as an optional add-on or matter of personal initiative, but as a core, nonnegotiable function. Equity should be as necessary and ubiquitous as the air we breathe.

 Expand our evidence to include *community data*. Generated by communities on their terms, *community data*—including stories, numbers, art, maps, and firsthand accounts—are credible and trusted information about everyday realities.[62] These forms of data reflect community-defined priorities, needs, and lived experiences, providing depth and context that institutional metrics alone cannot capture. While dominant institutions cannot collect this data directly, they can partner with and fund community organizations to support its generation and use. To advance equity, we must acknowledge that quantitative data—such as population surveys, administrative records, and epidemiological reports—are insufficient on their own. We can bridge different insights, like pairing survey results with quotes from listening sessions or including historical context alongside outcome metrics.

This can help us generate information that is more accurate, contextual, and community-centered.

 Budget and resource with an equity lens. Advancing equity means allocating resources based on need, history, and context—not dividing them evenly by default. We must intentionally direct greater funding to communities that have faced historic and ongoing injustices to ensure that all can reach universal outcomes. This requires connecting directly with people within communities, understanding how past and present policies—from redlining and Jim Crow to gerrymandering and school disinvestment—have shaped health and well-being, and embedding those realities into budget processes and decisions. Equitable budgeting also means resourcing meaningful community participation by including funds for honoraria, childcare, transportation, interpretation, and food—not as extras, but as essentials. These costs must be regularly built into grant proposals and internal planning. We must track how funds are used and prepare to adjust course so that they reflect our values, commitments, and universal goals.

 Invest in community leadership. We must fund community-based organizations with deep local ties and expertise in power building—not just well-resourced dominant institutions. This means adopting inclusive procurement policies that open competitive opportunities beyond familiar vendors, allow time for small business owners and community-serving organizations to apply, simplify application processes, and ensure fairness in proposal review and award distribution. There are also opportunities to provide better-structured support: multiyear grants, flexible funding, capacity-building, and feedback mechanisms that foster honest dialogue and accountability. We must value lived experience as expertise and elevate community leadership. For example, when communities generate and govern their own data, they reclaim the authority to name problems, set priorities, and shape solutions—challenging gatekeeping and shifting power. When communities lead the way, they have the power to create transformative change.

 Connect and co-create across sectors. Advancing equity goals requires building and maintaining authentic relationships with people beyond our immediate spheres, including those within schools, planning departments, community power-building organizations, labor unions, and disability justice organizations. These connections begin as *relationships* and grow into *partnerships* when we co-create initiatives and establish co-governance structures for shared decision-making. Trust grows through honesty and accountability, so we must create spaces for regular, candid feedback—both formal and informal—and act swiftly on what we hear with transparent communication about changes and gratitude for the learning. When people see their feedback directly shaping the work, relationships deepen and collective progress accelerates.

Ensure sustainability through onboarding and succession. Equity work should be built to last, enduring beyond changes in individual roles and organizational priorities. As new staff, partners, and collaborators join, we must orient them to the values, practices, and history that shape our work. This means developing onboarding guides, handbooks, and trainings that capture lessons learned and ground newcomers in shared commitments. At the same time, we must embed succession strategies into organizational planning, team structures, and equity initiatives to sustain momentum while preserving and growing institutional knowledge. This can help ensure continuity and progress even when people move on. If we proactively and intentionally plan for the future, we can ensure that equity work not only survives but also thrives.

 Recognize and resource equity leadership. Although equity should be part of everyone's role, this work often falls on the shoulders of marginalized staff, partners, and community members, whose labor and ingenuity are uncompensated. Those of us working within dominant institutions must make this work visible and structurally supported. From facilitating internal workgroups to participating on advisory committees, leading on equity takes time, skill, and responsibility. Equity work must be recognized through formal organizational roles, leadership pathways, and compensation. Our goal should be to ensure those driving positive organizational change are valued and their efforts are treated as essential to collective success.

By focusing on the routine, we can weave equity into the fabric of public health. This is not always glamorous work, but it's the kind that lasts. What begins as deliberate effort can, with time and intention, become second nature and eventually an institutional cornerstone. Actions that once seemed bold can become the new normal.

10. REIMAGINE PUBLIC HEALTH

Use imagination, discipline, and audacity to rewrite the rules. Redefine public health as a force for joy, justice, and liberation.

Public health is often described in technical terms: as a set of interventions, a field of data and research, or professionalized work that operates within government bureaucracy. But our practice is so much more. Public health is a collective promise: that we will take care of one another, we will create systems and structures that advance equity and justice, and we will work toward creating a world where everyone can flourish.

Reimagining public health means letting go of old assumptions—about what's possible, about who is worthy, and about where expertise lives. It means rejecting the notion that our work must be confined to narrow lanes or incremental reforms. This work requires boldness, creativity, and joy. It challenges us not only to confront unjust systems but also to dream up new ones that center care, accountability, reciprocity, interdependence, and possibility. When someone tells us, "We do it this way because that's the way it's always been done," we should take it as a challenge, not a constraint.

The injustices we face are not natural facts of the universe that we must accept. They are human-made and changeable, and we can change them for the better. Together, we can create a future that is generative, connected, and joyful.

We've seen glimpses of this future already: health care institutions funding community land trusts,[63] organizers developing crisis response programs rooted in community care,[64] and institutional survey practices being reimagined in partnership with research justice scholars and advocates.[65,66] We've also seen local governments use their authority to block harmful private development,[67] expand access to housing,[68] provide affordable public transit,[69] and declare sanctuary cities that protect immigrants.[70] These are not outliers—they are previews.

As civil rights leader and philosopher Grace Lee Boggs reminded us, "We are the leaders we've been looking for."[71] We have the collective power, passion, courage, and moral force to shape the future of public health—because it belongs to us. We can forge a movement that proudly embraces its social justice roots, that creates the conditions for all to flourish, and that centers and uplifts the marginalized—and ultimately, everyone.

The systems we're confronting are formidable, but they are built on rules—and rules can be rewritten. This is the next chapter. And it is ours to write together.

REFERENCES

1. Morrissette M. Nikole Hannah-Jones: Speaking frankly about progress, hope, and the present. *Minnesota Women's Press.* December 7, 2022. Accessed May 7, 2025. https://www.womenspress.com/nikole-hannah-jones-speaking-frankly-about-progress-hope-and-the-present
2. North Carolina Department of Natural and Cultural Resources. 1898 Wilmington coup. Accessed June 23, 2025. https://www.dncr.nc.gov/1898-wilmington-coup
3. Rierson SL, Schwimmer M. The Wilmington Massacre and coup of 1898 and the search for restorative justice. *Elon Law J.* 2022;14. Accessed June 23, 2025. https://papers.ssrn.com/sol3/Delivery.cfm/SSRN_ID4065959_code258113.pdf?abstractid=4065959&mirid=1
4. Equal Justice Initiative. The Wilmington Massacre of 1898. November 10, 2024. Accessed June 23, 2025. https://eji.org/news/wilmington-massacre-of-1898
5. Tulsa Race Massacre: What you didn't learn in history class. PBS. June 10, 2021. Accessed June 23, 2025. https://www.pbs.org/wnet/tulsa-the-fire-and-the-forgotten/2021/06/10/tulsa-race-massacre-what-you-didnt-learn-in-history-class
6. US Commission on Civil Rights. The US Commission on Civil Rights marks the 100th anniversary of the Tulsa Race Massacre. June 4, 2021. Accessed August 17, 2025. https://www.usccr.gov/news/2021/us-commission-civil-rights-marks-100th-anniversary-tulsa-race-massacre
7. Moreno C. Black Wall Street's second destruction. *Next City.* May 31, 2021. Accessed August 17, 2025. https://nextcity.org/features/black-wall-streets-second-destruction

8. Equal Justice Initiative. Justice Department finds Tulsa Massacre was a "coordinated, military-style attack." January 13, 2025. Accessed June 23, 2025. https://eji.org/news/justice-department-finds-tulsa-massacre-was-a-coordinated-military-style-attack

9. Darity WA Jr., García RE, Russell L, Zumaeta JN. Racial disparities in family income, assets, and liabilities: A century after the 1921 Tulsa Massacre. *J Fam Econ Issues.* 2024;45(2):256–275. doi:10.1007/s10834-023-09938-4

10. Equal Justice Initiative. Tulsa Massacre survivor Viola Ford Fletcher continues to call for justice. July 5, 2023. Accessed June 23, 2025. https://eji.org/news/tulsa-massacre-survivor-viola-ford-fletcher-continues-to-call-for-justice

11. Letang A. AAPI heritage: Remembering the Watsonville Riots of 1930. *KSBW.* May 21, 2021. Accessed June 26, 2025. https://www.ksbw.com/article/aapi-heritage-remembering-the-watsonville-riots-of-1930/36482159

12. US Department of Labor. Filipino labor leaders of the Delano Grape Strike Hall of Honor induction. 2024. Accessed August 15, 2025. https://www.dol.gov/general/aboutdol/hallofhonor/2024-filipino-farm-workers

13. Romasanta G. Why it is important to know the story of Filipino-American Larry Itliong. *Smithsonian Magazine.* July 24, 2019. Accessed August 15, 2025. https://www.smithsonianmag.com/smithsonian-institution/why-it-is-important-know-story-filipino-american-larry-itliong-180972696

14. Foy N. California farmworkers cope with wildfire smoke, pesticides, roaches and rodents, survey says. *CalMatters.* February 3, 2023. Accessed June 26, 2025. https://calmatters.org/california-divide/2023/02/farmworkers-conditions-california-report

15. Pasulka N. Ladies in the streets: Before Stonewall, transgender uprising changed lives. *NPR.* May 5, 2015. Accessed June 26, 2025. https://www.npr.org/sections/codeswitch/2015/05/05/404459634/ladies-in-the-streets-before-stonewall-transgender-uprising-changed-lives

16. Beltran T, Allen AM, Lin J, Turner C, Ozer EJ, Wilson EC. Intersectional discrimination is associated with housing instability among trans women living in the San Francisco Bay area. *Int J Environ Res Public Health.* 2019;16(22):4521. doi:10.3390/ijerph16224521

17. Baguso GN, Aguilar K, Sicro S, Mañacop M, Quintana J, Wilson EC. "Lost trust in the system": System barriers to publicly available mental health and substance use services for transgender women in San Francisco. *BMC Health Serv Res.* 2022;22(1):930. doi:10.1186/s12913-022-08315-5

18. Levin S. Compton's Cafeteria riot: A historic act of trans resistance, three years before Stonewall. *The Guardian.* June 21, 2019. Accessed June 26, 2025. https://www.theguardian.com/lifeandstyle/2019/jun/21/stonewall-san-francisco-riot-tenderloin-neighborhood-trans-women

19. Pilkington E. 'Timestamp on our minds': Philadelphia marks 1985 MOVE bombing that killed 11. *The Guardian.* May 13, 2025. Accessed August 15, 2025. https://www.theguardian.com/us-news/2025/may/13/philadelphia-1985-move-bombing

20. Puckett JL. MOVE on Osage Avenue. West Philadelphia Collaborative History. Accessed August 15, 2025. https://collaborativehistory.gse.upenn.edu/stories/move-osage-avenue

21. Kelly K. The history of the Black radical group MOVE and its infamous bombing by police. *Teen Vogue.* May 14, 2020. Accessed August 15, 2025. https://www.teenvogue.com/story/history-black-radical-group-move-infamous-bombing-by-police

22. Levenson M. Philadelphia health chief resigns over cremation of remains from MOVE bombing. *New York Times.* May 13, 2021. Accessed July 7, 2025. https://www.nytimes.com/2021/05/13/us/health-commissioner-philadelphia-move-bombing.html

23. Peterson J. The fires still burn. *The Philadelphia Citizen.* May 13, 2025. Accessed August 15, 2025. https://thephiladelphiacitizen.org/move-40-years

24. Snyder T. *On Tyranny: Twenty Lessons from the Twentieth Century.* Tim Duggan Books, 2017.

25. Minnesota Department of Health. Preventing violence using intersectionality. October 23, 2024. Accessed August 17, 2025. https://www.health.state.mn.us/communities/svp/data/intersection.html

26. Fakunle DO. Storytelling and public health 101. In: *Arts-Focused Approaches to Public Health Communications.* Public Health Communications Collaborative; February 29, 2024. Accessed June 27, 2025. https://www.slideshare.net/slideshow/artsfocused-approaches-to-public-health-communications/266583002#3

27. Kerubo J. What gentrification means for Black homeowners. *New York Times.* August 17, 2021. Accessed May 7, 2025. https://www.nytimes.com/2021/08/17/realestate/black-homeowners-gentrification.html

28. Willard K. Community, county leaders fight planned landfill in Silver Creek area of Tarrant County. *NBC 5 Dallas-Fort Worth.* November 20, 2023. Accessed May 7, 2025. https://www.nbcdfw.com/news/local/community-county-leaders-fight-planned-landfill-in-silver-creek-area-of-tarrant-county/3392982

29. Love H, Donoghoe M. Atlanta's 'Cop City' and the relationship between place, policing, and climate. Brookings. September 21, 2023. Accessed May 7, 2025. https://www.brookings.edu/articles/atlantas-cop-city-and-the-relationship-between-place-policing-and-climate

30. Smart Growth America. National Complete Streets Coalition. Accessed June 27, 2025. https://www.smartgrowthamerica.org/programs-and-coalitions/national-complete-streets-coalition/about

31. Bloomberg American Health Initiative. Addressing food insecurity through community schools in California. May 2, 2025. Accessed August 17, 2025. https://americanhealth.jhu.edu/news/addressing-food-insecurity-through-community-schools-california

32. Shape SSF 2040 General Plan. Mobility. City of South San Francisco. Accessed August 17, 2025. https://shapessf.com/mobility

33. Arao B, Clemens K. From safe spaces to brave spaces: A new way to frame dialogue around diversity and social justice. In: Landreman LM, ed. *The Art of Effective Facilitation: Reflections From Social Justice Educators.* Stylus Publishing; 2013:135–150.

34. Bow Valley Immigration Partnership. Brave space. September 20, 2021. Accessed August 14, 2025. https://bvipartnership.com/resources-blog/brave-space

35. Manuel T. *Strategic CaseMaking: The Field Guide for Building Public and Political Will.* TheCaseMade Press; 2020.

36. Hayes K, Kaba M. *Let This Radicalize You: Organizing and the Revolution of Reciprocal Care.* Haymarket Books; 2023.

37. North Carolina Department of Health and Human Services. Injury and Violence Prevention Branch: Suicide and self-inflicted injury data. May 14, 2025. Accessed June 28, 2025. https://injuryfreenc.dph.ncdhhs.gov/DataSurveillance/SuicideData.htm

38. Kaufman JA, Salas-Hernández LK, Komro KA, et al. Effects of increased minimum wages by unemployment rate on suicide in the USA. *J Epidemiol Community Health* 2020;74:219-224. doi:10.1136/jech-2019-212981

39. Occhipinti JA, Skinner A, Iorfino F, et al. Reducing youth suicide: Systems modelling and simulation to guide targeted investments across the determinants. *BMC Medicine.* 2021;19(1):61. doi:10.1186/s12916-021-01935-4

40. US Dept of Housing and Urban Development. Housing First: A review of the evidence. *Evid Matters.* 2023;Spring/Summer:2. Accessed August 16, 2025. https://archives.huduser.gov/portal/periodicals/em/spring-summer-23/highlight2.html

41. Tsemberis S. Housing First: Implementation, dissemination, and program fidelity. *Am J Psychiatr Rehabil.* 2013;16(4):235-239. doi:10.1080/15487768.2013.847732

42. US Environmental Protection Agency. Progress cleaning the air and improving people's health. March 19, 2025. Accessed August 17, 2025. https://www.epa.gov/clean-air-act-overview/progress-cleaning-air-and-improving-peoples-health

43. Lee K, Neighly M. The power of cash: How guaranteed income can strengthen worker power. Economic Security Project. May 1, 2023. Accessed August 23, 2025. https://economicsecurityproject.org/resource/the-power-of-cash

44. Wething H, Slopen M. Paid sick leave improves workers' health and the economy. Economic Policy Institute. January 30, 2025. Accessed August 17, 2025. https://www.epi.org/blog/paid-sick-leave-improves-workers-health-and-the-economy

45. Blum DG, Shahbaz S. Why inclusive laws and policies for LGBTQI+ people benefit us all. CID Voices Blog. Harvard Kennedy School Center for International Development. December 17, 2024. Accessed August 17, 2025. https://www.hks.harvard.edu/centers/cid/voices/why-inclusive-laws-and-policies-lgbtqi-people-benefit-us-all

46. Blossom P. What are the benefits of free school meals? Here's what the research says. University of Illinois. October 17, 2023. Accessed August 17, 2025. https://fshn.illinois.edu/news/what-are-benefits-free-school-meals-heres-what-research-says

47. Nemsick K. 5 ways whole communities can benefit from affordable housing. United Way Bay Area. March 14, 2024. Accessed August 17, 2025. https://uwba.org/blog/5-ways-whole-communities-can-benefit-from-affordable-housing

48. Centers for Disease Control and Prevention. Safety and effectiveness of syringe services programs. February 8, 2024. Accessed May 13, 2025. https://www.cdc.gov/syringe-services-programs/php/safety-effectiveness.html

49. Harris AP. Anti-colonial pedagogies: "[X] justice" movements in the United States. *Can J Women Law.* 2018;30(3):567-594. Accessed August 17, 2025. https://muse.jhu.edu/article/713416

50. Lathrop Y, Wilson MD, Lester TW. A 10-year legacy: The fight for $15 and a union movement. National Employment Law Project. November 29, 2022. Accessed June 27, 2025. https://www.nelp.org/insights-research/10-year-legacy-fight-for-15-union-movement

51. Biron CL. Free college tuition? More US communities say yes. *Context.* Thomson Reuters Foundation. February 26, 2025. Accessed August 17, 2025. https://www.context.news/socioeconomic-inclusion/free-college-tuition-more-us-communities-say-yes

52. Coates T. The case for reparations. *The Atlantic.* June 2014. Accessed August 17, 2025. https://www.theatlantic.com/magazine/archive/2014/06/the-case-for-reparations/361631

53. Villanueva E. *Decolonizing Wealth: Indigenous Wisdom to Heal Divides and Restore Balance.* Berrett-Koehler Publishers; 2018.

54. Booker L. Boston Ujima Project leverages collective power to build $5 million fund. *Boston Globe.* August 29, 2024. Accessed August 13, 2025. https://www.bostonglobe.com/2024/08/29/metro/boston-ujima-project-investment-fund

55. City of Evanston. Evanston local reparations. Accessed August 13, 2025. https://www.cityofevanston.org/government/city-council/reparations

56. Ramirez SA, cummings adp. Roadmap for anti-racism: First unwind the War on Drugs now. *Tul L Rev.* 2022;96:469–501. Accessed June 29, 2025. https://lawecommons.luc.edu/facpubs/716

57. Uggen C, Larson R, Shannon S, Stewart R, Lueder C. The denial of voting rights to people with criminal records. In: Budd KM, Lane DC, Muschert GW, Smith JA, eds. *Beyond Bars: A Path Forward From 50 Years of Mass Incarceration in the United States.* Policy Press; 2023:73–85.

58. Harper A, Ginapp C, Bardelli T, et al. Debt, incarceration, and re-entry: A scoping review. *Am J Crim Justice.* 2021;46(2):250–278. doi:10.1007/s12103-020-09559-9

59. Wildeman C, Wang EA. Mass incarceration, public health, and widening inequality in the USA. *Lancet.* 2017;389(10077):1464–1474. doi:10.1016/S0140-6736(17)30259-3

60. FXB Center for Health and Human Rights. Making the public health case for reparations: Landscape report. Harvard University. February 2022. Accessed August 13, 2025. https://content.sph.harvard.edu/wwwhsph/sites/2464/2022/02/Making-the-Public-Health-Case-for-Reparations-Final.pdf

61. Aly S, Diaby A, Drix J. The five dimensions of inside-outside strategy: A guide for public health and social movements to build powerful partnerships. Health in Partnership. April 30, 2025. Accessed May 19, 2025. https://www.healthinpartnership.org/resources/the-five-dimensions-of-inside-outside-strategy-guide

62. Mohsini M, Lopez A, Msibi K, haley d, Campos-Melchor P. Introducing community data. Coalition of Communities of Color. 2024. Accessed August 8, 2025. https://www.coalitioncommunitiescolor.org/research-and-publications/introducing-community-data

63. Hindman DJ, Pollack CE. Community land trusts as a means to improve health. *JAMA Health Forum.* 2020;1(2):e200149. doi:10.1001/jamahealthforum.2020.0149

64. Mitchell C, Badruzzaman RA. Mental health first: Evaluating Oakland and Sacramento's non-police crisis response program. Health in Partnership. July 1, 2025. Accessed August 18, 2025. https://www.healthinpartnership.org/resources/mental-health-first-evaluating-oakland-and-sacramentos-non-police-crisis-response-program

65. Bernal DW, Hagan MD. Redesigning justice innovation: A standardized methodology. *Stanford J Civ Rights Civ Libert.* 2020;16:335–372. Accessed August 17, 2025. https://law.stanford.edu/publications/redesigning-justice-innovation-a-standardized-methodology

66. Petteway RJ, López-Cevallos D, Mohsini M, et al. Engaging antiracist and decolonial praxis to advance equity in Oregon public health surveillance practices. *Health Aff (Millwood).* 2024;43(6):813–821. doi:10.1377/hlthaff.2024.00051

67. Piser K. Why industry city rezoning is failing. *City & State New York.* August 6, 2020. Accessed August 18, 2025. https://www.cityandstateny.com/politics/2020/08/why-industry-city-rezoning-is-failing/175744

68. Enterprise Community Partners; Wells Fargo Foundation; Ivory Innovations; Terner Labs. The case for innovation in housing: How local governments can drive solutions. Enterprise Community Partners. January 16, 2025. Accessed August 18, 2025. https://www.enterprisecommunity.org/learning-center/resources/case-innovation-housing-how-local-governments-can-drive-solutions

69. San Mateo County Transportation Authority. Reconnecting communities: Connect4SSF. Accessed August 18, 2025. https://www.smcta.com/connect4ssf

70. Catholic Legal Immigration Network. Sanctuary cities toolkit. March 2023. Accessed August 18, 2025. https://www.cliniclegal.org/toolkits/sanctuary-cities-toolkit

71. Bill Moyers Journal. Bill Moyers talks with Grace Lee Boggs. PBS. June 15, 2007. Accessed June 30, 2025. https://www.pbs.org/moyers/journal/06152007/watch3.html

Appendix A. Resources to Expand Your Knowledge

To support ongoing learning and strategic action, we've developed a selected list of resources organized by chapter. These resources include research, history, practical tools, guiding frameworks, and insights from respected and trailblazing leaders, scholars, and organizations.

This list is not comprehensive; many important and worthwhile resources are not included here, as the scholarship and practice of equity and justice continues to evolve. Instead, this list should be considered a starting point to dive deeper into topics that resonate—and to seek new knowledge and tools as they emerge.

CHAPTER 1: DEFINING WHAT'S AT STAKE

Articles and Essays

- Blackwell AG. The curb-cut effect. *Stanford Social Innovation Review*. Winter 2017. https://ssir.org/articles/entry/the_curb_cut_effect: Shows how policies designed for marginalized groups benefit everyone, offering a compelling case for equity-based policymaking.
- Fairchild AL, Rosner D, Colgrove J, Bayer R, Fried LP. The EXODUS of public health: What history can tell us about the future. *Am J Public Health*. 2010;100(1):54-63. doi:10.2105/AJPH.2009.163956: Tracks the American public health profession's shift from a social reform-centered model to a science-based identity.
- Global Health Europe. Inequity and inequality in health. August 24, 2009. https://globalhealtheurope.org/values/inequity-and-inequality-in-health: Clarifies the difference between inequity and inequality and their implications for public health.
- Krieger N, Birn AE. A vision of social justice as the foundation of public health: Commemorating 150 years of the spirit of 1848. *Am J Public Health*. 1998;88(11):1603-1606. doi:10.2105/AJPH.88.11.1603: Discusses major events in and around 1848 that affirm social justice as the foundation of public health.
- Yong E. How public health took part in its own downfall. *The Atlantic*. October 23, 2021. https://www.theatlantic.com/health/archive/2021/10/how-public-health-took-part-its-own-downfall/620457: Analyzes how public health weakened its own position by abandoning its broader social mission and how its future lies in reclaiming that origin.

Books

- Sins Invalid. *Skin, Tooth, and Bone: The Basis of Movement Is Our People—A Disability Justice Primer*. 2nd ed. Sins Invalid; 2019: Introduces the principles of disability justice, centering the voices of disabled, queer, and Black and brown people in the pursuit of collective liberation.
- Tobin-Tyler E, Teitelbaum JB. *Essentials of Health Justice: Law, Policy, and Structural Change*. 2nd ed. Jones & Bartlett Learning; 2022: Analyzes how law and policy structure health inequities and offers advocacy tools to promote systemic reform and health justice.
- Venkatapuram S. *Health Justice: An Argument from the Capabilities Approach*. Polity Press; 2011: Argues from a philosophical perspective that health is a fundamental human capability and moral entitlement, making it central to any theory of social justice.

Guides, Reports, and Tools

- Carey ML, Hewitt AA. Words matter: A guide to inclusive language around racial and ethnic identity. District of Columbia Office of Human Rights; Mayor's Office of Racial Equity. April 2023. https://ohr.dc.gov/page/ohrore-guide-inclusive-language-race-and-ethnicity: Offers practical guidance for respectful, equity-centered language when discussing race and ethnicity.
- powell ja, Menendian S, Ake W. Targeted universalism: Policy & practice. Othering & Belonging Institute, University of California, Berkeley. December 2022. https://belonging.berkeley.edu/targeted-universalism: Describes how to set universal goals while tailoring strategies to meet the needs of marginalized groups.

CHAPTER 2: "RACE," RACISM, AND THE STRUGGLE FOR EQUITY AND JUSTICE

Articles and Essays

- Coates T-N. The case for reparations. *The Atlantic*. May 21, 2014. https://www.theatlantic.com/magazine/archive/2014/06/the-case-for-reparations/361631: Makes the case that Black people in the United States are owed reparations, tracing how slavery, Jim Crow, and government-sanctioned housing discrimination created enduring systemic oppression.
- Jones CP. Levels of racism: A theoretic framework and a gardener's tale. *Am J Public Health*. 2000;90(8):1212-1215. doi:10.2105/AJPH.90.8.1212: Explores a framework for understanding racism on three levels using an extended allegory about a gardener who attempts to grow flowers in rich and poor soil.

- Tuck E, Yang KW. Decolonization is not a metaphor. *Decolonization Indig Educ Soc.* 2012;1(1):1–40. doi:10.25058/20112742.n38.04: Argues that decolonization must involve the repatriation of Indigenous land and life, challenging the widespread misuse of the term as a metaphor for social justice reforms within settler colonial frameworks.

Books

- Crenshaw K. *On Intersectionality.* New Press; 2019: Includes key essays and articles that have defined the concept of intersectionality.
- Estes N. *Our History Is the Future: Standing Rock Versus the Dakota Access Pipeline, and the Long Tradition of Indigenous Resistance.* Verso Books; 2019: Links the 2016 Standing Rock protests to centuries of Indigenous resistance, revealing how Indigenous struggles for land, water, and sovereignty are central to broader movements for justice.
- Lee E. *America for Americans: A History of Xenophobia in the United States.* Basic Books; 2019: Details the long history of how immigration has been persistently racialized across different groups and eras.
- McGhee H. *The Sum of Us: What Racism Costs Everyone and How We Can Prosper Together.* One World; 2021: Uses stories and evidence to reveal how racism undermines society as a whole and how solidarity can unlock shared prosperity.
- Rothstein R. *The Color of Law: A Forgotten History of How Our Government Segregated America.* W. W. Norton & Company; 2017: Describes how US government policies enforced and entrenched racial segregation.
- Simpson LB. *As We Have Always Done: Indigenous Freedom Through Radical Resistance.* University of Minnesota Press; 2017: Offers a vision of Indigenous resistance rooted in land, relational ethics, and resurgence, rejecting settler systems in favor of lived freedom and grounded normativity.
- Skloot R. *The Immortal Life of Henrietta Lacks.* Crown Publishers; 2010: Details the story of Henrietta Lacks, a Black woman whose cells were taken without her consent in 1951 and were used to create the first "immortal" human cell line—known as HeLa cells—used extensively for scientific research.
- Smith C. *How the Word Is Passed: A Reckoning With the History of Slavery Across America.* Little, Brown and Company; 2021: Explores how the legacy of chattel slavery continues to shape American identity and culture.
- Stannard DE. *American Holocaust: The Conquest of the New World.* Oxford University Press; 1992: Details the centuries-long colonialist genocide against Indigenous peoples across what is now known as North and South America.
- Strings S. *Fearing the Black Body: The Racial Origins of Fat Phobia.* New York University Press; 2019: Reveals how anti-fat prejudice emerged not from medical concerns

but from racist and sexist ideologies that pathologized Black bodies and upheld white supremacy.

- Wilkerson I. *Caste: The Origins of Our Discontents*. Random House; 2020: Frames racism in the United States as a caste system, tracing its deep historical and structural roots.

Guides, Reports, and Tools

- Lawrence K, Sutton S, Kubisch A, Susi G, Fulbright-Anderson K, Aspen Institute Roundtable on Community Change. Structural racism and community building. Aspen Institute. 2004. https://www.aspeninstitute.org/wp-content/uploads/files/content/docs/rcc/aspen_structural_racism2.pdf: Describes how "race" shapes the social, political, economic, and cultural institutions of our society and the necessity of adopting a more "race"-conscious approach to community building and social justice work.

CHAPTER 3: THE ROOT CAUSES OF HEALTH INEQUITIES

Articles and Essays

- ChangeLab Solutions. A blueprint for change makers: Achieving health equity through law & policy. March 27, 2019. https://www.changelabsolutions.org/product/blueprint-changemakers: Provides legal strategies and best practices for policymakers and communities to improve health outcomes and create equitable communities.
- Harris AP, Pamukcu A. The civil rights of health: A new approach to challenging structural inequality. *UCLA Law Rev*. 2020;67:758–832. https://www.uclalawreview.org/the-civil-rights-of-health-a-new-approach-to-challenging-structural-inequality: Calls for public health to partner with civil rights advocates and social justice movements to confront structural inequality and advance transformative change.
- Jones CP. Systems of power, axes of inequity: Parallels, intersections, braiding the strands. *Med Care*. 2014;52(10 suppl 3):S71–S75. doi:10.1097/MLR.0000000000000216: Examines the impacts of racism on health to identify parallels and intersections and uses a "cliff analogy" framework for distinguishing between five levels of health intervention.
- Kline S. Guaranteed income: A primer for funders. Asset Funders Network; Center for High Impact Philanthropy; Economic Security Project; Springboard to Opportunities. May 2022. https://assetfunders.org/resource/guaranteed-income-a-primer-for-funders: Explains what guaranteed income is, discusses its origins and evolution, and provides real-world case examples of guaranteed income efforts.
- Lopez RP. Public health, the APHA, and urban renewal. *Am J Public Health*. 2009;99(9):1603–1611. doi:10.2105/AJPH.2008.150136: Documents how public health institutions contributed to harmful urban renewal policies.

- Taylor NL, Porter JM, Bryan S, Harmon KJ, Sandt LS. Structural racism and pedestrian safety: Measuring the association between historical redlining and contemporary pedestrian fatalities across the United States, 2010–2019. *Am J Public Health.* 2023;113(4):420‑428. doi:10.2105/AJPH.2022.307192: Describes how the nearly century-old policy of redlining drives present-day pedestrian fatalities in the United States.
- Yearby R. Structural racism and health disparities: Reconfiguring the social determinants of health framework to include the root cause. *J Law Med Ethics.* 2020;48(3):518‑526. doi:10.1177/1073110520958876: Discusses how structural racism is the root cause of health inequities, which is missing from the social determinants of health framework used in public health.

Books

- Atiles J. *Crisis by Design: Emergency Powers and Colonial Legality in Puerto Rico.* University of Chicago Press; 2024: Exposes how US emergency laws and fiscal control mechanisms in Puerto Rico function as tools of colonial governance, manufacturing crisis and deepening structural inequality.
- Davidson A. *Social Determinants of Health: A Comparative Approach.* Oxford University Press; 2019: Outlines how structural factors drive global health inequities and how public health practitioners can address them.
- Johnson W, Kelley R, eds. *Race Capitalism Justice.* Haymarket Books; 2018: Explores how slavery and racial capitalism shape modern racial injustice and resistance movements.
- Marmot M. *The Health Gap: The Challenge of an Unequal World.* Bloomsbury Publishing; 2015: Describes how social determinants of health drive inequities and calls for action to address root causes.
- Walia H. *Border and Rule: Global Migration, Capitalism, and the Rise of Racist Nationalism.* Haymarket Books; 2021: Examines how borders function as tools of racial capitalism and nationalist control, connecting global migration systems to broader patterns of oppression and exclusion.

Guides, Reports, and Tools

- Health in Partnership. Health equity guide. https://healthequityguide.org: Offers strategies and case studies for embedding equity into public health practice.
- National Association of County & City Health Officials. Roots of health inequity. https://rootsofhealthinequity.org: Examines structural drivers of health inequities and the role of public health in dismantling them.
- United Nations General Assembly. *Universal Declaration of Human Rights.* United Nations; 1948: Affirms that "all human beings are born free and equal in dignity and

rights" and describes a global standard that has shaped modern human rights law and advocacy worldwide.

CHAPTER 4: TRANSFORMING MINDSETS AND NARRATIVES TO ADVANCE HEALTH

Articles and Essays

- Crenshaw K. Kimberlé Crenshaw on intersectionality, more than two decades later. Columbia Law School News. June 8, 2017. https://www.law.columbia.edu/news/archive/kimberle-crenshaw-intersectionality-more-two-decades-later: Reflects on the evolution of intersectionality and its relevance to contemporary movements for justice.
- Shorters T. From fixers to builders. *Stanford Social Innovation Review*. January 9, 2025. https://ssir.org/articles/entry/narrative-change-from-fixers-to-builders: Introduces asset framing as a communications strategy that defines people by their aspirations and contributions—rather than their challenges—to build more inclusive and effective narratives for social change.

Books

- Bailey M. *Misogynoir Transformed: Black Women's Digital Resistance.* New York University Press; 2021: Discusses misogynoir—a form of anti-Black racist misogyny—and explores how Black women, particularly queer and trans women, have used social media platforms to confront it.
- Coates T-N. *The Message.* One World; 2024: Examines how dominant narratives—including myths about nationhood, "race," and identity—are constructed to justify oppression and argues that courageous storytelling can disrupt these narratives.
- Desmond M. *Evicted: Poverty and Profit in the American City.* Crown Publishing; 2016: Reveals how eviction is not a consequence of poverty but a driver of it, challenging the myth that poor people are disposable and exposing the systemic exploitation at the heart of the US housing crisis.
- Farmer P. *Pathologies of Power: Health, Human Rights, and the New War on the Poor.* University of California Press; 2003. Argues that structural violence—rather than individual behavior—is the root cause of global health disparities, demanding a moral and political reckoning that affirms health as a human right.
- Geronimus AT. *Weathering: The Extraordinary Stress of Ordinary Life in an Unjust Society.* Little Brown Spark; 2023: Reveals how chronic exposure to systemic injustice—especially racism and classism—accelerates aging and deteriorates health among marginalized communities, reframing poor health outcomes as the physical toll of oppression.

- Gordon A. *What We Don't Talk About When We Talk About Fat.* Beacon Press; 2020: Reframes anti-fat prejudice as a systemic form of discrimination rooted in moral judgment, social exclusion, and institutional bias—not in objective health concerns.
- Meadows DH. *Thinking in Systems: A Primer.* Chelsea Green Publishing; 2008: Lays the groundwork for understanding and transforming complex systems by showing how feedback loops, structures, and paradigms drive system behavior and long-term change.

Guides, Reports, and Tools

- American Medical Association, American Association of Medical Colleges. Advancing health equity: A guide to language, narrative and concepts. https://www.ama-assn. org/system/files/ama-aamc-equity-guide.pdf: Provides a framing tool for public health professionals to move beyond "neutral" language and toward equity-informed communication.
- County Health Rankings & Roadmaps. Narratives for health. https://www. countyhealthrankings.org/strategies-and-solutions/narratives-for-health: Highlights storytelling as a tool to shift public understanding and support for health equity.
- FrameWorks Institute. Changing narratives and moving mindsets. https://www. frameworksinstitute.org/what-we-do/key-initiatives/changing-narratives-and-moving-mindsets: Offers resources that examine the relationship between narratives, mindsets, culture, and public policy.
- FrameWorks Institute. Fast frames: Introduction. February 1, 2024. https://www. frameworksinstitute.org/articles/fast-frames-introduction: Provides short videos on messaging techniques, including framing vulnerability and using visual context.

Networks and Hubs

- Radical Communicators Network. RadComms. https://www.radcommsnetwork.org: Connects a global community of social justice communicators that builds narrative power to support liberation movements.

CHAPTER 5: EQUITY AND JUSTICE ARE A MATTER OF POWER
Articles and Essays

- Gilman HR, Schmitt M. Building public trust through collaborative governance. *Stanford Social Innovation Review.* March 17, 2022. https://ssir.org/articles/entry/building_public_trust_through_collaborative_governance: Explores how co-governance can improve equity in decision-making.

- McGrath D, Goldberg H. Governing power. Grassroots Power Project. 2022. https://grassrootspowerproject.org/wp-content/uploads/2023/09/GPP_Book_09.22-SinglePage_Digital.pdf: Examines the necessity of grassroots political power to achieve structural change.
- Michener J. Health justice through the lens of power. *J Law Med Ethics*. 2022;50(4):656–662. doi:10.1017/jme.2023.5: Discusses how health justice requires political struggle, taking at least two forms: building power and breaking power.

Books

- Bobo KA, Kendall J, Max S. *Organizing for Social Change: Midwest Academy Manual for Activists*. 4th ed. Forum Press; 2010: Presents a practical framework for grassroots campaign planning, power analysis, and direct action.
- Ganz M. *People, Power, Change: Organizing for Democratic Renewal*. Oxford University Press; 2024: Offers a comprehensive framework for democratic organizing, emphasizing relationships, public narrative, strategy, and structure as the building blocks of collective power.
- Oluo I. *Be a Revolution: How Everyday People Are Fighting Oppression and Changing the World—And How You Can, Too*. HarperOne; 2024: Provides insights and accounts from people across the United States working to create systemic change in education, labor, media, health, housing, and beyond.

Guides, Reports, and Tools

- González R. *The Spectrum of Community Engagement to Ownership*. Facilitating Power. 2021. https://www.facilitatingpower.com/spectrum_of_community_engagement_to_ownership: Outlines shifts in power that organizations can make to move away from harmful community engagement practices and toward truly meaningful efforts that advance co-governance and community leadership in decision-making.
- Health in Partnership. Activities to deepen your power-building analysis. June 27, 2022. https://www.healthinpartnership.org/resources/activities-to-deepen-your-power-building-analysis: Provides hands-on activities and exercises that can help practitioners assess their power and influence and formulate their power-building strategies.

CHAPTER 6: MAKING AND MEASURING CHANGE

Articles and Essays

- Mann J. Human rights and the new public health. *Health Hum Rights*. 1995;1(3):229–233. doi:10.2307/4065135: Argues that integrating human rights into public health transforms the field by shifting focus from individual behavior to the societal structures that shape health outcomes.

- Pamukcu A, Harris AP. Health justice and the criminal legal system: From reform to transformation. *Bill of Health.* September 10, 2021. https://petrieflom.law.harvard. edu/2021/09/10/health-justice-criminal-legal-system: Applies a health justice framework to the criminal legal system, arguing that transformation requires divesting from punishment and investing in care and community well-being.

- Perry IA. Assessment, policy development, and assurance: Evolving the core functions of public health to address health threats. *AJPM Focus.* 2023;3(1):100172. doi:10.1016/j.focus.2023.100172: Describes the core functions of public health and how they have evolved to more explicitly address social inequities on population health.

- Schaffer K, Porter J. Show me the values: Centering communities and co-creation in an equity-driven evaluation. *J Public Health Manag Pract.* 2025;31(5):897–898. doi:10.1097/PHH.0000000000002187: Describes key questions evaluators should ask themselves as they plan and implement a values-based, equity-driven evaluation.

Books

- Alexander M. *The New Jim Crow: Mass Incarceration in the Age of Colorblindness.* Rev ed. The New Press; 2020: Explores how mass incarceration functions as a racial caste system in the United States.

- Martinez C, Mukerjee R, eds. *All This Safety Is Killing Us: Health Justice Beyond Prisons, Police, and Borders—Abolitionist Frameworks and Practices From Clinicians, Organizers, and Incarcerated Activists.* North Atlantic Books; 2025: Exposes how marginalized communities are vilified by "carceral safety" systems and calls for a radical break with these systems strategies in favor of ones grounded in grassroots organizing and abolition.

- Purnell D. *Becoming Abolitionists: Police, Protests, and the Pursuit of Freedom.* Astra House; 2021: Makes a personal and political case for abolishing policing and state-sanctioned violence and instead investing in care-based systems of public safety.

Guides, Reports, and Tools

- Chicago Beyond. Why am I always being researched? 2018. https://chicagobeyond. org/insights/philanthropy/why-am-i-always-being-researched: Challenges extractive research practices and offers actionable strategies for centering equity, community voice, and shared power in research and evaluation.

- Critical Resistance. *Abolitionist Toolkit.* May 14, 2020. https://criticalresistance.org/ resources/the-abolitionist-toolkit: Rejects punishment-based models of safety and justice, offering community accountability and transformative approaches to address harm.

- Ella Baker Center for Human Rights. Peer-to-peer resource organizing toolkit. 2021. https://ellabakercenter.org/resourceorganizing: Provides a step-by-step guide for community-based fundraising that centers reciprocity, accountability, and justice values, making resource mobilization accessible to organizers at all levels.
- Mohsini M, Lopez A, Msibi K, haley d, Campos-Melchor P. Introducing community data. Coalition of Communities of Color. 2024. https://www.coalition communitiescolor.org/research-and-publications/introducing-community-data: Defines the concept of *community data* and differentiates it from dominant data, interrogates what should count as trusted evidence, and offers principles for properly collecting and using community data.

Networks and Hubs

- Health in Partnership. Community safety: Health instead of punishment program. https://www.healthinpartnership.org/programs/community-safety: Provides a hub of resources for replacing criminalization with public health approaches to safety, justice, and well-being.

CHAPTER 7: ENVISIONING AND ACTUALIZING A BETTER WORLD

Articles and Essays

- Blackwell AG. How we achieve a multiracial democracy. *Stanford Social Innovation Review*. Spring 2023. https://ssir.org/articles/entry/how_we_achieve_a_multiracial_ democracy: Argues that building an inclusive, multiracial democracy requires redesigning systems to equitably function amid profound diversity.
- Harris AP, Pamukcu A. Health justice and Just Transition. *J Law Med Ethics*. 2022;50(4):674-681. doi:10.1017/jme.2023.7: Uplifts the Just Transition framework as a justice-driven strategy for public health, advocating for deeper collaboration with climate justice movements to confront racial capitalism and other structural drivers of health inequities.
- Krieger N. Public health, embodied history, and social justice: Looking forward. *Int J Health Serv*. 2015;45(4):587-600. doi:10.1177/0020731415595549: Discusses notable features of our current era and offers insights for ensuring that health equity is the guiding star to orient us all.
- Willis R. Reckoning: No bodily autonomy without gender liberation. *YES! Magazine*. March 27, 2025. https://www.yesmagazine.org/opinion/2025/03/27/reckoning-raquel-willis-gender-liberation: Calls for a cultural shift toward gender liberation, linking bodily autonomy, reproductive justice, and collective care.

Books

- Boggs GL. *The Next American Revolution: Sustainable Activism for the Twenty-First Century*. University of California Press; 2012: Blends political theory, lived experience, and practical wisdom to offer an approach to activism rooted in community, imagination, and deep systems change.
- brown am. *Emergent Strategy: Shaping Change, Changing Worlds*. AK Press; 2017. Blends science fiction, biomimicry, and movement organizing to offer a guide to adaptive change.
- Butler OE. *Parable of the Sower*. Four Walls Eight Windows; 1993: Explores adaptability and collective survival through a speculative novel set in a collapsing United States, where a young Black woman develops the Earthseed philosophy amid climate crisis and systemic injustice.
- Chambers B. *A Psalm for the Wild-Built* and *A Prayer for the Crown-Shy*. Tor Books; 2021 and 2022: Explores rest, purpose, sustainability, and interdependence through a hopeful speculative duology that offers quiet meditations on care in a postcapitalist world.
- Hannah-Jones N, ed. *The 1619 Project: A New Origin Story*. One World; 2021: Explores the legacy of slavery in the United States, illuminating key moments of oppression, struggle, and resistance through an anthology of essays, poetry, photographs, and other works of art.
- Hayes K, Kaba M. *Let This Radicalize You: Organizing and the Revolution of Reciprocal Care*. Haymarket Books; 2023: Aids and advises activists and organizers as they map their own journeys through the work of justice-making.
- Hemphill P. *What it Takes to Heal: How Transforming Ourselves Can Change the World*. Random House; 2024: Explores how personal healing and community transformation are interconnected.
- hooks b. *All About Love: New Visions*. HarperCollins; 1999: Explores love as a political and healing force necessary for justice and liberation.
- Kimmerer RW. *Braiding Sweetgrass: Indigenous Wisdom, Scientific Knowledge, and the Teachings of Plants*. Milkweed Editions; 2013: Weaves Indigenous knowledge, ecology, and storytelling into a vision of relational reciprocity and healing.
- Lorde A. *Sister Outsider: Essays and Speeches*. Crossing Press; 2007: Examines the interconnections between power, sexism, feminism, racism, and society.
- Sarsour L. *We Are Not Here to Be Bystanders: A Memoir of Love and Resistance*. 37 Ink; 2020: Recounts autobiographical experiences of of growing up as a Muslim Palestinian American feminist in Brooklyn, New York and becoming an activist in solidarity with marginalized communities nationwide.
- Shetterly ML. *Hidden Figures: The American Dream and the Untold Story of the Black Women Mathematicians Who Helped Win the Space Race*. William Morrow; 2016:

Reveals the true story of Black female mathematicians at NASA whose calculations helped fuel America's greatest achievements in space.

Networks and Hubs

- NDN Collective. Land Back. https://ndncollective.org/land-back: Provides resources, narratives, and organizing tools to support Indigenous-led efforts to reclaim land, restore sovereignty, and dismantle colonial systems through the Land Back movement.

CHAPTER 8: TEN WAYS TO PUT EQUITY AND JUSTICE INTO PRACTICE

Articles and Essays

- Daly HS, Martinchek K, Martinez R, Morgan JW, Farrell L, Falkenburger E. Exploring individual and institutional positionality. Urban Institute. December 15, 2023. https://www.urban.org/research/publication/exploring-individual-and-institutional-positionality: Encourages reflection on how positionality shapes analysis, action, and equity outcomes.

Books

- Heifetz RA, Linsky M, Grashow A. *The Practice of Adaptive Leadership: Tools and Tactics for Changing Your Organization and the World.* Harvard Business Press, 2009: Offers tools for leading through complexity by aligning values and strategy in the face of systemic challenges.
- Kim MM. *The Wake Up: Closing the Gap Between Good Intentions and Real Change.* Balance; 2021. Guides equity practitioners navigating internal and external systems change, with relevance for public sector leaders.
- Manuel T. *Strategic CaseMaking: The Field Guide for Building Public and Political Will.* The CaseMade Press; 2020. Provides a blueprint for "making the case" in ways that build public and political will.
- Snyder T. *On Tyranny: Twenty Lessons from the Twentieth Century.* Tim Duggan Books; 2017: Provides lessons and advice for surviving and resisting authoritarianism.
- Wingfield AH. *Gray Areas: How the Way We Work Perpetuates Racism and What We Can Do to Fix It.* Harper Business; 2023: Reveals why racial inequity persists in the workplace and provides actionable solutions for creating equitable, multiracial workplaces of the future.

Guides and Reports

- Aly S, Diaby A, Drix J. The five dimensions of inside-outside strategy: A guide for public health and social movements to build powerful partnerships. Health in Partnership. April 30, 2025. https://www.healthinpartnership.org/resources/the-five-dimensions-of-inside-outside-strategy-guide: Guides institutional and grassroots actors in building strong, aligned movements for health and justice.
- Anaissie T, Clifford D, Wise S, Cary V, Malarkey T. Liberatory design deck. National Equity Project. https://www.nationalequityproject.org/tools/liberatory-design-card-deck: Practically introduces a creative problem-solving approach to design with equity, co-creation, and reflection.
- Autistic Self-Advocacy Network. Holding inclusive events: A guide to accessible event planning. 2019. https://autisticadvocacy.org/resources/accessibility: Offers practical tips for making events accessible, explicitly framing accessibility as a matter of equity, dignity, and self-advocacy.
- Holler JL. Equity budgeting: A manifesto. Marion Voices: Folklife & Oral History Program. 2020. https://marionvoices.org/equity-budgeting: Frames budgets as ethical documents, using an arts and culture lens that extends across sectors to align financial decisions with justice and community accountability.

Networks and Hubs

- Public Health Awakened. https://publichealthawakened.org/about: Provides a national network of public health practitioners organizing for health, equity, and justice.
- Race Forward. Toolkits. https://www.raceforward.org/resources/toolkits: Provides a collection of practical guides and frameworks designed to help individuals and institutions advance racial equity across sectors, including government, media, education, and grassroots organizing.
- Racial Equity Tools. https://www.racialequitytools.org: Provides an expansive online library of resources—including planning guides, organizational self-assessments, curricula, and facilitation materials—to support individuals and organizations working toward racial justice across systems and communities.

Appendix B: Glossary

Abolition: A vision and practice for building a society where police and prisons are no longer needed. Abolition centers two core commitments: (1) it addresses the root causes of harm in society so that systems of policing and punishment become obsolete, and (2) it reimagines and creates new systems grounded in care, co-governance, accountability, and community well-being. Abolition draws its name and purpose from the 19th century movement to end chattel slavery. It connects to that legacy by dismantling modern systems of racial and social oppression and replacing them with community-based approaches that embrace human dignity.

Accountability: A personal and structural obligation to honor our commitments, to take responsibility for our decisions, and to face the consequences of our actions. Accountability is not about assigning blame but is instead about pursuing transformation and repair. It requires openness, honesty, and courage, especially in the face of harm or discomfort.

Anticipatory obedience: A term coined by historian and author Timothy Snyder that refers to the act of preemptively conforming to imagined demands of authority before any explicit directive is given. He warns: "Do not obey in advance. Most of the power of authoritarianism is freely given."[1(p17)]

Assurance: The holistic responsibility to guarantee that all public health interventions—policies, programs, services, and communication campaigns—are implemented *effectively* (ensuring interventions achieve their intended goals), *equitably* (actively rectifying injustices and providing resources according to need), *structurally* (by addressing the social determinants of health and the systems of oppression that shape how they are distributed), and *responsibly* (using approaches that foster trust and accountability rather than causing harm or instilling fear).

Assurance-centered evaluation: An approach to evaluation that places community needs at the center, shifts power, focuses on systems, and mutually benefits communities as well as the institutions funding the evaluation.

Audacity: The bravery to question the systems we have inherited and to dream beyond them.

Base: An organized, connected group of people who share common interests and goals, trust one another enough to act collectively—even under pressure—and whose leadership guides priorities and strategies.

Black Codes: A system of laws adopted by nearly all Southern states after the Civil War to restrict the rights of Black people, including their labor, voting rights, property ownership, and mobility. Enforced by all-white police and state militia forces, Black Codes were intended to largely restore the system of chattel slavery that had existed before the war.

Budget: A plan for managing funds, setting levels of spending, and financing expenditures. Budgets are aligned with policy decisions and direct how resources are allocated across programs and services. The budget process is the primary means by which organizations and agencies select among competing demands for the allocation of resources. Budgets reflect our values: They show where attention and effort will be directed—and what will be neglected. Budgets can even serve as policy statements in themselves, reflecting the values and priorities of communities and institutions.

Capitalism: An economic system in which private individuals and businesses own and control property as well as the means of production for goods and services. Capitalism relies on markets and competition to determine prices and wages.

Casemaking: The art and science of communicating persuasively to inspire support for a cause by presenting solutions in ways that resonate. It draws on storytelling, framing, data, and strategy to understand what moves people to act—and applies those insights in ways that allow for the strategic crafting and sharing of messages for systems change.

Chattel slavery: A colonial system of slavery, supported by the Transatlantic Slave Trade, that was practiced in all 13 British colonies in what would eventually become the United States. African people were purchased to become the personal property of their owners for all of their lives and for the entirety of their descendants' lives. Through chattel slavery, enslavement was permanent and inheritable. Children of an enslaved mother automatically inherited her status and were also enslaved for life. Enslaved people were considered a commodity that could be bought, sold, bequeathed, and traded like livestock or furniture.

Co-creation: A collaborative process that begins with community consent and centers shared decision-making. Co-creation draws on mutual respect and complementary strengths. Institutions contribute policy expertise, technical tools, implementation staff, and access to decision-making spaces. Communities bring lived experience, cultural knowledge, organizing power, and clarity about what justice looks like on the ground. Together, these assets can fuel solutions that are visionary, viable, and rooted in shared values.

Coded language: Words that seem neutral on the surface but carry hidden meanings—often to implicitly invoke stereotypes, perpetuate prejudice, and reinforce destructive power imbalances. Coded language operates under the guise of civility, professionalism, and common sense. It provides the speaker with plausible deniability while simultaneously allowing them to communicate ideas that would otherwise be called out as discriminatory, offensive, and socially unacceptable.

Collaborative governance or co-governance: A shared decision-making approach in which government agencies and community members—especially those historically excluded from power—work together to shape and implement public policies, programs, and the allocation of resources. In co-governance, communities are not merely consulted; they hold real authority and leadership. Governments act as partners and implementers of the community's will.

Collective care: A shared responsibility for one another's emotional, physical, and social well-being within communities, organizations, and movements.

Colonialism: A system and process through which one nation asserts control over another territory and its people that invariably involves violence, land dispossession, and political domination.

Colonization: The process of establishing foreign control over land and people through displacement and subjugation to extract land, labor, and resources. Colonization is a central mechanism of colonialism.

Colorblindness: An ideology that downplays or denies the role of structural racism in shaping opportunities and outcomes for people of color. Colorblindness can manifest in ways that include (1) denying the concept of "race" altogether (e.g., "We are all the same"); (2) ignoring or dismissing blatant racial discrimination based on skin color; (3) overlooking institutional racism, which includes the cumulative policies, practices, and norms that disadvantage people of color; and (4) disregarding the influence of *white privilege*, which refers to the unearned advantages and opportunities that come with being white.

Communities: People who are connected by shared experiences, identities, and geography. Because of its focus on entire communities, the term *public health* is synonymous with *community health*.

Community data: Coined by research justice advocates and scholars Mira Mohsini, Andres Lopez, Khanya Msibi, dallas haley, and Polet Campos-Melchor, these are forms of trusted and credible evidence that are generated by communities themselves and include all the ways communities express and document their everyday experiences and realities. *Community data* include stories, narratives, numbers, art, music, maps, oral histories, and firsthand accounts. These forms of data reflect people's lived experiences, priorities, and aspirations and must be produced on the terms of communities themselves. They offer critical context about what has happened in the past, what is happening in the present, where and to whom things are happening, and why it matters.

Community governance: A form of collective decision-making in which community members have full authority to make decisions and guide their implementation.

Community health: See *public health*. A term that emphasizes the well-being of communities overall, focusing on the interconnectedness of social, economic, and environmental factors and their impacts on health and flourishing. Community health is synonymous with *public health*, and the two terms can be used interchangeably. That said, *community health* can be particularly useful when communicating with the general public and with those in other professional fields to emphasize the people-focused and community-centered nature of public health work.

Community power: As defined by Lead Local, "the ability of communities most impacted by structural inequity to develop, sustain and grow an organized base of people who act together through democratic structures to set agendas, shift public discourse, influence who makes decisions, and cultivate ongoing relationships of mutual accountability with decision-makers that change systems and advance health equity."[2]

Concentrated, intergenerational poverty: A pervasive form of poverty that is entrenched, neighborhood- and community-wide, and difficult—oftentimes impossible—to escape. This is because systems of oppression and structural inequities drive racial segregation, community disinvestment, and other forms of subjugation to keep it intact. As a result, upward mobility is not only harder to achieve but also more fragile and fleeting.

Co-powered consent: A participatory approach to evaluation and consent wherein evaluation participants have influence over the evaluation's design and implementation. In an evaluation that embraces co-powered consent, evaluation participants can decide *if* they will participate in an evaluation, as well as *how* their participation will be structured in the first place.

Cultural racism: A form of racism that involves defining white cultural norms as the standard, while portraying or distorting the traditions and behaviors of people of color as abnormal, inferior, or pathological. Cultural racism operates by allowing people to avoid direct discussions of "race" by blaming seemingly "colorblind" or "race-neutral" proxies—like people's language, religion, immigration status, or participation in social safety net programs—as "problems" to be fixed, ultimately ensuring racist ideas can persist.

Data: Facts, statistics, and other basic units of information about people, places, communities, conditions, and systems. They are the building blocks that elected officials, policymakers, organizers, advocates, and others use to draw conclusions about how a community functions and the realities of people living within them. Data are collected all the time, often without our conscious awareness. On their own, data are raw information. They become meaningful when analyzed, interpreted, and placed in context—often by combining different data points or connecting them to a broader story.

Dignity: Every person's intrinsic value, worth, and deservingness of respect and fair treatment simply because they are human.

Disability justice: A movement that asserts that all bodies and abilities are equally valuable, and that people are not disabled by their bodies or minds; they are disabled by barriers built into environments, policies, and systems. It imagines a world where disabled people—especially disabled people of color, queer disabled people, and others at the intersections—lead the transformation of society.

Discipline: The daily practice of staying the course, ignoring distractions, and maintaining focus on our goals.

Discrimination: Treating people differently in ways that violate their dignity. Discrimination entrenches and exacerbates inequities—typically by benefiting already privileged groups at the expense of those who have been historically excluded and oppressed.

Disparate impact: Addresses policies that may appear "neutral" on paper but result in disproportionate harm to specific protected groups. Proving disparate impact does not require evidence of discriminatory intent—the emphasis is on effects, not motives.

Disparate treatment: Occurs when individuals or groups are intentionally treated differently based on their "race" or another legally protected identity, such as religion, gender identity, or disability status.

Disparity: A term that simply describes difference. Not all disparities are unjust. A disparity becomes an *inequity* when that difference is avoidable, unnecessary, and indefensible.

Dominant institutions: Organizations and institutions in our society that hold the most power, resources, and authority, such as governments, philanthropic organizations, universities, and corporations.

Enforcement: The mechanisms institutions use to ensure compliance with laws, rules, or policies. Governments primarily carry out the enforcement that shapes people's lives and structures the systems we live in. Although enforcement can involve monitoring, education, and accountability-centered action, it has historically and functionally relied on punitive and coercive strategies such as fines, arrests, and surveillance.

Equality: Refers to the sameness of all people. As a value or principle, it means that people have the same inherent worth—for example, by asserting the right to equal protection under the law. In practice, equality means treating everyone the same: providing the same resources, opportunities, or services regardless of people's starting points, needs, or circumstances. Equality, as an approach, assumes that everyone begins from a level playing field and requires the same support to succeed. But when applied in the context of addressing systemic oppression and structural inequity, this kind of uniform treatment can do the opposite—treating everyone equally can actually reinforce injustice. Equal treatment within unequal systems cannot produce equal outcomes. In fact, offering the same supports to people—regardless of their specific circumstances, histories, or needs—can perpetuate harm, widen unjust disparities, and exacerbate the root causes of inequity.

Equity: A principle that acknowledges that people face different barriers and circumstances and need different levels of support to achieve fair and just outcomes. Equity is grounded in the recognition that systemic injustices—such as discriminatory policies, unequal access to resources, and legacies of exclusion—have created vastly different starting points for people and entire communities. Rather than treating everyone as if their needs are the same, equity calls for meeting people where they are and giving them what they need to flourish. Equity has three requirements: (1) valuing all people and populations equally, (2) recognizing and rectifying historical and contemporary injustices, and (3) providing resources according to need. Equity becomes real through acknowledgment, accountability, and—most importantly—action.

Evaluation: The systematic assessment of the merit, worth, or significance of an intervention. As one of the 10 Essential Public Health Services, evaluation is an essential mechanism through which assurance is realized.

Fairness: A principle that means ensuring people are treated justly and have meaningful access to the resources and opportunities needed for health and flourishing.

Fakequity: Performative or inauthentic equity efforts that co-opt the language of equity without doing the work of shifting power, resources, or decision-making to those who have been marginalized. These efforts are destructive because they protect the status quo while giving the appearance of change. Ultimately, they deceive people, cause harm, and perpetuate distrust.

Flourishing: A broader and more expansive vision of health that means having what we need, both individually and collectively, to lead lives of purpose, agency, connection, and possibility. Flourishing is about more than survival or longevity; it's about living a life that feels meaningful. Flourishing invites us to move beyond deficit-based models of health and toward an expansive vision of thriving, connection, and self-determination. Flourishing is synonymous with *health*.

Food apartheid: Refers to the ways in which food is segregated so that "healthy, fresh food is accessible in wealthy neighborhoods while unhealthy food abounds in poor neighborhoods"[3]—a situation resulting from decades of policy and planning decisions that have perpetuated segregation and disinvestment, like Jim Crow and redlining.

Gender liberation: A movement that imagines a world where every person has the freedom to express, define, and live their gender without fear or violence. Gender liberation is about *bodily autonomy*: the right of all people to make decisions about their own bodies, lives, and futures.

Genetic ancestry: Refers to paths through which genetic material has been inherited. People are born with a genetic ancestry; they are socially assigned a "race."

Governance: Processes by which communities make collective decisions and distribute power and resources.

Governing power: The ability to control systems and decisions that shape lives.

Guaranteed income: Recurring cash payments that are distributed to members of a community, with no strings attached. A guaranteed income can create an income floor below which no one can fall. It can be targeted (for specific groups of people based on their needs) or universal (for everyone), but it ultimately ensures "those with the greatest need are prioritized for assistance."[4]

Health: See *flourishing*. Health is not truly described by the World Health Organization's definition of health as "a state of complete physical, mental, and social well-being and not merely the absence of disease or infirmity."[5] The presence of illness or disability does not automatically negate health. Many people navigate physical and mental health conditions every day while leading fulfilling lives rooted in meaning, connection, and dignity. A deficit-based lens overlooks the importance of joy, connectedness, and belonging, and it denies the complexity of people's lives and reinforces a narrow, medicalized view of what it means to be healthy. Health is a dynamic, self-defined experience shaped by care, community, and having access to the resources we need to live well, both individually and in relationship with others.

Health and quality-of-life outcomes: Overarching and culminating effects that reflect levels of physical, mental, emotional, and social well-being. Health and quality-of-life outcomes are not static; they change dynamically over time based on the conditions, systems, and environments that impact people's lives. Health and quality-of-life outcomes include physical and mental health; meaningful employment, living wages, and wealth; safe, stable, dignified, and desirable homes and opportunity-rich neighborhoods; educational attainment; access to affordable and high-quality goods and services; and community connectedness and civic participation.

Health equity: A term that applies the principle of equity to health and flourishing. It means ensuring that everyone, no matter who they are or where they come from, has a fair and just opportunity to live a full and meaningful life. Achieving health equity requires us to confront historical and ongoing injustices, provide resources according to need, and actively dismantle the social, economic, and systemic barriers to health.

Health inequities: Preventable differences in health outcomes that result from inequities in access to respectful, high-quality conditions necessary to flourish.

Health justice: A community-driven movement to dismantle systemic barriers to health and ensure resources are distributed according to need, so that everyone has an equal chance to live a flourishing, fulfilling life. The health justice movement recognizes that health is shaped by social, economic, and political conditions and seeks to transform these conditions to eliminate health inequities. Health justice embraces five commitments: urgency, connectedness, solidarity, law, and power.

Imagination: The courage to dream beyond what currently exists.

Implementation: The process of putting plans into motion, coordinating people and resources, and adapting to context to ensure meaningful and measurable impact. Implementation is where theoretical commitments to equity and justice are tested, translated into action, and operationalized through specific programs, policies, and practices.

Inequality: Describes a difference between individuals or groups. Not all inequalities are unjust. An inequality becomes an *inequity* when that difference is avoidable, unnecessary, and indefensible.

Inequity: A difference that is avoidable, unnecessary, and indefensible. Inequities should provoke moral outrage because they result from unjust systems and structures.

Informed consent: Participants are told the risks and benefits of a procedure, process, evaluation, or research study to help them determine if they are willing to participate of their own free will.

Inside–outside strategy: A long-term strategic approach that builds trust and collaboration between those working on the *inside* (within dominant institutions like government agencies, universities, and philanthropies) and those working on the *outside* (in community power-building groups, grassroots organizations, advocacy networks, and justice movements). Inside-outside strategies leverage the positionality of these institutions and the relationships that exist between people across institutions to inform a dynamic set of tactics that are collectively used to transform policies, systems, and practices that directly improve people's lives.[6] The endgame of an inside-outside strategy is to make these collaborations greater than the sum of their parts—to achieve wins for equity, justice, community power, and collective flourishing that we could not do alone or solely within our respective organizations.

Intersectionality: A concept rooted in Black feminist thought that describes how different forms of oppression overlap and compound one another. Intersectionality helps us understand how multiple systems work together to intensify inequities in opportunity and flourishing for people with multiple marginalized identities.

Jim Crow laws: State and local laws in the United States that legalized racial segregation and racial discrimination in all facets of daily life. Jim Crow laws restricted the movement of Black people in all public spaces, including schools, public transit, parks, and hospitals, forbidding interaction between Black and white people and denying Black people access to community resources and services. Jim Crow laws were a form of racial terror that were used to legally deny Black people the right to vote, gain employment, obtain an education, purchase homes and land, and much more. If these laws were even perceived to be violated in any way, Black people faced arrest, imprisonment, violence, and death.

Justice: A principle that embraces the three requirements of equity—valuing all people, addressing historical injustices, and redistributing resources based on need—while going further to fully transform systems and structures. Justice is focused on making permanent changes to systems and structures, and as a result is transformative in its scope and scale. Justice work creates policies and processes that cement shifts in power and generate conditions where opportunities to flourish are built into the very foundations of society. If equity is about leveling the playing field, justice is about changing the game entirely.

Just Transition: A vision-led framework grounded by the principle that a healthy economy and a healthy environment can and must coexist. It calls for a shift from an extractive, racialized economy—one that sacrifices people and planet in pursuit of ever-growing profits—to a generative economy rooted in dignity, sustainability, and shared prosperity.

Land Back: A movement envisions a future where Indigenous peoples reclaim stewardship over their ancestral lands and waters. Land Back is not only about physical territory; it is about acknowledging sovereignty, restoring relationships to land and culture, and dismantling colonial systems that continue to harm Indigenous communities and all other communities of color. Land Back emerges from centuries of Indigenous resistance—an ongoing fight for survival, sovereignty, and dignity in the face of colonialism.

Law: Codified and enforceable rules established by governments to regulate behavior, allocate power and resources, protect rights, resolve disputes, and set the terms for how government authority is used—including when it can compel or coerce. Although law is often portrayed as neutral and fair, in practice, it has long served to protect those in power, enforce social hierarchies, and authorize state-sanctioned force—deciding when and how that force is deemed "legitimate." While modern legal systems operate on the assumption that coercion and control are necessary features, we reject that premise. Instead, we envision a legal and political order rooted in care, consent, and collective accountability—where justice is cultivated not through domination but through relationships of mutual responsibility and repair. Laws can take various forms: ordinances and statutes passed by legislative bodies, regulations issued by administrative agencies, case law established through judicial decisions, and executive orders issued by presidents, governors, or other executive officials. All laws are policies, but not all policies are laws.

Learning: Our collective efforts to build shared knowledge and understanding about what's effective, what isn't, and why so we can make meaningful improvements.

Liberation: The realization of self-determination, justice, and collective flourishing. A liberated future is one in which all people have the freedom, power, and resources to live with dignity, make choices about their own lives, and participate fully in shaping their communities and the systems that govern them. In a public health context, liberation means people have open and abundant access to the resources, opportunities, and conditions necessary to lead a healthy and flourishing life on their own terms.

Lifestyle drift: A tendency in public health to narrowly focus on individual behavior rather than the root causes, systems, and structures that shape and constrain people's choices.

Marginalized: Being pushed to the margins of civic life, public narratives, and community belonging. The margins are metaphorical edges: peripheral places far from the concentrated centers of influence, visibility, and decision-making authority. As a result, marginalized people are excluded from having access to resources and opportunities, representation in influential institutions, a voice in public discourse, visibility in mainstream narratives, and the ability to shape policies that affect their lives.

Medical racism: Refers to the ways in which racial discrimination—whether conscious or not—is embedded in medical training, clinical guidelines, diagnostic tools, and patient care. It shows up in how pain is assessed, how symptoms are interpreted, who receives care, and how medical research is conducted and applied.

Mindset–narrative loop: A circular relationship that describes the interactions between *mindsets* and *narratives*. Dominant narratives reinforce and amplify dominant mindsets, and dominant mindsets shape the narratives we accept or reject. The mindset-narrative loop influences not only how individuals think but also how systems are structured, how policies are made, and how institutions operate.

Mindsets: Deeply held beliefs, attitudes, assumptions, and perspectives that shape how we think about the world.

Misogynoir: Describes the specific form of discrimination faced by Black women at the intersection of racism and sexism. Misogynoir captures the ways Black women are simultaneously hyper-visible and devalued.

Multiracial democracy: A form of democratic governance developed by and for people in a racially diverse society where everyone's basic rights and liberties are universally respected and protected. A multiracial democracy also calls for a transformation of democracy—the creation of a democracy in which all people, especially those who have been racialized and oppressed, have real decision-making power and the ability to shape policies and institutions that directly impact their lives.

Narratives: As defined by PolicyLink, "the big stories we tell ourselves about the world, rooted in our values, that influence how we process information and make decisions."[7(p10)]

Organizational policy: Refers to a written statement that sets out an agency or organization's position, decision, or course of action on specific issues and procedures. Organizational policies are designed to guide decisions and behaviors within an organization, shaping its operations, culture, and actions. They define how an organization engages with internal constituents (such as employees and members) and external constituents (such as clients, communities, and the public). Organizational policies influence a wide range of practices—from programmatic activities and ethical stewardship to operational processes and strategic planning.

People of color: People who have been racialized—that is, people upon whom the construct of "race" has been imposed and who bear the social, political, and economic burdens of racism.

Policy: Encompasses the decisions and actions taken by governments or organizations to address societal issues. Policies can also take the form of non-legally binding guidelines or informal practices that are instituted by governing bodies but may not be formally codified into law.

Policy violence: The act of making unjust policy choices in the face of abject need. This includes policy decisions that actively harm people by denying them resources and rights, as well as a failure or outright refusal of governments to adopt essential policies in the face of clear need. Policy violence is an effective means of perpetuating systems of oppression like structural racism, classism, and racial capitalism.

Political power: The ability to vote, organize, influence policy, and shape civic life.

Positionality: The ways our insights and beliefs are informed by intersecting contexts like our backgrounds, professional experiences, and lived realities. Positionality is always unique and context-dependent: How others see us depends on their own positionalities and may shift across time, place, environment, and relationships. Just as it influences how we're perceived, it also shapes how we perceive and the perspectives we bring to our work—affecting whose voices we amplify, whose needs we prioritize, and how we interpret information.

Power: The ability to influence outcomes, make decisions, and control one's own destiny. Power determines who has the ability to act to ultimately shape the trajectory of their lives and determine their futures.

Power building: What communities do to organize, mobilize, and strengthen their own collective capacity to govern, advocate, and act.

Power sharing: When dominant institutions deliberately cede control, step back from the center, and support communities in leading. Shifting power is possible through power sharing.

Power shifting: Changing who has authority, decision-making control, and access to resources.

Practice: An informal or customary procedure or norm that shapes how things are done within an organization or community. Unlike formal policies, practices are not always written down or legally mandated. They evolve over time and often reflect shared habits, expectations, and cultural norms.

Preemption: The ability of a higher level of government (such as a state or federal government) to override or limit the authority of a government at a lower level, like a city or county.

Public health: See *community health*. The science and art of ensuring that entire communities have what they need to flourish. Public health is ultimately "anything related to the acknowledgement, appreciation, understanding, and advancement of human health and well-being."[8] Public health embraces four commitments: scale, prevention, root causes, and justice. Public health is synonymous with *community health*, and the two terms can be used interchangeably.

Punitive preemption: A form of governance where higher levels of government not only override local authority but also block policies that protect public health—and threaten to punish the lower government and its leaders in the process. Also known as *abusive preemption.*

Qualitative data: Rich information that includes stories, interviews, conversations, group discussions, and testimonials.

Quantitative data: Numeric metrics and statistics like percentages, rates, and counts.

"Race": A human-made idea and social construct that was developed to categorize people solely by their physical appearance. It forms the basis of a false and rigid hierarchy of human value grounded in the belief that darker skin colors are inferior, while lighter, "whiter" skin colors are superior. Despite its pernicious existence in every aspect of our society, the concept of "race" has no factual, biological, or genetic basis.

Racial capitalism: Describes the ways in which our economic system is set up to extract value from the exploitation of racialized people. Racial capitalism structures economic opportunity and labor along racial lines. It relies on land extraction, labor exploitation, and racial hierarchy to generate wealth for the few at the expense of the many.

Racial health gap: The well-documented pattern in the United States of Black and brown people, as a whole, living shorter, sicker lives than white people.

Racialized: Refers to how people are categorized and treated based on the socially constructed idea of "race." In systems shaped by white supremacy, this process has generally been used to define and control people of color by assigning meaning to their perceived "race" and using that assigned meaning to justify unfair treatment. Racialization isn't about individual identity or choice; it's about how systems label people, shape perceptions, and distribute power.

Racial wealth gap: A profound and persistent disparity in assets, income, and intergenerational wealth between white households and households of color.

Racism: A system of structuring opportunity and assigning value based on how people look (their "race") that unfairly disadvantages some individuals and communities, unfairly advantages other individuals and communities, and undermines our realization of the full potential of the whole society through the waste of human resources.

Reciprocity: An ethical principle that emphasizes mutual respect, shared benefit, and fitting response to others' contributions. It is widely recognized across disciplines—including philosophy, public health, and social psychology—as a norm that sustains fairness, trust, and cooperation.

Redlining: Originated as a discriminatory federal policy that started in the 1930s, but has since come to describe the broader system of racialized disinvestment carried out across public and private sectors. Under the New Deal, the federal government—through agencies like the Federal Housing Administration and the Home Owners' Loan Corporation (HOLC)—designated neighborhoods as "hazardous" for investment if Black people, other people of color, or immigrants lived there. HOLC collaborated with state and local government officials, bankers, realtors, and appraisers to create graded and color-coded maps to illustrate the perceived "desirability" of neighborhoods. These color-coded maps determined where banks would issue loans, where businesses could invest, and where government resources would be allocated. The grades and color codes were based on "race": White neighborhoods received the highest grades and were systematically approved for public and private loans and investments. However, neighborhoods where Black people, immigrants, and other people of color resided were assigned the lowest grade, which was color-coded red on maps, and systematically denied public and private loans and investments. This came to be known as redlining.

Redress: The act of rectifying past harms and injustices that begins with truth and moves to action. Truth-telling is the first act of redress; it creates the foundation for accountability, trust, and collective action. Redress then requires tangible and meaningful actions: returning land, reinvesting in communities harmed by policy violence, dismantling exclusionary systems, and shifting power to those long denied it. Redress is not about punishment; it is about making amends for the past to liberate our future.

Research: Efforts to create new knowledge and the innovative use of existing knowledge to generate new concepts, methodologies, and insights. It involves the analysis, synthesis, and interpretation of data to produce actionable learnings and to guide informed decision-making.

Resource mobilization: The practice of organizing, advocating for, and attracting new funding, partnerships, and political support to build lasting abundance—not simply manage scarcity.

Resources: Tangible commitments of money, materials, labor, relationships, and infrastructure that can be mobilized to advance a goal.

Restorative justice: A community-centered practice that brings together those who have been harmed and those responsible—whether individuals or institutions—to engage in facilitated, ongoing dialogue that acknowledges the harms committed, promotes accountability, and works toward meaningful repair.

Root causes avoidance: The tendency of many public health organizations and interventions to focus on surface-level factors like health behaviors or individual risk, while ignoring—or outright refusing—to name or address the underlying systems that shape these behaviors in the first place.

Root Causes Roadmap: A multilayered framework that illustrates how and where these connections exist, identifies intervention points to disrupt systems of oppression, and lays out tools to promote community health and well-being. The Root Causes Roadmap allows us to zoom out and see the dynamic interrelationships between the forces, tools, and outcomes connected to community health. These include *systems of oppression, structural inequities, tools for systems change, the social determinants of health,* and *outcomes for health and flourishing.*

Scientific racism: A form of racism that involves the co-optation, abuse, and distortion of science to uphold a fictional hierarchy of human value and to legitimize the myth of white racial superiority.

Self-determination: The ability of individuals and communities to define and pursue their own vision of health, safety, and well-being on their own terms. In international law, it is recognized as a collective right of peoples to determine their political status and control their economic, social, and cultural development. In public health, it functions as both a principle and a practice rooted in respect for autonomy, lived experience, community power, and the right to direct one's own future.

Settler colonialism: A form of colonialism that involves the ongoing process of taking land, even when it is clearly occupied or owned by others. Settler colonialism requires that anyone living on the land before the arrival of settler colonists—usually Indigenous peoples—is removed or eliminated and replaced entirely with a permanent settler society.

Seven Generations Value: A core value of the Haudenosaunee Confederacy that requires us to consider how our present-day decisions will impact those who follow us, as we are merely borrowing the world from future generations.

Shifting power: Changing who has authority, decision-making control, and access to resources.

Social construction (or social construct): "An idea or collection of ideas that have been created and accepted by the people in a society. These constructs serve as an attempt to organize or explain the world around us."[9] A social construct is not an immutable truth, but rather a creation of human thought and belief.

Social determinants of health: An interconnected web of conditions and contexts that shape our health by influencing the opportunities, resources, and choices available to us in our daily lives. The social determinants of health include, but are not limited to, economic stability; education; neighborhoods, housing, and the built environment; public health and health care; resources, goods, and services; and social and community contexts.

Social movements: Collective efforts by groups of people to challenge existing conditions, demand change, and reshape society. Also referred to as *movements*.

Solidarity: Empathy in action that compels us to actively show up and stand alongside others, even when their struggles are not our own. Solidarity recognizes that injustices are interconnected and relationships must be grounded in mutual respect, shared fate, and collective liberation.

State-sanctioned violence: Refers to violence that occurs when a government, through its authorities—such as police or military—uses force, intimidation, or repressive actions against its citizens, often claiming to be upholding law and order or protecting citizens' interests, even if such actions violate human rights. State-sanctioned violence can also include the refusal of a government and its agents (such as police, government attorneys, and judges) to uphold or enforce existing laws intended to protect marginalized groups from violence and intimidation, serving to further subjugate and oppress marginalized groups. Also called *state violence* or *state-sponsored violence*.

Structural inequities: Large-scale, patterned, and entrenched disadvantages that shape people's everyday lives. They include structural discrimination, inequities in income and wealth, inequities in opportunity, inequities in political power, and governance that limits meaningful participation.

Structural racism: A form of racism that encompasses "the totality of ways in which societies foster racial discrimination through mutually reinforcing systems of housing, education, employment, earnings, benefits, credit, media, health care, and the criminal [legal and carceral system]. These patterns and practices in turn reinforce discriminatory beliefs, values, and distribution of resources."[10(p1453)] These systems and structures interact, evolve, and reinforce each other over time to entrench racism and sustain the privileges associated with "whiteness" and the disadvantages associated with "color."[11] Structural racism operates at a broad level and has a far-reaching impact on population health.

Systems change: The process of shifting the underlying conditions that hold a complex problem in place.

Systems of oppression: The root causes of health inequities. They are the entrenched social, economic, and political structures that distribute power and resources unfairly, creating advantages for some groups while marginalizing others. Systems of oppression include white supremacy, structural racism, colonialism, racial capitalism, and more—all of which produce conditions and contexts that govern how well and how long people live. These interconnected systems of oppression are ubiquitous, operating at all levels and across all sectors to shape policies, institutions, and social norms to determine who has access to the resources and opportunities they need to flourish. The inequities they create not only harm marginalized groups but also undermine the overall health and well-being of society.

Targeted universalism: A concept that means setting universal goals for everyone and using tailored strategies to help different groups achieve these goals based on their unique needs, preferences, circumstances, and contexts.

Tools for systems change: Powerful levers and mechanisms that can directly influence every layer of the *Root Causes Roadmap*—which include systems of oppression (the root causes of health inequities), structural inequities, social determinants of health, and outcomes for health and flourishing communities. The tools for systems change include laws, policies, practices, budgets, collaborative governance or co-governance, and data and research. The tools for systems change interact dynamically with every layer of the Roadmap, shaping health outcomes, social determinants of health, structural inequities, and systems of oppression—and also being shaped by them in turn.

Transmisogynoir: Describes the compounded harm Black trans women face from racism, sexism, and cissexism.

Transmisogyny: Names the intersectional harms of *traditional sexism* (which devalues femininity) and *oppositional sexism* (which enforces rigid gender norms and punishes those who defy them).

Trust: A principle that refers to being seen as honest, reliable, reciprocal, and accountable—not only as an individual but also as a representative of an organization and a professional field at large.

Universal goal: A fair and just outcome that everyone deserves.

Weathering: A term that describes how chronic exposure to structural racism, social marginalization, and economic hardship wears down the body over time, accelerating aging and increasing the risk of chronic illness and early death.

White supremacy: An ideology and system that upholds whiteness as superior. It underpins and drives structural racism. White supremacy is often portrayed as an extremist ideology associated with hate groups like the Ku Klux Klan and neo-Nazis. In reality, white supremacy is a system that has been woven into the very fabric of our structures, institutions, policies, and cultural norms. It is both mundane and pervasive, shaping the structure and function of all of our systems—including our economic, housing, education, employment, and criminal legal systems, and more—to maintain that hierarchy. White supremacy was the driving force behind the creation of the false hierarchy of human value, where "whiteness" sits at the top of the social, economic, and political order and "color" sits at the bottom.

REFERENCES

1. Snyder T. *On Tyranny: Twenty Lessons From the Twentieth Century.* Tim Duggan Books; 2017.
2. Lead Local Collaborative. Glossary. Accessed August 2, 2025. https://www.lead-local.org/glossary
3. Walker J. 'Food desert' vs. 'food apartheid': Which term best describes disparities in food access? University of Michigan School for Environment and Sustainability. November 29, 2023. Accessed May 12, 2025. https://seas.umich.edu/news/food-desert-vs-food-apartheid-which-term-best-describes-disparities-food-access
4. Kline S. Guaranteed income: A primer for funders. Asset Funders Network; Center for High Impact Philanthropy; Economic Security Project; Springboard to Opportunities. May 2022. Accessed August 4, 2025. https://assetfunders.org/wp-content/uploads/Guaranteed-Income_Primer-for-Funders_May-2022.pdf
5. World Health Organization. Constitution of the World Health Organization. Accessed May 12, 2025. https://www.who.int/about/governance/constitution
6. Aly S, Diaby A, Drix J. The five dimensions of inside-outside strategy: A guide for public health and social movements to build powerful partnerships. Health in Partnership. April 30, 2025. Accessed May 19, 2025. https://www.healthinpartnership.org/resources/the-five-dimensions-of-inside-outside-strategy-guide
7. McAfee M, Dunn V. Governing for all: An equity narrative playbook for policymakers. PolicyLink; 2022. Accessed June 3, 2025. https://www.policylink.org/sites/default/files/Governing%20for%20All%20Playbook.pdf
8. Fakunle DO. Storytelling and public health 101. In: *Arts-Focused Approaches to Public Health Communications.* Public Health Communications Collaborative; February 29, 2024. Accessed June 27, 2025. https://www.slideshare.net/slideshow/artsfocused-approaches-to-public-health-communications/266583002#3
9. National Museum of African American History and Culture. Historical foundations of race. May 31, 2020. Accessed June 1, 2025. https://web.archive.org/web/20240929122221/https://nmaahc.si.edu/learn/talking-about-race/topics/historical-foundations-race
10. Bailey ZD, Krieger N, Agénor M, Graves J, Linos N, Bassett MT. Structural racism and health inequities in the USA: Evidence and interventions. *Lancet.* 2017;389(10077):1453-1463. doi:10.1016/S0140-6736(17)30569-X
11. Lawrence K, Sutton S, Kubisch A, Susi G, Fulbright-Anderson K, Aspen Institute Roundtable on Community Change. Structural racism and community building. Aspen Institute. 2004. Accessed May 13, 2025. https://www.aspeninstitute.org/wp-content/uploads/files/content/docs/rcc/aspen_structural_racism2.pdf

About the Authors

Jamila M. Porter, DrPH, MPH (she/her) is an award-winning researcher, evaluator, and public health practitioner whose work focuses on transforming the interconnected social, environmental, and power structures that impact health. She is an outspoken leader, writer, researcher, and public speaker on a range of issues, including the root causes of health inequities, the social determinants of health, data and transportation justice, policy evaluation, community power-building, and public health practice. Dr. Porter is chief of staff at the de Beaumont Foundation, where she bolsters the work of teams across the foundation and ensures that equity and justice are organizational priorities. She is also the principal investigator of Modernized Anti-racist Data Ecosystems (MADE) for Health Justice—an initiative that is partnering with communities, local governments, and advocates to accelerate the development of health-focused local data ecosystems that center principles of antiracism, equity, justice, and community power. Dr. Porter's experience spans multiple sectors, including philanthropy, nonprofit, consulting, and international development. She earned her bachelor's degree in communication and health policy and administration from Wake Forest University, her MPH from Mercer University School of Medicine, and her DrPH from the University of Georgia College of Public Health.

Aysha Dominguez Pamukcu, JD (she/they) is a nationally recognized movement strategist, attorney, and policy advocate who builds cross-sector coalitions and drives ambitious justice agendas. Her work reflects a deep commitment to solidarity and multi-movement organizing. As Director of the Policy Fund at the San Francisco Foundation, Aysha leads a network of local governments and communities co-designing policy solutions that promote housing justice and shared prosperity. She also founded Movement Praxis to help organizations practice trust-based philanthropy and equity-centered policy advocacy. Aysha is honored to have collaborated closely with movement leaders across public health, human rights, civil rights, and climate justice—including co-creating the *civil rights of health* framework. She serves on nonprofit boards and in local government, championing equity and community-driven change. A proud parent and partner, Aysha draws inspiration from these roles to enrich her advocacy.

Index

Page numbers followed by *b, f,* and *t* indicate boxes, figures, and tables, respectively. Numbers followed by *n* indicate footnotes.

community governance, 171
community health, 16
community power, 23, 167–182
    accountability in, 223
    in assurance-centered approach, 191
    building of, 249–251
    in co-governance, 97, 178–180, 182
    core principles in, 176
    defer to stage in, 170*f*, 171, 173, 180
    definition of, 168
    and empowerment, 163
    in health justice, 31
    resource decisions in, 176–177
    Spectrum of Community Engagement to Ownership,
        168–174, 170*f*, 182, 250
    transportation example, 171–173
community services, 89, 91
Complete Streets, 98, 241
Compromise of 1877 ending Reconstruction, 149
Compton's Cafeteria Riot (CA), 234*b*
confidentiality in evaluations, 201
conflicts, in inside–outside strategies, 257
consent
    co-powered, 200–202
    FRIES model of, 201
    informed, 201
co-powered consent, 200–202
corporate influence
    and accountability, 29
    as dominant institutions, 25*b*
    in election spending, 120
    on equity-centered interventions, 26
    fakequity in, 25*b*
    on food access, 35
    on health as personal responsibility mindset,
        140–141
    on housing, 29
courage, value of, 238
COVID-19 pandemic, 60, 97, 213
    eviction protection during, 119
    medical racism in, 63*b*
    Pansy Collective during, 225*b*
    "race" and ethnicity data in, 63*b*, 97
    root causes of health outcomes in, 63*b*, 97
Crenshaw, Kimberlé, 56
Crime Bill (1994), 121–122
criminalization
    of abortion, 150
    of addiction, 121
    in "broken windows" policing, 122
    of homelessness, 121, 189
    of people of color, 145
    of poverty, 120
    in punitive enforcement, 189
    of queer people, 120, 234*b*
criminal legal system, 12, 29, 120–122
    false hierarchy of human value in, 56
    fines and fees in, 29, 122, 188, 189
    incarceration in. *See* incarceration
    punitive enforcement in, 188–192. *See also*
        punitive enforcement

as unjust by design, 152
    use of term, 152
Critical Race Theory, 150, 150*n*
cultural affirmation, 165
    foods in, 1, 34, 167*b*
cultural identity, 3, 11
cultural racism, 67–68
Curb-Cut Effect, 38–39, 245

D

daily work for equity and justice, 232–262
    communication and problem framing in, 232,
        242–246
    imagination and reimagination in, 232, 261–262
    inside–outside strategies in, 232, 254–258
    integration as routine, 232, 258–261
    learning about community legacies in, 232,
        233–236
    power shifting and sharing in, 232, 249–251
    resource organization and mobilization in, 232,
        251–254
    root causes and systems as focus in, 232, 239–242
    solidarity in, 232, 246–249
    values in, 232, 236–239
data, 95–96, 97
    accountability agreements on, 202
    census, 52*b*, 119
    community, 94, 199–200, 205, 259–260
    co-powered consent to collection and use of,
        201–202
    intersectional analysis of, 240
    qualitative, 194–195, 196*b*, 259–260
    quantitative, 199, 259
    "race" as variable in, 48, 61*b*, 70, 97, 195*b*
decision-making
    accountability for. *See* accountability
    in assurance-centered approach, 191, 193, 194,
        198, 200, 202
    in community, 170–171
    data-driven, 96
    equity in, 40
    exclusion from, 85–86
    fakequity in, 25*b*
    in gender liberation, 218
    in governance processes, 87, 92, 95, 171, 257, 260
    in health justice, 30, 31
    inequity in, 34, 85, 86, 89
    in leading with values, 237, 238
    mindsets in, 134
    in multiracial democracy, 217
    power in. *See* power
    on resource allocation, 95, 252, 253, 260
    on universal goals, 38
    values in, 236, 237, 238, 239
Deferred Action for Childhood Arrivals (DACA), 101,
    101*n*
defer to stage
    in co-governance, 180, 250
    in self-determination, 170*f*, 171, 173
Delano Grape Strike, 234*b*